Functional Assessment and Outcome Measures for the Rehabilitation Health Professional

Sharon S. Dittmar, PhD, RN
Professor, School of Nursing
Clinical Professor, Department of Rehabilitation Medicine
School of Medicine and Biomedical Sciences
University at Buffalo
State University of New York

and

Glen E. Gresham, MD
Professor and Chairman
Department of Rehabilitation Medicine
School of Medicine and Biomedical Sciences
University at Buffalo
State University of New York

With a Foreword by

Carl V. Granger, MD
Professor, Rehabilitation Medicine
Director, Center for Functional Assessment Research
Department of Rehabilitation Medicine
School of Medicine and Biomedical Sciences
University at Buffalo
State University of New York

Supported by the US Department of Education, National Institute on Disability and Rehabilitation Research and The Rehabilitation Research and Training Center on Functional Assessment and Evaluation of Rehabilitation Outcomes, University at Buffalo, State University of New York
Sponsor ID No. H133B30041

AN ASPEN PUBLICATION®
Aspen Publishers, Inc.
Gaithersburg, Maryland
1997

Library of Congress Cataloging-in-Publication Data

Functional assessment and outcome measures for the rehabilitation
health professional / edited by Sharon S. Dittmar and Glen E.
Gresham; with a foreword by Carl V. Granger.
p.   cm.
Includes bibliographical references and index.
ISBN 0-8342-0929-2
1. Handicapped—Functional assessment. 2. Outcome assessment
(Medical care) I. Dittmar, Sharon S. II. Gresham, Glen E.
[DNLM: 1. Rehabilitation—standards. 2. Disability Evaluation.
3. Outcome Assessment (Health Care)—standards. WB 320 F978 1997]
RM930.8.F85   1997
617′.03—dc21
DNLM/DLC
for Library of Congress
97-7201
CIP

Orders: (800) 638-8437
Customer Service: (800) 234-1660

About Aspen Publishers • For more than 35 years, Aspen has been a leading professional publisher in a variety of disciplines. Aspen's vast information resources are available in both print and
electronic formats. We are committed to providing the highest quality information available in the
most appropriate format for our customers. Visit Aspen's Internet site for more information resources, directories, articles, and a searchable version of Aspen's full catalog, including the most
recent publications: **http://www.aspenpub.com**
Aspen Publishers, Inc. • The hallmark of quality in publishing
Member of the worldwide Wolters Kluwer group

Editorial Resources: Lenda Hill
Library of Congress Catalog Card Number: 97-7201
ISBN: 0-8342-0929-2

Printed in the United States of America

1 2 3 4 5

Table of Contents

Contributors

Laura A. Cushman, PhD
Associate Professor
University of Rochester Medical Center

Gary S. Danford, PhD, MA
Associate Professor
School of Architecture
University at Buffalo
State University of New York

Sharon S. Dittmar, PhD, RN
Professor
School of Nursing
Clinical Professor
Department of Rehabilitation Medicine
School of Medicine and Biomedical Sciences
University at Buffalo
State University of New York

Glen E. Gresham, MD
Professor and Chairman
Department of Rehabilitation Medicine
School of Medicine and Biomedical Sciences
University at Buffalo
State University of New York

Kenneth J. Ottenbacher, PhD, OTR/L
Vice Dean and Professor
School of Allied Health Sciences
University of Texas Medical Branch at Galveston

Marcia J. Scherer, PhD, MPH
Senior Research Associate and Director of Consumer
    Evaluations
Center for Assistive Technology
University at Buffalo
State University of New York

Marietta P. Stanton, PhD, RN, C
Associate Professor
School of Nursing
University at Buffalo
State University of New York

Edward H. Steinfeld, DArch, MArch
Professor
School of Architecture
University at Buffalo
State University of New York

Lucy T. Vitaliti, PhD
Rehabilitation Engineering and Assistive Technology
    Society of North America (RESNA)
Project Director, Assurance of Quality in Assistive
    Technology
Service Provision Grant

Foreword

The terms functional assessment, rehabilitation programs, and outcomes are closely intertwined. *Functional assessment* is the method used to describe abilities and limitations individuals experience so that performance of the necessary activities of daily living can be measured. *Rehabilitation programs* help individuals change their behaviors in ways that support greater independence in physical, emotional, social, vocational, and avocational tasks. *Outcomes* are changes and achievements representing benefits of the rehabilitation program. Functional assessment alone cannot define those benefits, but measurement of function over time clearly contributes to their definition.

For individuals with severe disability, fundamental tasks of daily living involve self-care, sphincter control, transfer from bed to chair or chair to standing, locomotion, communication, and interaction with other persons. Other of life's tasks are more varied and not as readily specified. The rehabilitation program incorporates methods for restoring function, adapting to new ways of functioning, or compensating for residual limitations. Functional assessment provides the clinician with tools to measure individuals' status in functioning at the beginning of, during, at the conclusion of, and as a follow-up to a rehabilitation intervention. Assessment results support determination and documentation of functioning and allow explicit description of benefits for a course of treatment.

The two primary outcome measures of rehabilitation are change in functional status toward more independence in activities of daily living and enhancement of options for restoring quality to daily living.

Instruments used for functional assessment should meet psychometric (biometric) standards; that is, validity, reliability, feasibility, and precision.

Lawton (1971) was the first to define functional assessment as "any systematic attempt to measure objectively the level at which a person is functioning in any of a variety of areas" (p. 465). Joe (1984) observed that

> current methods for defining and treating disabilities are, however, dismayingly primitive . . . medical labels also do a disservice to disabled persons by failing to take into account the interaction of one's strengths and weaknesses with their particular environments. . . . assessing an individual's functional performance in a specific environment would give professionals and policymakers a far better understanding of how to target services to the real needs of disabled persons. . . . [and] functional assessment also directs proper attention to the possibility of modifying the environment in ways that enable functionally impaired persons to adapt to or compensate for their limitations, thus increasing their potential for living independently. (pp. vii–viii)

In its evolution, functional assessment is emerging from the shadows to become an area for productive scientific inquiry with possibilities for short-term translation into clinical utility. As this occurs, it is expected that there will be a uniform language for describing disablement and outcomes that will significantly benefit persons with disability by improving the effectiveness and efficiency of their rehabilitation programs.

Carl V. Granger, MD
Professor, Rehabilitation Medicine
Director, Center for Functional
    Assessment Research
232 Parker Hall
State University of New York at Buffalo
3435 Main Street
Buffalo, NY 14214

REFERENCES

Joe, T. (1984). Foreword. In C.V. Granger & G.E. Gresham (Eds.), *Functional assessment in rehabilitation medicine* (pp. vii–viii). Baltimore: Williams & Wilkins.

Lawton, M.P. (1971). The functional assessment of elderly people. *Journal of the American Geriatrics Society, 19*, 465–491.

Preface

For many years, rehabilitation team members have searched for valid, reliable, precise, and practical instruments with which to measure rehabilitation outcomes. Through use of standardized functional assessment instruments and methods, documentation of outcomes of care becomes reproducible from both one rehabilitation professional to another and one setting to another. Benefits can also be quantified and related to costs. Functional assessment and evaluation of rehabilitation outcomes can assist students in the rehabilitation health professions, clinicians, and researchers to be more effective in helping persons with disabilities attain and maintain a satisfactory quality of life.

This book will serve the needs of many rehabilitation disciplines in their continuing efforts to document and quantify the functional status of individuals before, during, and after rehabilitation intervention. Rehabilitation students, clinicians, and researchers in medicine, nursing, physical therapy, occupational therapy, speech-language-hearing pathology, psychology, rehabilitation administration, social work, rehabilitation engineering, rehabilitation counseling, nutrition, public health, and architecture may use this book as a resource for instruments to measure variables associated with disability and societal limitation (formerly known as handicap). Administrators, public health officials, and accreditors may use instruments in this book as a basis to justify third-party payment, evaluate rehabilitation programs and facilities, and determine appropriate levels of care.

Content of the book is geared to rehabilitation professionals prepared at the baccalaureate and master's degree levels. Emphasis is on measurement of activities of daily living with some attention to cognition and functional communication as measures of disability. Less emphasis is placed on measures of societal limitation because state-of-the-art instruments in this dimension are, in general, still being developed.

This book contributes to the goals specified by the National Institute on Disability and Rehabilitation Research as priorities for the University at Buffalo Rehabilitation Research and Training Center for Functional Assessment and Evaluation of Rehabilitation Outcomes. In addition, it contributes specifically to the measurement of goals for independence, empowerment, and maximum human functioning and health.

Chapter 1 provides an overview of functional assessment and evaluation, including a conceptual model for functional assessment, background leading to the development of functional measurement instruments, models for a functional approach to care, uses of functional assessment and evaluation instruments, requisites for an operational functional assessment and evaluation system, and an introduction to one specific instrument.

Chapter 2 addresses the criteria for selection and administration of functional status measures to help students and rehabilitation team members identify their needs and make a knowledgeable decision as to whether a formalized functional assessment instrument should be used. Approaches to collecting data about functional status are discussed. This chapter also describes factors to consider when readers develop a new functional assessment instrument, as well as how to retrieve existing instruments.

Chapter 3 includes a discussion of measurement in rehabilitation and biometric properties of instruments, including validity, reliability, and sensitivity. The importance of statistical power in rehabilitation outcome research is explained. Common methods of measurement scaling and implications of measurement error for establishing reliable and valid measurement procedures are also discussed.

Chapter 4 describes selected instruments including specific domains, categories and numbers of items, validity, reliability, scaling, norms (when available), revised forms, and applications to individuals and programs plus comments about their uses in clinical and research settings.

Chapter 5 addresses differences and similarities in, as well as advantages and disadvantages of, general health, disease-specific, and functional status measures.

Chapters 6, 7, and 8 address important factors in assessing the degree to which individuals function within society. The environment as a mediating factor in functional assessment is discussed in Chapter 6. Theoretical considerations, a case study in developing measures, issues in measurement, and a study of environments are discussed. In Chapter 7, a functional approach to the assessment of psychological and psychosocial factors in rehabilitation is addressed. The chapter begins with a case study discussed in terms of an individual's motivation and coping and the importance of timing in measuring these two variables. Theoretical frameworks, including psychological, developmental, and cognitive theories, are discussed. Sources for instruments to evaluate psychological status are identified.

Chapter 8 addresses a growing area of interest in assessment; that is, the assessment of technological factors in rehabilitation. Assistive devices for upper and lower extremity functional limitations, importance of matching persons with the most appropriate technology, description of available outcome measures for assistive technology service delivery, individual incentives and disincentives to assistive technology use, and measurement of outcomes from several dimensions of self are included.

Appendix A consists of selected functional assessment instruments, chosen for display because of their common usage. References for each instrument are given after the instrument description.

Appendix B includes a list of resources for further information about functional assessment and evaluation.

Currently, rehabilitation practitioners and researchers must sort through several references to find commonly used functional assessment and evaluation instruments. Then they spend further time determining the validity, reliability, sensitivity, and sensibility of these instruments, as well as assessing the appropriateness of each instrument for their specific needs. It is hoped that this book will be a timesaver for service providers, investigators, and students, as well as act as an impetus for further research in the measurement of impairment, disability, and societal limitation.

Sharon S. Dittmar, PhD, RN
Glen E. Gresham, MD

Acknowledgments

The editors acknowledge the assistance of the following graduate students for writing reviews of instruments:

Susan D. Meyers, BS, RN
Self-rating Depression Scale
Frenchay Activities Index

Mary A. Cosmas, BS, OTR/L
Frenchay Activities Index
Beck Depression Inventory

Gretchen E. Gross-Kralj, BS, OTR/L
Jebsen Test of Hand Function
Pediatric Evaluation of Disability (PEDI)

Dianne P. McFall, BS, RN
Klein–Bell ADL Scale
Instrumental Activities of Daily Living

Patricia A. Sperle, MS
WeeFIM®
Pediatric Evaluation of Disability (PEDI)

The editors also acknowledge the following persons for use of the summary describing field testing of the American Speech-Language-Hearing Association's instrument titled "Functional Assessment of Communication Skills for Adults":

Carol M. Frattali, PhD
Cynthia K. Thompson, PhD
Audrey L. Holland, PhD
Cheryl B. Wohl, BA
Michelle M. Ferketic, MA

CHAPTER 1

Overview: A Functional Approach to Measurement of Rehabilitation Outcomes

Sharon S. Dittmar

BEHAVIORAL OBJECTIVES

After completing this chapter, the reader will be able to
- discuss the concept of function.
- relate the background leading to development of functional assessment and evaluation instruments.
- describe models for a functional approach to rehabilitative care.

- explain uses of functional assessment and evaluation instruments in rehabilitation.
- outline requisites of an operational functional assessment and evaluation system.
- describe a widely used functional assessment instrument.

The way in which a person functions despite disease and impairment is of major interest in rehabilitation. In this chapter, the concept of function is discussed, and models for a functional approach to documentation of rehabilitation are presented. Background in the development of instruments to measure degree of independent function is also given. Both uses of instruments for functional assessment and evaluation and requisites for an operational functional assessment system are discussed. Finally, an example of an instrument to measure function is discussed. Measurement is used synonymously throughout with assessment and evaluation.

CONCEPT OF FUNCTION

As stated in the Foreword, Lawton (1971) provided one of the earliest definitions of functional assessment, relating that it was "any systematic attempt to measure objectively the level at which a person is functioning, in any of a variety of areas such as physical health, quality of self-maintenance, quality of role activity, intellectual status, social activity, attitude toward the world and self, and emotional status" (p. 465). According to Moinpour, McCorkle, and Saunders (1988), the concepts of *physical functioning* and *functional*

status have been used interchangeably, as well as equated to other terms such as *health status*, *level of impairment*, and *disability*.

The World Health Organization ([WHO], 1947) defines health status as "a comprehensive state of physical, mental, and social well-being and not merely the absence of disease or infirmity" (p. 1). Liang and Jette (1981) distinguish functional status from *disease activity*—which refers to a biologic state and health status—by stating that it "is an individual's performance in activities of daily living" (p. 80).

Harris, Jette, Campion, and Cleary (1986) operationalize function in relation to specific tasks. They divide skills into basic activities of daily living (BADL) and instrumental activities of daily living (IADL) needed to perform in an environment. They identified five components of BADL: walking inside, performing bed-to-chair transfers, getting on and off the toilet, putting on and taking off shoes, and putting on and taking off socks. Other researchers have measured many other components of BADL such as aspects of self-care (e.g., bathing, dressing, sphincter control, eating, and mobility). Lawton (1971) identified IADL as ability to use the telephone, shopping, food preparation, housekeeping, laundry, mode of transportation, taking responsibility for own medications, and ability to handle finances.

To accomplish the above-mentioned skills, a person must be able to think about the activities in logical sequence; distinguish left from right; be oriented to time, place, person, and self; organize self physically and mentally for performance; and understand the consequences for self and society of varying degrees of performance. A person might physically be able to dress himself or herself but not understand societal reaction to wearing his or her pants as a shirt. Consequently, necessary interventions and level of care for the person who is unable to dress appropriately differ greatly from those for the person who dresses as expected by society. In this book, *function* is conceptualized as a person's ability to perform BADL and IADL; think about and plan these basic and instrumental tasks within his or her own environment, whether that be home, institution, or community; and assume roles expected by society.

A term related to physical status and the medical model is *pathophysiology*, which refers to "any interruption of or interference with normal physiological and developmental process or structures" (U.S. Department of Health and Human Services, [HHS], 1993, p. 32). Another term related to the medical model is *impairment*, which refers to "any loss or abnormality at the organ or organ system level of the body. Impairment may include cognitive, emotional, physiological, or anatomical structure or function and includes all losses or abnormalities, not just those attributable to the initial pathophysiology" (HHS, 1993, p. 36). Impairments may be temporary, permanent, or progressive. Terms related to functional status include *functional limitation, disability, societal limitation* (formerly known as handicap), *functional assessment*, and *functional evaluation*. These terms are defined as follows:

- Functional limitation is a "restriction or lack of ability to perform an action in the manner or within the range consistent with the purpose of an organ or organ system" (HHS, 1993, p. 36).
- Disability is an inability or "limitation in performing tasks, activities, and roles to levels expected within physical and social contexts" (HHS, 1993, p. 37).
- Societal limitation (formerly known as handicap) is a "disadvantage resulting from impairment and the ensuing disability which limits the fulfillment of an individual's social role" (Susset & Raymond, 1984, p. 325).
- Functional assessment is "a method for describing abilities and activities in order to measure an individual's use of the variety of skills included in performing the tasks necessary to daily living, vocational pursuits, social interactions, leisure activities, and other required behaviors" (Granger, 1984, p. 24). For purposes of this book, functional assessment refers to any systematic attempt to measure objectively ability at the person level

including BADL, IADL, mental status, communication, and sensorimotor ability. It also refers to ability to function at the societal level, including performing roles in the family and during leisure time, as well as at work and school and in the person's own environment albeit home, institution, or community.
- Functional evaluation is the measurement of function in several specific domains.

DEVELOPMENT OF FUNCTIONAL ASSESSMENT AND EVALUATION INSTRUMENTS

Rehabilitation has long been associated with measurement of specific functions and quality of life as the aggregate of all functions. With the holistic approach to the individual prominent after World War II, a comprehensive assessment—including physical, functional, psychosocial, and vocational factors—became the norm. Thus, in addition to physical function, attention was given to how the individual interacted with others and the environment. Only recently have rehabilitation professionals given adequate attention to how individuals intellectually process information and think about the world. Quality of life issues have received increased attention as the costs and effects of advances in science and technology, as well as what these advances mean to the individual and society in terms of health and well-being, have been examined.

One of the responsibilities of rehabilitation team members is to assess physical, psychosocial, vocational, and cognitive functions of an individual with a disability. Although much attention has been given to the objective measurement of physical status, little attention has been given to the objective measurement of how a person functions with remaining abilities despite impairment. The increasing number of persons with impairments and the cost of providing services to these individuals have resulted in attention to the need for evaluation and classification of functional abilities before, during, and after rehabilitation service delivery from individual, family, and societal perspectives.

The medical model of cause, pathology, and manifestations of disease is generally considered to be limited to identification of characteristics of *disease*, rather than *function*. When using a medical model for approaches to care, all too often individuals with disabilities are encouraged to maintain, rather than give up, the sick role. Thus they are frequently exempt from what are considered normal social activities and responsibilities, as well as less likely to be motivated to take charge of their personal and social affairs with any degree of independence. Their ability to function within their institutional or home environments is frequently not assessed.

In one of the first attempts to reconcile various performance criteria with disease classifications, Moskowitz and

McCann (1957) used a systematic functional classification scheme developed by the Canadian Army and subsequently adopted by the United States Army during World War II. In its original application, this classification system was based on rigid standards geared to the performance levels of young men. To determine functional abilities of chronically ill and aged individuals, Moskowitz and McCann adapted the classification scheme used in Canada and referred to it as the PULSES Profile. This adapted measure is still used today to evaluate objectively the functional abilities of United States Army troops (see Appendix A, Exhibit A–4).

Further impetus for the development of functional assessment and evaluation measures came as a result of five factors:

1. Difficulties arising in using diagnostic terms for the provision of care or rehabilitative services for institutionalized chronically ill and aged persons. In nursing home care, diagnostic labels did not offer the kind of information needed by nonphysician care providers to plan rehabilitation programs.
2. Need to prescribe patient rehabilitation interventions for persons with physical and cognitive disabilities. In this instance, data are needed to provide rehabilitation therapies in both hospital and nursing home settings, as well as in home care and outpatient programs.
3. Need to determine the amount of individual benefit from the Workers' Compensation Board.
4. Need to justify national expenditures for Social Security Income payments to persons with disabilities.
5. Need to justify national expenditures for Medicare and state expenditures for Medicaid.

MODELS FOR A FUNCTIONAL APPROACH TO CARE

A need for standard terminology in rehabilitation exists. Historically, specialists in rehabilitation medicine (Nagi, 1965; Topliss, 1978; Wood, 1980) have attempted to establish common terms. Their work led to the World Health Organization's publication of the *International Classification of Impairments, Disabilities, and Handicaps (ICIDH)* (1980). More recently, Stineman and Granger (1994) have depicted the terminology of the *ICIDH* in a conceptual model for functional assessment (Figure 1–1). In this model, some of the commonly used terms in rehabilitation are related to origin of conditions, resulting conditions, attachment of labels to these conditions, a way of examining characteristics of the conditions, and interventions appropriate for each conceptual formulation.

Figure 1–1 shows that key terms have been attached to three conditions. The first condition, pathology at the organ level, is defined by anatomical, physiological, mental, and psychological deficits, which can be explained by specific diagnostic descriptors resulting in impairment (e.g., weakness of muscles, requiring medical and restorative therapy). An impairment does not necessarily mean that a disease is still present.

The second condition, behavioral manifestations at the person level, is characterized by performance deficits within the physical and social environments, which result in difficulty with tasks or disability (sometimes called a functional limitation). Examples of disability would be limited abilities in performance of self-care and mobility; recreational, vocational, and economic activities; as well as communication and the fulfilling of social roles. Disability is minimized through the use of adaptive equipment and therapeutic relearning of activities of daily living (ADL).

The third condition, role assignment at the societal level, is represented by environmental and societal deficits influenced by social norms and social policies leading to the label handicap, which results from a social disadvantage for a given individual (Stineman & Granger, 1994) and is henceforth referred to as societal limitation.

Societal limitations (handicaps) are characterized by a difference between what an individual can do or how he or she appears and how particular groups expect a person to perform. Societal limitation is influenced strongly by existing societal values and institutional arrangements. It is minimized through social policy support and reduction in physical and attitudinal barriers. Handicapping conditions or conditions that create societal limitation include inaccessible buildings and negative public attitudes. Individuals affected by impairment, disability, and societal limitation need long-range coordination of services to improve and maintain their functional abilities (Stineman & Granger, 1994). The term *handicap* is no longer used in the language of federal agencies or by persons with disabilities.

Whiteneck (1994) expanded WHO's model (1980) to include secondary impairment, secondary disability, and secondary handicap, all of which lead to perceived health, perceived activity limitation, and perceived role limitation, respectively. All areas of perception yield an individual's quality of life. Both societal limitations and individual characteristics affect handicap (now known as societal limitation) (see Figure 1–2).

In this model, Whiteneck discusses the need for broader health status measures to "track individuals over time," thus determining how successfully rehabilitation has controlled lifetime secondary impairments (p. 1074). In theory, he believes that instruments such as the Functional Independence Measure (FIM^SM) discussed later in this chapter and Appendix A, should be able to document changes in ADL over time. In turn, instruments such as the CHART: Craig Handicap Assessment and Reporting Technique and Community Integration Questionnaire "should be able to track the cumu-

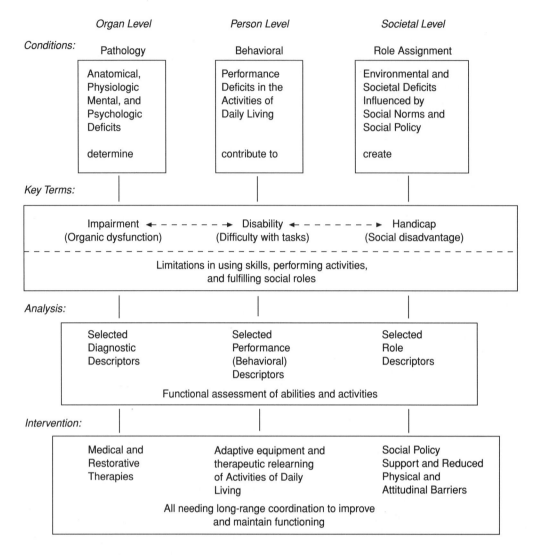

Figure 1–1 Outcome measurement in rehabilitation. *Source:* Reprinted with permission from M.G. Stineman and C.V. Granger. Outcome Studies and Analysis: Principles of Rehabilitation That Influence Outcome Analysis, in G. Fesfenthal, S.J. Garrison, and F. Steinberg, eds., p. 516, *Rehabilitation of the aging and elderly patient*, © 1994, Williams & Wilkins Co.

lative impact of primary and secondary handicaps" (Whiteneck, 1994, p. 1074).

Whiteneck (1994) points out that, in addition to objective measurements, individuals with disability have subjective perceptions regarding health, activity limitations, and role limitations. Although these perceptions are related to the more objective measurements of impairment, disability, and societal limitation (handicap), these perceptions are distinct. The National Institutes of Health now recommends the measurement of patient perceptions of specific impairments and more global perceptions of perceived health as appropriate outcome measures in clinical trials (Furberg & Schuttinga, 1990). Quality of life is evolving as a comprehensive subjec-

tive measurement of well-being, which is "comprised of subjective perceptions in broad domains" (p. 1075). A strength resulting from this model is the logical connection between rehabilitation interventions and the ultimate concern with quality of life (Whiteneck, 1994).

The National Center for Medical Rehabilitation and Research (NCMRR) (HHS, 1993) summarized the approaches to classification proposed by WHO (1980), Nagi (1965), and the Public Health Service Task Force. The NCMRR then added its own conceptualization (see Table 1–1), and its Advisory Board developed a model to describe the medical rehabilitation process (see Figure 1–3). In Table 1–1, the classification schema proposed by WHO, Nagi, and the Public

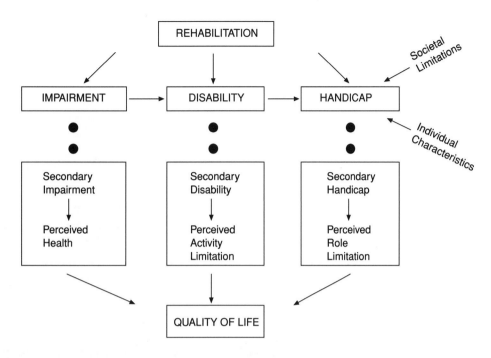

Figure 1–2 A model of rehabilitation outcomes that builds on the concepts of impairment, disability, and handicap from the World Health Organization's model of disablement (1980). *Source:* Reprinted with permission from G.G. Whiteneck. The 44th Annual John Stanley Coulter Lecture, Measuring What Matters: Key Rehabilitation Outcomes, *Archives of Physical Medicine and Rehabilitation, Vol. 75*, p. 1075, © 1994, W.B. Saunders.

Health Service (PHS) Task Force are compared according to impact on the person with a disability and impact on others. The NCMRR classification schema is then outlined, followed by definitions of pathophysiology, impairment, functional limitation, disability, and societal limitation.

In the model presented in Figure 1–3, the person is viewed as the primary focus of the rehabilitation process. Also considered are personal background factors, such as organic, psychosocial, and environmental aspects of the person before disability. The health care environment and society as a whole are considered as having an impact on the rehabilitation process. Quality of life is affected by survival, productivity, and social and work relationship issues. This model incorporates bidirectional arrows to depict the complexities, feedback loops, and integrating aspects of the process across the life span. According to the Advisory Board of NCMRR, "the systems approach is an essential feature of medical rehabilitation research and, ultimately, all health care delivery" (HHS, 1993, p. 27).

The Advisory Board of NCMRR rejected a linear model of pathology, impairment, functional limitation, disability, and societal limitation because members believed that progression is not always sequential, nor unidirectional. Rather, it is a complex feedback loop that "integrates the whole person as an entity who must adjust to problems in many of

these areas simultaneously" (HHS, 1993, p. 31). (Refer to Figure 1–3.)

As a final consideration, Granger raises questions regarding the art and science of rehabilitation. He asks, "What is the essence of rehabilitation? How objective are we in determining the success of rehabilitation? What are the personal, social, and economic costs in determining burden of care? Science is yet lacking in answering these questions" (C.V. Granger, personal communication, March 1995). He proposes an organizing and unifying model to guide research (see Figure 1–4) in answering these questions (Granger et al., 1996). The model stems from Maslow's theory of human motivation (Maslow, 1968). This model fits well with existing theoretical frameworks, including von Bertalanffy's open systems model (1968) and Lewin's (Bennis, Benne, & Chin, 1961) planned change theory.

Granger's model proposes that an individual's fulfillment and quality of living are a result of striking a balance between functional opportunities and functional requirements (or demands) portrayed on the right and left sides of his model, respectively (Figure 1–4). "Functional opportunities are expressed in physical, cognitive, and emotional terms. In order to achieve fulfillment and to maximize the quality of daily living, there must be a balance between improved opportunities through individual health and functioning (*on the*

Table 1–1 Terminology in Disability Classification

Classification Schema Proposed by	Impact on Person with Disability				Impact on Others	
WHO	Disease	Impairment	Disability	Handicap Disadvantage in Life Roles		
Nagi Disability in America Model	Pathophysiology	Impairment	Functional Limitations	Disability		
Public Health Service Task Force	Underlying Cause	Organ Level	Person Level	Interaction of Environment on Person	Family	Community
NCMRR	Pathophysiology	Impairment	Functional Limitation	Disability Limitation	Societal Limitation	

Pathophysiology: Interruption or interference with normal physiological and developmental processes or structures.

Impairment: Loss or abnormality of cognitive, emotional, physiological, or anatomical structure or function, including all losses or abnormalities, not just those attributable to the initial pathophysiology.

Functional Limitation: Restriction or lack of ability to perform an action in the manner or within the range consistent with the purpose of an organ or organ system.

Disability: Inability or limitation in performing tasks, activities, and roles to levels expected within physical and social contexts.

Societal Limitation: Restriction attributable to social policy or barriers (structural or attitudinal), which limits fulfillment of roles or denies access to services and opportunities that are associated with full participation in society.

Source: Reprinted from U.S. Department of Health and Human Services, *Research Plan for the National Center for Medical Rehabilitation Research,* NIH Pub. No. 93–3509, March, 1993, National Institutes of Health, National Institute of Child Health and Human Development, Bethesda, Maryland.

left) and the reduction or removal of life's barriers (*on the right*)" (Granger et al., 1996, p. 240). The ultimate goal of medical rehabilitation then becomes, in Maslow's terms, self-actualization—the full use of the human capacities to perceive, feel, create, and love in the form of fulfillment through the everyday efforts to challenge barriers and overcome them. Although the opportunities and requirements identified as challenges to the quality of daily living are not directly measurable, the factors that determine the opportunities and requirements are subject to description and measurement. Thus a number of instruments have been developed in rehabilitation to measure these factors.

USES OF FUNCTIONAL ASSESSMENT AND EVALUATION INSTRUMENTS IN REHABILITATION PROGRAMS

Functional assessment and evaluation instruments are used for a number of reasons. Measures are applied to deter-

mine rehabilitation outcomes for both individuals and program management. Instruments to determine functional progress or lack of progress can be used (1) internally to improve quality of programs or (2) externally by third-party payers for reimbursement and accreditation purposes. Data are used to plan rehabilitation interventions, determine effectiveness of treatment, maintain continuity of care, and develop and improve treatment resources.

In planning rehabilitation interventions, patient problem lists are developed as a result of the systematic assessment of function. For instance, on initial assessment team members may note impaired mobility manifested by the individual's inability to transfer due to right-sided hemiparesis. Rehabilitation interventions might be to teach a patient to use pull ropes, use his or her left leg and arm to come to a sitting position, and practice balance exercises at the side of the bed before progressing to a standing position and transfer to a chair.

Data from functional assessment can be used to determine clinical changes in the above-mentioned example by com-

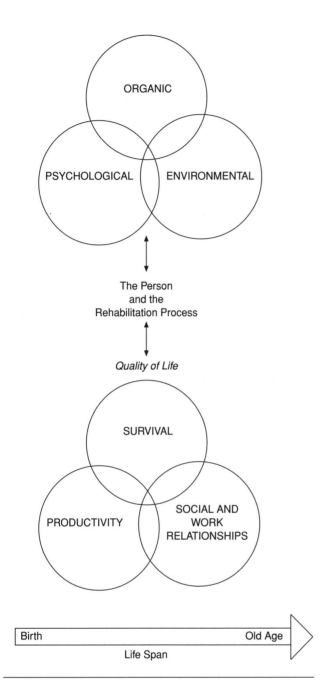

Figure 1–3 The rehabilitation process: A systems approach. *Source:* Reprinted from U.S. Department of Health and Human Services, *Research Plan for the National Center for Medical Rehabilitation Research*, NIH Pub. No. 93–3509, March, 1993, National Institutes of Health, National Institute of Child Health and Human Development, Bethesda, Maryland.

paring scores in transfer before and after these interventions. Benefits of clinical intervention could also be demonstrated in terms of cost for a personal care aide to assist in transfer versus independent transfer. Further, data could also be used

in utilization review to determine the least restrictive environments and most cost-effective levels of care.

Tracking the progress of all patients with hemiparesis through a system of care helps rehabilitation program personnel determine strengths and weaknesses of discipline-specific and rehabilitation team interventions. Data can then contribute to decisions for changing interventions to improve outcomes. Functional measurement can also be used to ensure that a program of care is addressing issues most likely to improve quality of life for a person with a disability by facilitating individual case management.

The needs of a defined population such as a group of patients with right-sided hemiparesis—who, at the time of admission to a rehabilitation program, cannot execute self-transfer—can be related to the assessment and analysis of function from a sample of individuals with that impairment and functional limitation. In addition, staffing needs for number and type of rehabilitation team personnel can be related to the levels of independence in the patients observed. If and when health care resources are rationed, needs can be prioritized when examined in relation to aggregate outcomes.

Treatment resources can also be improved when objective data are used to measure function. Deficiencies in care can be identified and improvements planned and implemented when functional assessment is used in program evaluation. Quality improvement procedures and rehabilitative care audit studies are used to gather data for improving resources. Another method of improving treatment resources is through establishing comparability of patient groups through research studies and using the findings to affect national standardized clinical guidelines such as those developed by professionals on committees of government agencies and professional organizations.

A WIDELY USED COMPREHENSIVE FUNCTIONAL ASSESSMENT INSTRUMENT: CASE OF THE FIM℠

In 1983 a task force, funded by the US Department of Education, National Institute of Handicapped Research (NIHR), later known as the National Institute on Disability and Rehabilitation Research (NIDRR) and sponsored by the American Congress of Rehabilitation Medicine and the American Academy of Physical Medicine and Rehabilitation, began to develop a uniform data system for medical rehabilitation. Task force members were charged with developing a minimum data set of key functions in a form that could be easily administered. Reliability, validity, and suitability for administration by any discipline were to be determined for any functional assessment instrument developed. This project was housed in the School of Medicine and Bio-

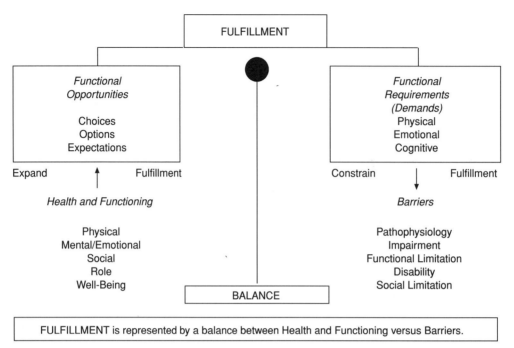

Figure 1–4 *Source:* Reprinted with permission from C.V. Granger et al., Quality and Outcome Measures for Rehabilitation, in *Physical Medicine and Rehabilitation*, R.L. Braddom, ed., p. 240, © 1996, W.B. Saunders Company.

medical Sciences at the University at Buffalo, State University of New York.

The instrument developed by this task force, after review of extant functional assessment instruments, is known as the FIM^SM (see Table 1–2). The biometric properties of this instrument were tested for several years at various facilities serving patients with disabilities throughout the United States. The FIM^SM is designed to measure level of independence in self-care, sphincter control, transfers, locomotion, communication, and social cognition. Each variable within these categories (some of which are also domains) is scored on a one to seven scale, with the higher scores indicating more independence and less assistance. When the instrument was tested in the field by clinicians in all rehabilitation disciplines, these professionals indicated that a one to seven scoring system would give them more precise information than a one to four scale to evaluate patient progress and the rehabilitation program overall. Input regarding this instrument was also sought and obtained from every professional organization representing rehabilitation disciplines. With input from these groups and field testing of the instrument, the

FIM^SM was revised *(Guide for the Uniform Data Set for Medical Rehabilitation [Adult FIM^SM], Version 4.0, 1993).*

The Adult FIM^SM is now used in more than 700 facilities in the United States and in more than 15 foreign facilities. The United States UDS_MR^SM database contains more than 1.2 million patient records and adds 200,000 new cases annually (C.V. Granger, personal communication, September 24, 1996). More than 150 articles have appeared in the professional literature discussing this instrument's psychometric properties and application. (See Chapter 4 and Appendix A for further description of the FIM^SM.)

CONCLUSION

The concept of function, need for and development of functional measurement instruments, models for a functional approach to care, and uses of functional assessment data have been discussed. The FIM^SM has been initially described. In Chapter 2, issues related to selecting and administering functional assessment and evaluation instruments are addressed.

Table 1–2 Functional Independence Measure^{SM}

Adult FIM^{SM}

LEVELS		NO HELPER / HELPER
	7 Complete Independence (Timely, Safely) 6 Modified Independence (Device)	NO HELPER

	Modified Dependence
	  5 Supervision
	  4 Minimal Assist (Subject = 75% +)
	  3 Moderate Assist (Subject = 50% +)
	
	Complete Dependence
	  2 Maximal Assist (Subject = 25% +)
	  1 Total Assist (Subject = 0% +)
		HELPER

	ADMIT	DISCHARGE	FOLLOW-UP
Self-Care			
A. Eating	☐	☐	☐
B. Grooming	☐	☐	☐
C. Bathing	☐	☐	☐
D. Dressing—Upper Body	☐	☐	☐
E. Dressing—Lower Body	☐	☐	☐
F. Toileting	☐	☐	☐
Sphincter Control			
G. Bladder Management	☐	☐	☐
H. Bowel Management	☐	☐	☐
Transfers			
I. Bed, Chair, Wheelchair	☐	☐	☐
J. Toilet	☐	☐	☐
K. Tub, Shower	☐	☐	☐
Locomotion	Walk / Wheelchair / Both ☐	Walk / Wheelchair / Both ☐	Walk / Wheelchair / Both ☐
L. Walk/Wheelchair			
M. Stairs	☐	☐	☐
Motor Subtotal Score	☐	☐	☐
Communication	Auditory / Visual / Both ☐	Auditory / Visual / Both ☐	Auditory / Visual / Both ☐
N. Comprehension			
O. Expression	Vocal / Nonvocal / Both ☐	Vocal / Nonvocal / Both ☐	Vocal / Nonvocal / Both ☐
Social Cognition			
P. Social Interaction	☐	☐	☐
Q. Problem Solving	☐	☐	☐
R. Memory	☐	☐	☐
Cognitive Subtotal Score	☐	☐	☐
Total FIM	☐	☐	☐

Note: Leave no blanks; enter 1 if patient not testable due to risk.

Copyright © 1993 Uniform Data System for Medical Rehabilitation, a division of U B Foundation Activities, Inc.

Source: Reprinted with permission from Uniform Data System for Medical Rehabilitation, a division of U B Foundation Activities, Inc. *Guide for the Uniform Data Set for Medical Rehabilitation (Adult FIM^{SM})* Version 4.0, State University of New York, Buffalo, © 1993, Buffalo, NY.

REFERENCES

Bennis, W.G., Benne, K.D., & Chin, R. (1961). *The planning of change.* New York: Holt, Rinehart & Winston.

Furberg, D.C., & Schuttinga, J.A. (Co-chairmen). (1990). Quality of life assessment: Practice, problem, and promise. Proceedings of a workshop, October 15–17, 1990. Washington, DC: U.S. Department of Health and Human Services, Public Health Service, National Institutes of Health.

Granger, C.V. (1984). A conceptual model for functional assessment. In C.V. Granger & G.E. Gresham (Eds.), *Functional assessment in rehabilitation medicine.* Baltimore: Williams & Wilkins.

Granger, C.V., Kelly-Hayes, M., Johnston, M., Deutsch, A., Braun, S.L., & Fiedler, R.C. (1996). Quality and outcome measures for medical rehabilitation. In R.L. Braddom (Ed.), *Physical medicine and rehabilitation* (pp. 239–254). Philadelphia: W.B. Saunders.

Guide for the uniform data set for medical rehabilitation (Adult FIM^SM), version 4.0. (1993). Buffalo, NY: State University of New York.

Harris, B.A., Jette, A.M., Campion, E.W., & Cleary, P.D. (1986). Validity of self-report measures of functional disability. *Topics in Geriatric Rehabilitation, 1*(3), 31–41.

Lawton, M.P. (1971). The functional assessment of elderly people. *Journal of the American Geriatric Society, 19*(6), 465–481.

Liang, M.H., & Jette, A.M. (1981). Measuring functional ability in chronic arthritis: A critical review. *Arthritis and Rheumatism, 24*(1), 80–86.

Maslow, A. (1968). *Toward a psychology of being* (2nd ed.). Princeton, NJ: Van Nostrand.

Moinpour, C.M., McCorkle, R., & Saunders, J. (1988). Measuring functional status. In M. Frank-Stromborg (Ed.), *Instruments for clinical nursing research* (pp. 23–45). Norwalk, CT: Appleton & Lange.

Moskowitz, E., & McCann, C.B. (1957). Classification of disability in the chronically ill and aging. *Journal of Chronic Disease, 5,* 342–346.

Nagi, S.Z. (1965). *Disability and rehabilitation.* Columbus: Ohio State University Press.

Stineman, M.G., & Granger, C.V. (1994). Outcome studies and analysis: Principles of rehabilitation that influence outcome analysis. In G. Fesfenthal, S.J. Garrison, & F. Steinberg (Eds.), *Rehabilitation of the aging and elderly patient* (pp. 511–516). Baltimore: Williams & Wilkins.

Susset, V., & Raymond, P.M. (1984). Prognosis and prediction: From patient to policy. In C.V. Granger & G.E. Gresham (Eds.), *Functional assessment in rehabilitation medicine* (pp. 324–342). Baltimore: Williams & Wilkins.

Topliss, E. (1978). The disabled. In P. Brearly & E. Topliss (Eds.), *The social context of health care.* London: Martin Robertson.

U.S. Department of Health and Human Services. (1993, March). *Research plan for the National Center for Medical Rehabilitation Research* (NIH Publication No. 93–3509). Bethesda, MD: National Institutes of Health, National Institute of Child Health and Human Development.

von Bertalanffy, L. (1968). *General system theory: Foundations, development, applications* (rev. ed.). New York: George Braziller.

Whiteneck, G.G. (1994). The 44th Annual John Stanley Coulter Lecture: Measuring what matters—Key rehabilitation outcomes. *Archives of Physical Medicine and Rehabilitation, 75,* 1073–1076.

Wood, P.H.N. (1980). The language of disablement: A glossary relating to disease and its consequences. *International Rehabilitation Medicine, 2,* 86–92.

World Health Organization (1947). Constitution of the World Health Organization. *Chronicle of the World Health Organization.* Geneva: Author; p. 1.

World Health Organization. (1980). *International classification of impairments, disabilities, and handicaps.* Geneva: Author.

CHAPTER 2

Selection and Administration of Functional Assessment and Rehabilitation Outcome Measures

Sharon S. Dittmar

BEHAVIORAL OBJECTIVES

After completing this chapter, the reader will be able to
- describe considerations in choosing functional assessment instruments.
- discuss approaches to obtaining data about functional status.
- explain arguments for and against the reader's developing his or her own functional assessment instrument.
- locate existing functional assessment instruments.

In this chapter, issues in selecting functional assessment and evaluation measures, approaches to obtaining data about functional status, arguments for and against the reader's developing his or her own instruments, and helpful hints for locating functional assessment instruments are discussed.

SELECTION OF FUNCTIONAL ASSESSMENT AND EVALUATION MEASURES

As a professional and reader of this book, choosing a method to assess and evaluate individuals' progress over time in your rehabilitation program involves much thought, planning, and study. The selected functional assessment and evaluation system must demonstrate that the rehabilitation service provision is effective. Regardless of the system selected, the rehabilitation team should be able to show that

- communication is improved among team members, including the patient and his or her family.
- relationships exist between areas of functional limitation and types of service provided.
- outcomes of care are improved.
- individual patients or groups of patients, in which outcomes did not improve and who might need changes in rehabilitation services, can be easily identified. It should also be possible to examine these services for positive and negative outcomes.

In addition, the system chosen must strike a balance between ideal objectives and acceptable cost. Hence, it must be practical for the professional and the facility while still achieving the program objectives and documenting outcomes for internal and external evaluators.

The following 19 questions must be answered to determine the appropriate choice in selecting a functional measure:

1. Which functions will be measured?
2. Does the instrument account for cultural and ethnic diversity?
3. Are data being gathered for research or clinical purposes?
4. Are there plans for publishing the measurement findings?
5. Which members of the team will be observing and scoring which functions, or will each member of the team be scoring all functions?
6. At what times in the rehabilitation trajectory will the functional assessment and evaluation be completed?
7. What type of inservice will be given regarding the process; and at what times, to whom, and by whom will these programs be delivered?
8. Where will the instruments be kept?
9. How will inter-rater reliability be established?

10. Will one instrument suffice for all purposes, or will more than one instrument be needed to determine outcomes?
11. What will be done with the data?
12. What will the patient and his or her family be told about this procedure?
13. How will data be used in further education of the patient and his or her family?
14. Will the data be used in team conference, and if so, how?
15. Is there an established protocol to adjust interventions when function does not improve?
16. What kind of follow-up will be done with staff to ensure continued interest and quality improvement of the process?
17. How will data be used in continued education of staff?
18. In what ways can staff contribute to improving the methods of data collection and use?
19. What will be done with aggregate data to evaluate the rehabilitation program?

Any instrument used to assess and evaluate performance must meet the following criteria:

• Be readily available.
• Have measurement properties of validity, reliability, and sensitivity.
• Seem sensible and feasible to use in the situation.
• Ideally be formatted so that data can be used individually and in the aggregate for education, practice, and research.
• Be attractive and concise, requiring minimum time to administer while giving maximum information about performance.

The form should also have a relatively uncluttered appearance and provide capability to explain or augment responses in a narrative explanation. Ideally, it should be displayed in the patient's record, and the patient should have a copy.

Functional assessment instruments must be appropriate for the domains to be measured. For example, inpatients who are paraplegic or paraparetic will have to learn bed mobility, management of sphincters, transfer, and wheelchair management or functional ambulation. Thus, any chosen functional instrument must include self-care and mobility.

Levels of competence must also be considered when choosing a functional assessment instrument. What criteria will be used to measure a person's ability? Competence is usually measured against a set of norms in a specific society at a specific point in time. However, certain co-cultures may have different sets of norms, and competence must be related to differences in cultural practices. For example, for some co-cultures total baths are taken everyday, whereas in other cultures total baths are taken only once a week and partial bathing is carried out on a daily basis. Thus, observation of performance competence must be consistent with the cultural practices of the group being observed or cultural diversity must be considered when scoring performance (Moinpour, McCorkle, & Sanders, 1988).

Another consideration in selecting functional and evaluation measures is deciding whether to score usual performance or capacity for performance. Under structured conditions, an individual may perform at optimum capacity. In other situations, depending on factors such as environment, weather, mood, and life demands, the person may not function at optimum level (Moinpour et al., 1988).

Most measures of functional status are designed to elicit selected demographic information. Demographic information—such as gender; birth date; living arrangements before hospitalization; prehospital vocational category; discharge living arrangement; payment source for rehabilitation; ethnicity; admission date; discharge date; and program interruption, transfer, and return date—is often collected at the time of instrument administration. In addition, an outcome measurement can be designed to collect extensive information on diagnosis, including impairment group, date of onset, and etiologic diagnosis (code in the *International Classification of Diseases, Ninth Edition, Clinical Modification*). Follow-up assessment may also include living arrangements, such as type of dwelling and with whom living; vocational status; information source; method of follow-up; health maintenance; therapy; and current diagnoses. Thus, when instruments are designed to collect these data, all necessary demographic information for clinical and research purposes at specific points in time is available.

Many instruments have technical manuals to guide administration. Any measures intended for widespread use should be accompanied by a technical manual or instructions. According to Johnston, Keith, and Hinderer (1992), standards for technical manuals include the following:

1. Technical manuals should describe the intended use of the measure and should provide supporting evidence of the properties of the measure, including reliability and validity for recommended uses.
2. The qualifications of users, the circumstances of use, and the major limitations to use should be described.
3. If an assessment instrument is intended to measure functional capacity, the number of trials allowed to reach criterion should be specified.
4. Promotional material, advertising, and manuals should neither state nor suggest that a measure can do more than is supported by research evidence. (p. S–12)

The following seven guidelines are offered for selecting a functional assessment instrument:

1. Know the purpose for which function is being measured.
2. Know what domains are to be measured.
3. Know categories within domains that are to be measured.
4. Know the biometric (psychometric) properties of the chosen instrument, including type of validity, reliability, and precision (sensitivity); internal consistency; scaling; and norms for scaling.
5. Know with what sample the biometric (psychometric) properties were established.
6. Know that no single instrument can meet all assessment needs; clinical judgment is very important in assessment.
7. Continuously seek out improved instruments to measure function.

APPROACHES TO COLLECTING DATA ABOUT FUNCTIONAL STATUS

There are a number of ways rehabilitation team members can collect data about functional status. The oldest and most widely tested approach to data collection is observation. Seeing what a person can do and determining his or her grade on a scale often yield very reliable and accurate information to the educated and experienced clinician. Inconsistencies in education and experience, however, may lead to lack of a uniform database for evaluation across programs, as well as to inappropriate prescription of rehabilitation services as a result of these evaluations.

Another method of functional status data collection, which is practical and cost effective, is use of self-reports. Consumers can report on their own functional status in person through a structured interview or by telephone. In three survey research studies conducted by Sudman (1966) with the use of the telephone method, findings suggested that using the telephone reduced costs without decreasing cooperation or accuracy. In a more recent study, Harris, Jette, Campion, and Cleary (1986) found that the agreement level between self-report and observed performance on the Functional Status Index was high in a sample of 47 elderly patients with hip fracture. Advantages of the self-report are that it is the "easiest, fastest, and most inexpensive direct method of assessing functional disability" (Harris et al., 1986, p. 32). Conversely, direct observation of functional tasks is time consuming, costly, and limited to relatively simple activities. It also frequently requires transport of a patient to a testing site or transport of standardized equipment to a patient's home (Harris et al., 1986). Others (Nelson et al., 1983) have found clinically and statistically relevant differences between professional and patient ratings of physical and emotional function when independent judgments are made.

Whether self-reports of activities are obtained by telephone or with personal contact does not seem to have a significant effect on the measurement of outcomes. Rintala and Willems (1991) did not find significant differences when they compared reports obtained by trained observers and self-reports of 27 persons with spinal cord injury who used the Self-Observation and Report Technique. They concluded that the telephone was a more efficient and convenient mode of data collection and could be used with confidence.

Research findings to date seem to indicate that self-reports by telephone follow-up are cost effective with minimal sacrifice of accuracy, particularly when simple activities are judged in persons with few and less severe functional limitations. When more complex tasks are scored in persons with more severe functional limitations, however, professional judgment seems to be more reflective than self-report of actual functional status.

Whether administered by one team member or a number of team members, the users of the instrument should have the necessary training, experience, and professional qualifications to use the instruments. Users of instruments need to adhere to training guidelines specified in technical manuals or instructions. They should also know the populations for whom the measure was designed and be able to justify logically application of the measure to the population they are assessing. They should also know the population and conditions from which normative data were collected to judge whether these data are applicable to individuals they are testing. In addition, users should know the environmental conditions, equipment requirements, and procedures for correct administration and scoring of measures they use, as well as potential effects if these factors are altered (Johnston et al., 1992). When more than one team member is administering the instrument, inter-rater reliability must be established.

In certain situations, modifications of the instrument or the testing situation may be necessary. For instance, individuals with vision impairments "may need large print, Braille, tape recorded instructions, or to have instructions read aloud to them. Items using visual stimuli to measure knowledge acquired by other senses may be unnecessarily difficult for visually impaired people. . . . Similarly, hearing impaired individuals may have problems understanding language" (Johnston et al., 1992, p. S–16). Other special circumstances that could affect test administration include temporary factors in the environment such as renovation or transient factors for the individual such as tracheotomies and orthoses. When users test culturally diverse populations or non–English-speaking populations, modifications must also be made. With any modifications the validity of inferences may be questioned. According to Johnston et al. (1992), professionals must rely on logic, experience, and understanding of functional performance and testing procedures to distinguish between test modifications that are acceptable and those that affect validity (p. S–16).

The following nine points serve as guidelines to use when administering functional assessment instruments:

1. Remember that self-administered instruments, observational instruments, and structured interviews may yield different results. All approaches to measurement may be needed.
2. If a self-administered instrument is to be used, determine the person's mental status first before proceeding.
3. When a self-administered instrument or a structured interview is to be used, ask what the person *has done* (e.g., "When did you last transfer from tub to chair"?), rather than what the person might be able to do (e.g., "When do you think you will be able to transfer from tub to chair?").
4. Know that details must be obtained in self-administered questionnaires.
5. Know the person being evaluated, including his or her cultural beliefs and values, feelings about specific health practices, and attitudes about quality of life issues. All these areas must be considered when measuring function and determining interventions.
6. Know that approaches to measurement of function (telephone interview with self-report, cross-sectional assessments of groups, longitudinal assessment of individuals and groups, observation, structured interview) vary depending on degree of actual and potential disability.
7. Know that data collection methods should be standardized.
8. Consider that some diseases are progressive or intermittent and function can be expected to change over time.
9. When modifications are made for special circumstances, know that cautionary statements about inferences and decisions based on such measures should be issued unless these measures have been validated under these special circumstances.

READER'S DEVELOPMENT OF OWN FUNCTIONAL ASSESSMENT INSTRUMENTS

Sometimes professionals may feel it necessary to develop their own instrument. For example:

1. They may want to improve on the instrument currently available for their assessment purposes.
2. The instrument available for their assessment purposes does not have established validity, reliability, or sensitivity.

3. The instrument available for their assessment purposes is not practical for the situation.
4. No instrument is available for the domains and categories to be measured.
5. No instrument is available for the specific population.
6. The professionals may want to establish themselves as developers of measurement instruments in the academic or clinical sphere.

A number of different instruments have been used to measure many aspects of health and function in the rehabilitation disciplines. Regardless of the reasons to develop a new instrument, certain caveats must be heeded. Resources must be available to study and enhance reliability and validity of any instrument developed. If an established measure is revised, standards for test development must apply to the revisions. Johnston et al. (1992) stated the standards for test development in their classic special education issue of the *Archives of Physical Medicine and Rehabilitation*. These standards require that

1. developers of a measure have the responsibility for providing users with sufficient description and specification to enable users to determine its appropriateness for particular purposes,
2. developers of a measure have the responsibility for providing users with scientific evidence appropriate to its particular uses, and
3. measures intended only for research purposes that lack sufficient development for widespread routine use should be clearly labeled for research use. (p. 2–12)

The editors of this book (Dittmar and Gresham) were members of a clinical team when a new unit was opened to treat patients with spinal cord injuries at a local county hospital. A standardized instrument was needed to measure progress of individuals affected by tetraplegia. A review of the literature revealed that an instrument sensitive to the progress of these individuals was not available. Thus an instrument was developed with the purpose of showing that individuals with tetraplegia progressed in different ways (for example, individuals with tetraplegia can progress by learning to instruct others about how to care for them) than persons with use of one or more extremities. The resulting Quadriplegic Index of Function (QIF) was developed in 1979 (Gresham, Labi, Dittmar, Hicks, Joyce, & Stehlik, 1986). This measure is still undergoing studies for validity, reliability, and sensitivity.

Development of standardized measures is a time-consuming, meticulous, and expensive process. Many times an instrument that seems to have promise is taken over by a commercial company with the economic resources to support multisite studies of biometric (psychometric) properties. A thorough review of the many extant measures that might be applicable to a given situation should be conducted first to ensure that standardized instruments are not already available for the specific testing purposes.

RETRIEVAL OF EXISTING FUNCTIONAL ASSESSMENT INSTRUMENTS

Functional assessment and evaluation instruments can be located through a number of sources and resources (see Appendix B). A computer software program titled "Health and Psychological Instruments (HAPI) Online" is available in many universities and hospitals. This program can be used to search for instruments to measure a particular domain, as well as for information about a specific instrument. Moreover, traditional methods such as use of textbooks listing and outlining details about an instrument can also be used. A review of *Dissertation Abstracts International* may uncover useful instruments and thus provide a valuable resource in addition to published literature. Permission to use any information about validity, reliability, and other biometric (psychometric) properties of the specific instrument may be granted by the authors. Communication among researchers who are in the process of developing instruments can be most helpful. Discussions about new instruments may arise in networking sessions at conferences related to a professional's specialty or subspecialty area, in conversations with other researchers by telephone, and through correspondence on electronic mail and computer bulletin boards. The information highway is a new technology to help professionals stay up to date with many developments in specific fields (Burns & Grove, 1993). Libraries and reference librarians continue to be resources for clinicians and researchers as they search for the best instrument to measure functional outcomes related to their purposes.

CONCLUSION

The considerations in choosing a functional assessment instrument, as well as several approaches to collecting data about functional assessment, have been offered. Guidelines for both selecting and administering measures have been listed. Reasons for and pitfalls of developing one's own measures have been discussed. Finally, suggestions have been given for further information about measuring functional status. Further resources are described in Appendix B. In Chapter 3, methodological issues in measuring functional status are addressed.

REFERENCES

Burns, N., & Grove, S.K. (1993). *The practice of nursing research* (2nd ed.). Philadelphia: W.B. Saunders.

Harris, B.A., Jette, A.M., Campion, E.W., & Cleary, P.D. (1986). Validity of self-report measures of functional disability. *Topics in Geriatric Rehabilitation, 1*(3), 31–41.

Gresham, G.E., Labi, M.L.C., Dittmar, S.S., Hicks, J.T., Joyce, S.Z., & Stehlik, M.A.P. (1986). The Quadriplegia Index of Function (QIF): Sensitivity and reliability demonstrated in a study of thirty quadriplegic patients. *Paraplegia, 24*(1), 38–44.

Johnston, M.V., Keith, R.A., & Hinderer, S.R. (1992). Measurement standards for interdisciplinary medical rehabilitation [Special issue]. *Archives of Physical Medicine and Rehabilitation, 73*(12–S), S3–23.

Moinpour, C.M., McCorkle, R., & Sanders, J. (1988). Measuring functional status. In M. Frank-Stromborg (Ed.), *Instruments for clinical nursing research* (pp. 23–45). Norwalk, CT: Appleton & Lange.

Nelson, E., Conger, B., Douglass, R., Gebhart, D., Kirk, J., Page, R., Clark, A., Johnson, K., Stone, K., Wasson, J., & Zubkoff, M. (1983). Functional health status levels of primary care patients. *Journal of the American Medical Association, 249*, 3331–3338.

Rintala, D.H., & Willems, E.P. (1991). Telephone versus face-to-face mode for collecting self-reports of sequences of behavior. *Archives of Physical Medicine and Rehabilitation, 72*(7), 482–486.

Sudman, S. (1966). New uses of telephone methods in survey research. *Journal of Marketing Research, 3*, 163–167.

Methodological Issues in Measurement of Functional Status and Rehabilitation Outcomes

Kenneth J. Ottenbacher

BEHAVIORAL OBJECTIVES

After completing this chapter, the reader will be able to
- define how measurement is used in rehabilitation.
- discuss the importance of reliability and identify three types of reliability used in rehabilitation.
- describe the importance of validity and identify methods for establishing validity in rehabilitation.
- identify commonly used methods of measurement scaling.

- describe the implications of measurement error for establishing reliable and valid measurement procedures.
- discuss the importance of measurement sensitivity in rehabilitation outcome research.

In their article, "Measurement Standards for Interdisciplinary Medical Rehabilitation," Johnston, Keith, and Hinderer (1992) state that "rehabilitation emphasizes function, and so must address the problems inherent in the measurement of human performance" (p. S–4). Addressing the problems inherent in measurement of function is a complex task for rehabilitation health professionals. The first step is to identify research and outcome questions of critical importance to the field of rehabilitation. Johnston and Granger (1994) have proposed several questions of importance to rehabilitation, one of which poses a key consideration: "How do you measure quality and outcomes in medical rehabilitation?" (p. 296).

The focus of this chapter is on issues related to this critical question. The chapter is divided into six sections, and the material is designed to introduce and illustrate each of these key areas. Readers interested in more comprehensive coverage should consult the references at the end of the chapter for a more detailed examination of design and analysis issues in rehabilitation measurement.

DEFINITION OF MEASUREMENT IN REHABILITATION

Measurement is a process that results in the consistent assignment of individual characteristics or objects so they can be classified, ordered, or counted (Wade, 1992). Rothstein and Echternach (1993) note that the object of measurement in rehabilitation is to assign a label that is useful in planning and delivering intervention. The label signifies the quantity or the category to which something belongs. Rothstein and Echternach contend measurement *quantifies* a trait or object by assigning a label that indicates amount and *qualifies* by assigning a label that places objects, persons, or characteristics in a category. The assessment of range of motion in the elbow joint of a person receiving rehabilitation is an example of quantitative measurement. The number of degrees on the goniometer (e.g., 75°) indicates the amount of range of motion in the elbow. In contrast, Rothstein and Echternach classify evaluation of a person's muscle strength and labeling it as poor as an example of qualitative measurement. The ability to quantify and classify human performance is fundamental to rehabilitation measurement.

In this chapter, the terms *measurement* and *measure* are used in a generic sense to denote "assessment and evaluation procedures, tests, mechanical devices, observational procedures, and any other procedures that attach a number, ordination, or categorization to an observation" (Johnston et al., 1992, p. S–5).

The measurement process in clinical environments involves four steps:

1. Identifying a concept to be measured.
2. Specifying an indicator of the concept.
3. Defining operationally data necessary for measurement, so they can be quantified or classified into a variable.
4. Determining reliability and validity of the assessment process.

A *concept* is a verbal or symbolic representation of the phenomenon the researcher (or clinician) is interested in. It may refer to characteristics of the rehabilitation process, persons being served, therapist–patient interactions, or ecological and environmental phenomena. Concepts are the building blocks of any language; they are essential for professional communication and research. Some concepts are abstract and contain many ideas within them (e.g., quality of life or community integration); other concepts are concrete (e.g., degrees of range of motion or walking).

The instruments described in this book are designed to provide information about the concepts associated with functional status or functional independence. Granger (1984) describes *functional independence* as the person's ability to perform the tasks necessary for daily living, vocational pursuits, social interactions, leisure activities, and related behaviors. This is only a conceptual definition. A rehabilitation specialist interested in measuring functional independence needs some way to quantify or classify this concept of functional independence. Without such ability, it is impossible to determine the extent of any functional limitation, how functional ability changes over time, or whether an intervention will be successful in maintaining or improving functional independence. Thus to collect this information requires that functional independence be defined operationally.

When an operational definition is developed it must include (1) indicators used to obtain information about functional independence as well as (2) how that information was obtained, scored (quantified), and interpreted (classified).

One possible indicator of functional independence is examination of the person's skill in selected activities of daily living (ADL), such as feeding, dressing, grooming, toileting, and personal hygiene. Another might include examination of instrumental ADL such as vocational or leisure activities.

Examination, as well as satisfaction of the second component of an operational definition—that is, obtaining the in-

formation and then scoring and interpreting the results and thus making the concept measurable—can be accomplished with the assessment instruments reviewed in the remainder of this book.

One example is the Functional Independence Measure (FIM℠) (*Getting Started with the Uniform Data System for Medical Rehabilitation [Adult FIM℠]*, 1995), a widely used method for operationally defining function (Hamilton, Granger, Sherwin, Zielezny, & Tashman, 1987). The FIM℠ includes 18 items divided into motor (13 items) and cognitive (five items) domains. Each level of scoring (one through seven) is defined; for example, 7 = complete independence, 3 = moderate assist, and 1 = total assist. The scores on the FIM℠ represent a measure of overall performance in ADL and provide concrete indication of functional independence. The measurement orientation for the FIM℠ is based on the World Health Organization's *International Classification of Impairments, Disabilities, and Handicaps* (see Chapter 1).

There are many possible operational definitions for functional independence, each focusing on different aspects of complex conceptual variables. And different instruments can be used to determine the specific operational definition. For example, the Barthel Index is a widely used instrument to examine ADL. Although similar in many ways to the FIM℠, the Barthel Index does not assess function in the areas of communication and cognition (as does the FIM℠). Thus it provides a different operational definition of functional independence than that provided by the FIM℠. It is important to note that operational definitions are not inherently right or wrong. They simply provide different orientations and perspectives on concepts that are difficult to define. Operational definitions facilitate communication, replication, comparison, and the ability to accumulate a scientific knowledge base, and they are necessary to define a complex concept such as functional independence.

The utility of an operational definition is reflected in the reliability, validity, and sensitivity of the information obtained. Imprecise definitions (instruments) that cannot be used consistently (poor reliability) or are not related to the concept being examined (poor validity and sensitivity) are useless, and they contribute to confusion in clinical decision making. Estimates of reliability, validity, and sensitivity indicate whether there is a shared understanding of the concept. The ability to develop reliable, valid, and sensitive measures of functional independence is a high priority for rehabilitation researchers and clinicians. The remainder of this chapter examines issues associated with achieving this goal.

LEVELS OF MEASUREMENT AND VARIABLES

A *variable* is a measurable dimension of a concept (e.g., dressing as a dimension of functional independence). A variable is an indicator of a concept that is translated by means of an operational definition into one of four basic levels of measurement: nominal, ordinal, interval, or ratio. These four levels are referred to as scales of measurement and form a continuum on the basis of different types of information. Table 3–1 summarizes the properties of, and provides examples for, each level of measurement.

The simplest level of measurement is that of classification, the nominal scale. This level contains two or more categories that are mutually exclusive and exhaustive. For example, a person may be classified as either right-handed, left-handed, or ambidextrous. *Mutually exclusive* means that the person can be assigned only to one category. *Exhaustive* refers to inclusiveness of the possible range of responses; that is, everyone must fit into one of three categories: right-handed, left-handed, or ambidextrous (mixed).

Ordinal measurement scales contain the properties of nominal scales plus the additional characteristic that the scores can be rank ordered. For example, a therapist might examine a person with postpolio syndrome and rate the muscle strength in a lower extremity muscle group as trace, poor, fair, good, or normal. These five categories may be assigned numbers, with trace = 0 and normal muscle strength = 4. The assignment of numbers to these ordered categories, however, does not designate equal distances between each category. That is, the difference between 1 and 2 is not necessarily the same as the distance between 3 and 4. Other symbols (e.g., a, b, c or I, II, III) can be used to convey the order of the classification and indicate what some researchers and clinicians would regard as qualitative information.

Interval measurement scales include the properties of ordinal scales plus that of distance; that is, equal distance between adjacent categories. In assessing a patient with a spinal cord injury, a rehabilitation worker may be interested in the number of social contacts the person has had outside the home during a week. The number of social contacts is an interval-level variable (assuming, of course, a consistent method of recording frequency of social contacts over time is used). Ratio measurement scales contain the properties of interval scales plus that of a natural origin; that is, a fixed or absolute zero point. Calendars have arbitrary origins. The point at which one starts recording events is arbitrary. There is no absolute zero point where time does not exist. Thus the variable of social contact in the described example is associated with an arbitrary zero point and does not have a natural origin (absolute zero).

The distinction between interval and ratio scales is a relatively minor one for practical purposes of measurement. Values from interval and ratio scales can be added and averaged. Values from nominal and ordinal scales do not have arithmetic properties; that is, they cannot be added, subtracted, multiplied, or divided.

Controversy has developed in rehabilitation regarding the appropriate methods to analyze ordinal data collected from functional assessment instruments. Many of the most popular methods of evaluating functional capabilities use data that are ordinal in nature. For example, the items on the FIM℠ rate a person's performance by using an ordinal scale that ranges from complete dependence (assigned a score of 1) to complete independence (assigned a score of 7). These ordinal scale values are frequently averaged and compared with the use of a variety of statistical procedures. Merbitz, Morris, and Grip (1989) have argued that functional assessment instruments that use ordinal-level information produce scores that are easily misinterpreted and often misapplied in rehabilitation settings. Other authorities have argued that the nominal, ordinal, interval, and ratio classification system is inherently flawed and that decisions regarding how data should be analyzed must be based on the nature of the research question, rather than on the level of data. Velleman and Wilkinson (1993) suggest the scale types nominal, ordinal, interval, and ratio are not attributes of the data but, rather, depend on the research questions the data are intended to provide answers for. They describe several examples demonstrating that the scale type can change as a result of data transformation or how the information helps in interpreting the data, as well as related to the function of the question the researcher chooses to ask.

Table 3–1 Levels of Measurement Commonly Found in Rehabilitation Investigations

Level of Measurement	*Properties*	*Examples*
Nominal	Classification in categories.	Male, female. Left-handed, right-handed.
Ordinal	Order or ranking among categories.	Social class. Degree of burns (1st, 2nd, 3rd degree).
Interval	Equal distance between points or numbers but no absolute zero.	Temperature in degrees Fahrenheit. Calendar time.
Ratio	Equal distance between points or categories and the existence of an absolute zero.	Degrees of range of motion. Number of minutes of therapy.

The issue of whether ordinal data collected in a structured manner can be used to make statistical inferences is complex. One approach adopted by several investigators in rehabilitation has been to transform ordinal data by using methods of Rasch analysis (Wright & Linacre, 1989). Rasch analysis assumes that the consequence of any encounter between a person and a test item is governed by the difference between the ability of the respondent and the difficulty of the item on a latent trait dimension. A *latent trait dimension* is the abstract continuum associated with a construct (e.g., strength). Ability scores for persons are computed by transforming raw scores (total number of items answered correctly) to the same natural logarithmic latent trait scale used to measure item difficulty.

The Rasch model produces measures on a logit scale. The logit unit of measurement is the natural log of the odds of a correct response. The process of Rasch scaling transforms raw score data obtained from items and persons into log units. This transformation allows the researcher to interpret the person and item information by using the same units of measure. Once the scores for the persons and items have been transformed with Rasch scaling, other information about the persons and items can be obtained by using a variety of statistical methods.

RELIABILITY IN REHABILITATION MEASUREMENT

Despite the type of scale used to obtain a measure, the reliability of the information collected is a key component of the assessment process. Portney and Watkins (1993) state that "reliability is fundamental to all aspects of clinical research, because without it we cannot have confidence in the data we collect, nor can we draw rational conclusions from those data" (p. 53). *Reliability* refers to the extent to which there is consistency in responses on repeated applications of the measurement instrument. Repeated applications may be obtained over time (test–retest reliability) or by different raters (inter-rater reliability).

The terms reliability and agreement are frequently used interchangeably. There are, however, important technical differences between these two terms for the researcher and clinician to understand. *Reliability* indicates the degree of association or co-variation between two variables. A measure of reliability will be high if there is relative or proportional agreement between two variables. *Agreement*, in contrast, is the extent to which measurement procedures yield the same results across individuals or over time. Agreement requires that the values between two variables (raters or time) be the same.

The data presented in Table 3–2 illustrate the distinction between reliability and agreement. The table includes data for two raters. The scores for these two raters are not the same, but the relative ordering (co-variation) is not changed across the raters. That is, the person rated highest by the first rater is also rated highest by the second rater, and the person rated lowest by rater one is also rated lowest by rater two. No exact agreement exists between the two sets of scores. However, if a Pearson product-moment correlation coefficient (*r*) is computed, the *r* value is 1.00, indicating perfect reliability across the two raters. The Pearson *r* value is high because there is excellent co-variation across the two raters even though the absolute agreement is poor.

Johnston et al. (1992) have identified three types of reliability commonly encountered in rehabilitation research: inter-rater (agreement), test–retest (also referred to as stability), and internal consistency. *Inter-rater reliability* refers to the extent to which two or more independent observers of the same phenomenon agree in their observations. For example, newborn infants are routinely evaluated to assess their physical activity, muscle tone, color, and reflex responses immediately after birth. This rating is referred to as the Apgar score. The inter-rater reliability of the method used to obtain an Apgar score could be determined by having two raters independently score a group of infants with the defined Apgar criteria. The inter-rater reliability (agreement) would be obtained by computing the appropriate reliability statistic by using the scores of the raters.

Test–retest reliability provides the researcher or clinician with information on the consistency of scores over time. Skin calipers are frequently used to measure percent body fat before and after intervention for persons enrolled in weight reduction programs. The scores from two (or more) administrations are then analyzed to determine the consistency over time. An important issue in establishing test–retest reliability

Table 3–2 Illustration of Reliability and Agreement with the Use of a Sample Set of Data* for Two Raters (Inter-rater)

Subject	Scores for Rater 1	Scores for Rater 2
1	10	100
2	20	200
3	30	300
4	40	400
5	50	500
6	60	600
7	70	700
8	80	800
9	90	900
10	100	1000
Mean (SD)	50 (10)	500 (100)

Pearson product-moment correlation (*r*) = 1.00.
*Data reflect good reliability (co-variation) but poor agreement (consensus).

is the time between testing. The duration between first and second administration of the test will depend on the nature of the variable being assessed. In the skin caliper example, it would be reasonable to assume that percent body fat should not change over a period of one to three days. Two or three days would be an appropriate retest interval in this example.

Information on test–retest reliability (stability) is particularly important in investigations in which the purpose is to analyze change over time. If there is a change in performance from beginning of intervention to end of treatment, it is hoped that the change reflects a true improvement in ability and is not the result of measurement error. If the test–retest reliability for the instrument is high, the probability that change in performance was due to measurement error will be small. This situation, of course, does not ensure that the change was due to treatment, but a reliable instrument can reduce the possibility that improvement was due to measurement error. This concept will be illustrated in a later section of this chapter.

The final type of reliability discussed by Johnston et al. (1992) is internal consistency. *Internal consistency* refers to the degree to which items in an assessment instrument are related to each other. High internal consistency means that the items are closely related and presumably measuring the same construct. For example, an assessment of a person's ADL might include 10 items assessing ability to dress himself or herself, 10 items examining ability to feed oneself, and 10 items assessing ability to communicate. A test for internal consistency would examine the correlation among all individual items as well as the correlation among individual items and subgroups of items. The results should indicate that the 10 dressing items are more closely related to each other than they are to any of the items evaluating communication. Specialized test statistics are available to provide a quantitative index of the internal consistency of items and subsets of items. Measures of internal consistency are often important in determining whether the test is measuring the appropriate construct (concept) or whether individual items should be revised or eliminated.

VALIDITY IN REHABILITATION MEASUREMENT

Validity is the degree of correspondence between the concept being measured and the variable used to represent the concept. An instrument is valid when the test actually measures what it is intended to measure. Validity implies accuracy as well as relevance of response. The more concrete the concept, the easier it is to obtain valid responses because the correspondence being sought between the concept and the variable is usually clear. For example, the information collected on age or blood type of patients can be verified easily by comparing the information with data in an official document or medical record. In contrast, a concept such as community integration is more abstract and therefore more difficult to verify. Definitions of community integration may show large differences, and items that reflect community integration are not consistently agreed on by researchers or clinicians.

Validity can be divided into two different forms: content and empirical. *Content validity* reflects the validity of the content of the instrument used to measure the concept. The content of the instrument should relate logically to the concept; that is, items should be relevant and representative of all possible areas indicative of the concept. For instance, a valid functional assessment instrument for ADL should include items that measure all areas of ADL, and these items should range from easy to difficult. A functional assessment instrument used to measure ADL that does not include any items evaluating dressing ability would have poor content validity.

Empirical validity refers to the verification of logical predictions based on accurate measurement of the concept. Predictions are made about relationships to external criteria. The criteria can include comparisons with current or future expectations, as well as with complex theoretical speculations. Empirical validity is often divided into three subsets: concurrent, predictive, and construct validity. Some investigators combine concurrent and predictive validity and refer to these two collectively as criterion-oriented validity (Johnston et al., 1992).

Concurrent Validity

Concurrent validity reflects the relationship between two instruments designed to measure the same construct (concept). A therapist measuring knee range of motion in a patient with a spinal cord injury may use a standard goniometer and compare the values with findings obtained from radiographic examination of the knee. The correlation derived from comparing the two sets of results provides a quantitative index of concurrent validity.

Predictive Validity

Predictive validity is verification of a relationship between the variable and an external criterion in the future. If children who score poorly on *The Miller Assessment of Preschoolers (MAP)* (Miller, 1986) at age 2 years are later found to have difficulty in school (indicated by poor grades and below average performance on teacher reports), support is provided for the predictive validity of *The Miller Assessment of Preschoolers (MAP)*. A quantitative index of predictive validity is frequently obtained by computing correlation coefficients between the two measures separated by the required time interval.

Construct Validity

Construct validity is the degree to which an instrument measures the theoretical construct (concept) it was designed to measure. Construct validity assumes that the concepts of interest are embedded in theory. Construct validity is established by piecing together a network of relationships. As a simple example, a theory of quality of life may lead to a hypothesis about a positive relationship between quality of life and functional ability. That is, the better the quality of life a person experiences, the more likely he or she will have high levels of functional independence. Verification of the hypothesis would add to the validity of the variable measuring the concept; that is, quality of life. The process of establishing construct validity is complex because there may be a large number of potential theoretical predictions, and it may be impossible to verify all of them for a particular variable. The development of construct validity is a continuous process and often requires numerous studies examining various theoretical predications related to the variable of interest.

MEASUREMENT BIAS

Measurement bias reduces reliability and validity. Bias is discussed here to increase the reader's awareness of factors that could reduce the value of information obtained in assessing and monitoring patient problems and progress toward rehabilitation intervention goals. Types of bias that can occur during the measurement process are bias in

- format of the instrument,
- instructions for use of the instrument,
- predispositions of the respondents, and
- measurement environment.

The content of an instrument used to collect data can bias the information it is designed to elicit. For example, items in a rating scale may be phrased so that respondents tend to answer in one way rather than another. That is, there may be an element of social desirability apparent in the items. A rehabilitation worker may not provide the same instructions to different patients completing a questionnaire or survey, or the examiner may not consistently answer questions correctly.

Other aspects of the environment may contribute to measurement bias. A therapist might be inconsistent in his or her use of an instrument by, for example, not placing the goniometer in the same place for each measurement trial. External distractions or noise present during the pretest, but not at the posttest, might reduce the instrument's reliability.

Training in the use of instruments is essential with an emphasis on consistency in application across patients as well as over time with the same individuals. Sources of systematic error (bias) are reduced when instruments are carefully constructed and adequately pilot tested before clinical use.

MEASUREMENT SENSITIVITY

One indicator of measurement sensitivity is the number of values that can be reliably discriminated for a given variable. In a nominal scale, the reliable discrimination of three categories is more sensitive than the reliable discrimination of two categories. For a variable such as muscle tone, the categories of trace, poor, fair, good, and normal provide more information than the categories of normal versus abnormal. In general, ordinal scales are more sensitive than nominal scales (if they are reliable) because ordinal scales are able to discriminate rankings of importance among categories as well as in the categories themselves. The key components of sensitivity are reliable discrimination and the number of categories or values for a variable. A rating scale for quality of life with 10 levels (or values) is not more sensitive than a rating scale with three levels, unless there is evidence that the patient can reliably discriminate among the 10 levels. The notion of sensitivity is especially important when a rehabilitation specialist is attempting to measure change. If the variable is not sufficiently sensitive, it may not register change.

A second indicator of measurement sensitivity is the ability to document reliable change in performance over time. Two or more measurements are necessary to determine whether changes occur and whether they are persistent. The first step in measuring change is to ensure that the instrument to be used has adequate reliability (test–retest reliability). Without demonstrated test–retest reliability, changes from one administration of the instrument to the next could be the result of random measurement error. Jacobson, Follette, and Revenstorf (1984) refer to change as a reliable difference in values for a variable over two or more points in time. They have proposed the *reliability change index* (RCI) to determine reliable changes over time for specific variables. To compute the RCI, the clinician must have the following information:

1. patient's preintervention or pretest score
2. patient's posttest score after treatment
3. standard error of measurement (*SEM*) for the instrument.

The *SEM* represents the spread or distribution of repeated performances for a given individual. The *SEM* is influenced by the reliability of the test and may be computed from the following equation:

$$SEM = SD \sqrt{1-r} \qquad (1)$$

where *SD* is the standard deviation for the test and *r* is correlation representing the test–retest value.

The RCI is computed as follows:

$$RCI = (X_2 - X_1)/SEM \qquad (2)$$

where X_2 is the postintervention score, X_1 is the preintervention score, and *SEM* is the standard error of measurement as defined earlier. For example, a patient receiving intervention for a deficit in ADL may have an initial FIM^SM score of 75. After rehabilitation treatment, the patient's FIM^SM score at discharge might be 85. If the *SEM* for the instrument is 5, Equation 2 can provide the reliability change index: RCI = 85 − 75/5 = 2.0. Jacobson et al. (1984) argue that the RCI should be interpreted by using a unit normal distribution, where a value of ±1.96 would be unlikely to occur ($p < .05$) without actual change.

The index proposed by Jacobson et al. (1984) provides a statistical indication of change that is not likely to be the result of random error. The RCI, however, does not include information regarding the clinical importance of the change. This information is vital in making an inference regarding the practical importance of the change. In the earlier example, the therapist using the RCI knows that the change of 10 points on the FIM^SM (from 75 to 85) was probably not due to chance (measurement error); that is, the increase from 75 to 85 points on the FIM^SM represents real change in performance. The RCI does not tell the therapist whether the 10-point improvement was due to the rehabilitation treatment or whether the 10-point increase is clinically important. The answer to the first question will be determined by the type of research design used to collect pretest and posttest data. The answer to the second question cannot be determined statistically. This answer will require knowledge of what the patient and his or her family believe are important functional skills, along with information on the cost required to obtain these skills.

A third approach to sensitivity in measurement is designed to determine the ability of new or revised tests to replace well-established assessments. This approach was developed by epidemiologists for comparing the relative accuracy and agreement among diagnostic tests, but its use has expanded to a number of related areas. The approach focuses on determining specificity and sensitivity of an assessment procedure. *Specificity* is the extent to which an instrument rules out a disorder or dysfunction when it is actually present. This is commonly referred to as a false-negative finding. *Sensitivity* is the extent to which an instrument or assessment process detects a disorder when it is truly present. A sensitive instrument is one with few false positives. A false positive occurs when a disorder or dysfunction is identified when there is actually no disorder.

The process of identifying false positives and false negatives implies that there is an established criterion against which to compare the results. This criterion is referred to as the gold standard and represents an accepted or established method of measuring an event or characteristic. The logic of the approach is based on a 2 × 2 contingency table, as displayed in Table 3–3. This table shows the results of a new or revised test when compared to those of a well-established instrument (the gold standard). Each of the cells is designated with a letter, a, b, c, and d. The sensitivity and specificity values of an assessment are determined by comparing the number of responses in each cell with the use of a defined set of formulas.

An example will help illustrate the use of the model presented in Table 3–3. In Table 3–4, the Functional Independence Measure for Children, referred to as the WeeFIM®, is a new instrument designed to assess functional abilities in children (*Guide for the Uniform Data Set for Medical Rehabilitation for Children (WeeFIM®, Version 4.0—Community/Outpatient*, 1993)). The WeeFIM® contains 18 items examining the following areas: self-care, sphincter control, transfers, locomotion, communication, and social cognition. The test can be administered by interview or direct observation and takes 15 to 20 minutes to complete. In contrast, the

Table 3–3 Model To Compare Results from New (Revised) Test to Those from Well-Established Test (Gold Standard) and Compute Sensitivity and Specificity of New Test

Sensitivity = [a/(a + c)] × 100
Specificity = [d/(b + d)] × 100

Vineland Adaptive Behavior Scales (Sparrow, Balla, & Cilcchetti, 1984) are designed to assess personal and social sufficiency in children and adults. The *Vineland Scales* are a well-established and widely used assessment that can be considered the gold standard in the area of measuring adaptive behavior. They are administered in a semistructured interview and assess four domains: communication, daily living skills, socialization, and motor skills. The standard version of the *Vineland Scales* requires 30 to 60 minutes to administer (Sparrow et al., 1984).

The hypothetical data in Table 3–4 are used to examine the specificity and sensitivity of the WeeFIM® (new test) compared to the *Vineland Adaptive Behavior Scales* (gold standard). Decisions regarding dysfunction are based on scores of one or more standard deviations below the mean. The sensitivity for the data in Table 3–4 is 0.88, indicating that the WeeFIM® correctly identified 88% of the children and the dysfunction as defined by scores of more than 1.00 SD below the mean. The specificity for the WeeFIM® is 0.78, suggesting that this test correctly identified the absence of dysfunction 78% of the time. The overall agreement between the two assessments is obtained by using the following equation:

$$\text{Agreement} = (a + d)/N \times 100 \qquad (3)$$

where a is the number of agreements, d is the number of disagreements, and N represents the total number of cases. Thus, with the use of data in Table 3–4, the percentage of agreement would be $(15 + 18)/40 \times 100 = 82.5\%$. This figure gives the percentage of direct agreements between the two tests. (See also equation at bottom of Table 3–4.) Results of the analysis reveal that the WeeFIM® sensitivity is relatively high, indicating that few children who have no dysfunction are inappropriately labeled as having delayed functional skills (false positives). The WeeFIM® is less efficient in detecting false negatives; that is, identifying those children who truly have dysfunction (as determined by the *Vineland Scales*) but who score within the normal range of the WeeFIM®.

The described sensitivity and specificity analysis goes beyond a simple correlation. Correlations, although valuable, reflect the overall relation between tests; they do not indicate the proportion of true and false positives or true and false negatives. The use of likelihood ratios permits the determination of whether dysfunction is actually present, given specific test results. The sensitivity and specificity approach can be used to help establish assessments that contribute accurate data to the rehabilitation process.

CONCLUSION

In describing the importance of interdisciplinary assessment in rehabilitation, Johnston et al. (1992) note that, "we must improve our measures to keep pace with developments in general health care. If we move rapidly and continue our efforts, we can move rehabilitation to a position of leadership in health care" (p. S–3). The ability to develop new as-

---

Table 3–4 Example of Sensitivity and Specificity for WeeFIM® (New Test) and *Vineland Adaptive Behavior Scales* (Gold Standard)

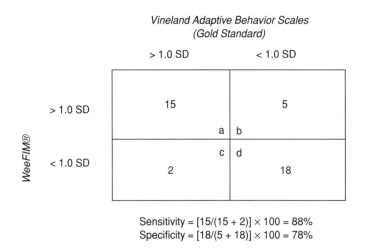

Sensitivity = [15/(15 + 2)] × 100 = 88%
Specificity = [18/(5 + 18)] × 100 = 78%

Percentage of agreement equation: (a + d)/N × 100 = % agreement; where
a = number of agreements, d = number of disagreements, and N = total number
of cases. (See Portney & Watkins, 1993, p. 516.)

sessment instruments and understand existing tests will be absolutely critical to the future development of medical rehabilitation. Without assessment expertise rehabilitation practitioners will be unable to meet the demands of efficiency, accountability, and effectiveness that are certain to increase in the future.

The interaction between reliable, valid, and sensitive instruments and professional accountability has been operationalized by Hamilton et al. (1987). They have proposed a model (see Figure 3–1) for estimating the care (cost) efficiency in rehabilitation on the basis of recovery of function after disease or injury. The model contains two primary components: a measure of functional skill (*y* axis) and the cost of rehabilitation (*x* axis). Cost of rehabilitation is estimated on the basis of time spent (length of stay) in a rehabilitation program. The trajectory of the line beginning at the *y* axis represents optimal function, which is interrupted by the onset of disease, accident, or injury. After onset of disability or disease (e.g., stroke), the person's functional skills are dramatically impaired. This reduction in functional skills is indicated by the sharp drop in the line representing functional ability. During the period of hospitalization and rehabilitation, the person's level of functional ability gradually returns. The rate of return depends on many factors, one of

which is the effectiveness of the rehabilitation intervention provided. Eventually, the person's level of functional skill begins to plateau and the person is discharged to the community. With the use of this model, care (cost) efficiency is estimated by dividing the increase in function (depicted by values on the *y* axis) by the cost incurred as the result of rehabilitation (i.e., cost of hospitalization and rehabilitation, which is depicted on the *x* axis). The care efficiency index obtained from this analysis depends on the reliability, validity, and sensitivity of the measure of functional performance (*y* axis). Without valid, reliable, and sensitive measures of functional ability, the care efficiency index will be impossible to determine accurately, and effectiveness and efficiency of rehabilitation services will remain unknown.

In today's rapidly changing health care environment, there are many variables related to service delivery and cost containment that rehabilitation specialists cannot control. Interpretation of assessment procedures and development of treatment programs, however, are still the direct responsibility of rehabilitation practitioners. Information concerning reliability, validity, and sensitivity will help practitioners meet this professional responsibility and ensure that consumers of rehabilitation services receive the best available evaluation and treatment.

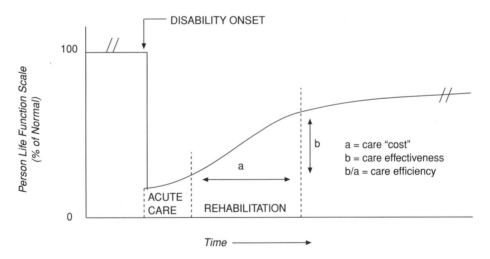

Figure 3–1 Care efficiency. *Source:* Reprinted with permission from B.B. Hamilton et al., in *Rehabilitation Outcomes: Analysis and Measurement,* M.J. Fuhrer, ed., p. 193, © 1993, Paul H. Brookes.

REFERENCES

Getting started with the uniform data system for medical rehabilitation (Adult FIM^SM). (1995). Buffalo, NY: State University of New York.

Granger, C.V. (1984). A conceptual model for functional assessment. In C.V. Granger & G.E. Gresham (Eds.), *Functional assessment in rehabilitation medicine* (pp. 14–25). Baltimore: Williams & Wilkins.

Guide for the uniform data set for medical rehabilitation for children (WeeFIM®), version 4.0—community/outpatient (1993). Buffalo, NY: State University of New York.

Hamilton, B.B., Granger, C.V., Sherwin, F.S., Zielezny, M., & Tashman, J.S. (1987). Uniform data system for medical rehabilitation. In M.J. Fuhrer (Ed.), *Rehabilitation outcomes: Analysis and measurement* (p. 139). Baltimore: Paul H. Brookes.

Jacobson, N.S., Follette, W.C., & Revenstorf, D. (1984). Psychotherapy outcome research: Methods for reporting variability and evaluating clinical significance. *Behavior Therapy, 15*, 336–352.

Johnston, M.V., & Granger, C.V. (1994). Outcomes research in medical rehabilitation: A primer and introduction. *American Journal of Physical Medicine and Rehabilitation, 73*, 296–303.

Johnston, M.V., Keith, R.A., & Hinderer, S.R. (1992). Measurement standards for interdisciplinary medical rehabilitation. [Special Issue.] *Archives of Physical Medicine and Rehabilitation, 73* (12–S), S3–23.

Merbitz, C., Morris, J., & Grip, J.C. (1989). Ordinal scales and foundations of misinference. *Archives of Physical Medicine and Rehabilitation, 70*, 308–312.

Miller, L.J. (1986). *The Miller Assessment for Preschoolers (MAP)*. Littleton, CO: Foundation for Knowledge in Development.

Portney, L.G., & Watkins, M.P. (1993). *Foundation of clinical research: Applications to practice*. Norwalk, CT: Appleton & Lange.

Rothstein, J.M., & Echternach, J.L. (1993). *Primer on measurement: An introductory guide to measurement issues*. Alexandria, VA: American Physical Therapy Association.

Sparrow, S., Balla, P., & Cilcchetti, D. (1984). *Vineland Adaptive Behavior Scales, Interview edition: Survey form manual*. Circle Pines, MN: American Guidance Service.

Velleman, P.F., & Wilkinson, L. (1993). Nominal, ordinal, and ratio topologies are misleading. *The American Statistician, 47*, 65–72.

Wade, D.T. (1992). *Measurement in neurological rehabilitation*. New York: Oxford Medical Publications.

Wright, B.D., & Linacre, J.M. (1989). Observations are always ordinal; measurements, however, must be interval. *Archives of Physical Medicine and Rehabilitation, 70*, 857.

CHAPTER **4**

Instruments Used To Assess Function and Measure Outcomes in Physical Rehabilitation

Glen E. Gresham and Sharon S. Dittmar

BEHAVIORAL OBJECTIVES

After completing this chapter, the reader will be able to
- categorize instruments used to measure outcomes in physical rehabilitation.
- give examples of specific instruments within each of three conceptual areas.

- discuss biometric properties of instruments described and displayed in Appendix A.

Functional assessment and evaluation instruments are designed for different purposes. Each instrument discussed in this chapter addresses a domain or a constellation of domains that constitute a specific "universe of function" (Labi & Gresham, 1984, p. 89) of persons with disabilities. The World Health Organization's *International Classification of Impairments, Disabilities, and Handicaps (ICIDH)* (1980) is used to address the three conceptual areas in physical rehabilitation: impairment (organ level), disability (person/activities level), and handicap (overall status of the disabled person in his or her specific environmental and psychosocial context). Throughout this book, handicap is referred to as societal limitation.

Since impairments, per se, are traditionally considered medical diagnostic descriptors, specific impairment measures are not included in this chapter. Instruments that measure impairment, such as the National Institutes of Health Stroke Scale (Brott & Reed, 1989) and the Canadian Stroke Scale (Cote, Battista, Wolfson, & Hachinski, 1988; Cote, Battista, Wolfson, Boucher, Adam, & Hachinski, 1989) are available in the general medical literature and beyond the scope of this book.

The emphasis in this chapter follows that of all fields of physical rehabilitation: description and measurement of disability or functional limitations in task performance at the person level. Many of the instruments discussed are used in

both inpatient and outpatient settings. If an instrument is designed for only one setting, it is specified in the description. In addition, many of the instruments—particularly in the comprehensive subcategory—measure both basic activities of daily living (BADL) and instrumental activities of daily living (IADL). The type of activities of daily living (ADL) measured is stated in the description of each instrument. The subcategories of functional assessment instruments described in this chapter are given below. Also discussed are examples of the few available measures of societal limitation (measures of handicap), as defined by the *ICIDH* model. Commonly used instruments in physical rehabilitation are described and displayed in Appendix A.

CATEGORIES OF FUNCTIONAL ASSESSMENT INSTRUMENTS TO MEASURE DISABILITY

Comprehensive Functional Assessment Instruments

The domains for functional assessment instruments that measure disability include many or all aspects of a person's life. Some of the more important and frequently used functional assessment instruments address several but not all domains of a person's function. The best known example is the Functional Independence Measure (FIM℠) (Granger, Hamilton, Keith, Zielezny, & Sherwin, 1986), which measures BADL, social cognition, and functional communication. Other instruments in this category address many domains and are sometimes referred to as global instruments (Gresham & Labi, 1984). Measures within this subcategory document overall disability regardless of impairment. The choices of measurement domains obviously reflect the needs and priorities of rehabilitation centers and professionals as they quantify function in specific groups of patients. Other examples are the Edinburgh Rehabilitation Status Scale (Affleck, Aitken, Hunter, McGuire, & Roy, 1988), The Functional Life Scale (Sarno, Sarno, & Levita, 1973), the Patient Evaluation and Conference System (PECS) (Harvey & Jellinek, 1981), the PULSES Profile (Moskowitz & McCann, 1957), and the Rankin Scale (Rankin, 1957).

Measures of ADL, Including IADL and BADL

Instruments that measure ADL are limited to the performance of self-care activities and may or may not include mobility (locomotion). They may also measure BADL, IADL, or both. It is commonly agreed that self-care and mobility are central to the determination of functional status (Moinpour, McCorkle, & Sanders, 1988). Activities of daily living have been a category in *Index Medicus* since 1968 (Gresham & Labi, 1984). These instruments are usually applicable to all impairments. Examples of BADL scales are the Barthel Index (Mahoney & Barthel, 1965), the Katz Index of ADL (Katz, Ford, Moskowitz, Jackson, & Jaffe, 1963), Kenny Self-Care Evaluation (Schoening, Anderegg, Bergstrom, Fonda, Steinke, & Ulrich, 1965), Klein-Bell Activities of Daily Living (Klein & Bell, 1982), and the Time Care Profile (Halstead & Hartley, 1975). A well-known IADL instrument is the Instrumental Activities of Daily Living Scale (Lawton, 1971; Lawton & Brody, 1969).

An Outpatient Functional Status Monitoring Instrument

A new instrument to monitor outpatient functional status has been developed by researchers at the State University of New York at Buffalo. The Medical Rehabilitation Follow-Along (MRFA℠) was developed to assess and monitor the functional status of patients with disability problems after discharge (Granger, Ottenbacher, Baker, & Sehgal, 1995). A description of this instrument can be found in Appendix A.

Measures of Cognitive Function and Affect

Cognitive Function

Instruments that measure cognitive function address the thinking and learning abilities of persons with physical dis-

abilities, regardless of the specific impairments. Scales to measure mental status were traditionally constructed to determine orientation to time, place, and person, as well as to assess memory and ability to perform intellectual tasks of varying degrees of difficulty (Lawton, 1971). Examples of tests of cognitive function are the Agitated Behavior Scale (ABS) (Corrigan, 1989) and the Mini-Mental State Examination (MMSE) (Folstein, Folstein, & McHugh, 1975).

Affect

Measurements of affect are used to address the state of mind or mood of individuals with disabilities. Among those widely used are scales to measure depression. These scales are used increasingly with rehabilitation patients, especially those with stroke. Examples are the Hamilton Rating Scale for Depression (Hamilton, 1960), the Self-rating Depression Scale (Zung, 1965), the Depression Status Inventory (Zung, 1972), and the CES–D (Center for Epidemiologic Studies Depression) Scale (Radloff, 1977).

Functional Communication Instruments

Functional communication instruments address the individual's ability to communicate with others. Speech articulation, language, and hearing as well as compensatory methods to accomplish these, are measured. However, emphasis, as stated, is on *functional communication*. One example of a functional communication instrument is the *Communicative Abilities in Daily Living* (Holland, 1980). (See Table A–8 for characteristics of selected functional communication instruments.) This instrument was developed and validated at the University of Pittsburgh through a two-year contract from the National Institute of Neurological and Communicative Disorders and Stroke. The ASHA (American Speech-Language-Hearing Association) Functional Assessment of Communication Skills for Adults (ASHA FACS) is an example of a more recent scale developed for a specific purpose; that is, measurement of communication in everyday contexts in adults with communication disorders (Frattali, 1992).

Tests of Sensorimotor Function

Sensorimotor scales are designed to measure sensation and motor ability. One example of a sensorimotor scale is the Fugl-Meyer Assessment (Fugl-Meyer, Jääskö, Leyman, Olsson, & Steglind, 1975). This instrument has been used to assess recovery of motor function and balance in individuals who have sustained a stroke leading to hemiparesis. Another example is the Standardized Test of Patient Mobility, a test that addresses a patient's ability to perform specific tasks as well as the time required and ease of performance (Jebsen, Trieschmann, Mikulic, Hartley, McMillan, & Snook, 1970).

Test of Hand Function

Because hand function involves motion, sensation, strength, edema, and pain, these factors should be assessed before rehabilitation therapy for individuals with hand problems. Because of the intricacy of these assessments, a separate subcategory is included to assess hand function. The example given is the Jebsen Test of Hand Function, which is designed to test seven aspects of various hand activities (Jebsen, Taylor, Trieschmann, Trotter, & Howard, 1969).

Medical Diagnosis–Specific Functional Assessment Instruments

Most functional assessment instruments used in the medical rehabilitation context were intentionally designed to be applicable to all categories of medical diagnoses. The emphasis is on performance of functional activities, not on the underlying impairments (whether injury or disease). There are, however, a number of functional assessment instruments that were developed to meet the needs of clinicians and investigators working with a specific disease or constellation of closely related diseases. Examples given in Appendix A are for persons with arthritis, stroke, traumatic brain injury, and quadriplegia.

Functional Assessment Instruments Used with Specific Age Groups

Functional assessment instruments designed for specific age groups address either pediatric or geriatric populations and are usually subsets of one of the other categories listed in this section. One example is the WeeFIM®, a pediatric functional independence measure (McCabe & Granger, 1990). Other examples of instruments for specific age groups are the *Pediatric Evaluation of Disability Inventory (PEDI)* (Haley, Faas, Coster, Ludlow, Haltiwanger, & Andrellos, 1989), the Older Adults Resources and Services (Duke University Center for the Study of Aging and Human Development, 1978), and the Rapid Disability Rating Scale (RDRS) (Linn, 1967).

The functional problems of persons with vision and hearing impairments are not addressed because of the complex interrelationships between these specific impairments and a variety of disabilities addressed in this book.

CATEGORIES OF FUNCTIONAL ASSESSMENT INSTRUMENTS TO MEASURE SOCIETAL LIMITATION

Measurements of societal limitation address four areas: family functioning, vocational/leisure function, community integration, and quality of life.

Family Functioning

Functional assessment instruments for family functioning are designed to measure the complex function of the family as a whole, rather than the individual contributions of each family member (although information is often collected from individual family members). One example is the McMaster Family Assessment Device (Epstein, Baldwin, & Bishop, 1983).

Vocational/Leisure Function

An instrument used to assess the domain of work is the Functional Assessment Inventory (Crewe & Athelstan, 1980). There are many commercially available instruments to assess work and leisure.

Community Integration

The CHART: Craig Handicap Assessment and Reporting Technique (Whiteneck, Charlifue, Gerhart, Overholser, & Richardson, 1992), an instrument designed to determine integration of persons with spinal cord injury; the Community Integration Questionnaire (Willer, Ottenbacher, & Coad, 1994), a measure originally used for persons with traumatic brain injury but now being studied with other impairment groups; and Activity Pattern Indicators (Brown, Gordon, & Diller, 1984), a more general measure of community integration, are included as examples in Appendix A.

Quality of Life

The Sickness Impact Profile (Gilson, Gilson, & Bergner, 1975) was chosen as an instrument to illustrate a measure of overall physical and psychosocial health independent of diagnostic criteria.

REFERENCES

Affleck, J.W., Aitken, R.C., Hunter, J.A., McGuire, R.J., & Roy, C.W. (1988). Rehabilitation status: A measure of medicosocial dysfunction. *The Lancet, 1,* 230–233.

Brott, T., & Reed, R.L. (1989). Intensive care for acute stroke in the community hospital setting: The first 24 hours. *Stroke, 20*(5), 694–697.

Brown, M., Gordon, W.A., & Diller, L. (1984). Rehabilitation indicators. In A.S. Halpern & M.J. Fuhrer (Eds.), *Functional assessment in rehabilitation* (pp. 187–203). Baltimore: Paul H. Brookes.

Corrigan, J.D. (1989). Development of a scale for assessment of agitation following traumatic brain injury. *Journal of Clinical and Experimental Neuropsychology, 11*(2), 261–277.

Cote, R., Battista, R.N., Wolfson, C., Boucher, J., Adam, J., & Hachinski, V. (1989). The Canadian Neurological Scale: Validation and reliability assessment. *Neurology, 39*(5), 638–643.

Cote, R., Battista, R.N., Wolfson, C.M., & Hachinski, V. (1988). Stroke assessment scales: Guidelines for development, validation, and reliability assessment. *Canadian Journal of Neurological Sciences, 15*(3), 261–265.

Crewe, N.M., & Athelstan, G.T. (1980). Appendix II: Functional Assessment Inventory. In B. Bolton & D.W. Cook (Eds.), *Rehabilitation client assessment* (pp. 289–296). Baltimore: University Park Press.

Duke University Center for the Study of Aging and Human Development (1978). *Functional assessment: The OARS Methodology.* Durham, NC: Duke University.

Epstein, N.B., Baldwin, L.M., & Bishop, D.S. (1983). The McMaster Family Assessment Device. *Journal of Marital and Family Therapy, 9*(2), 171–180.

Folstein, M.F., Folstein, S.E., & McHugh, P.R. (1975). A "Mini-Mental State": A practical method for grading the cognitive state of patients for the clinician. *Journal of Psychiatric Research, 12*(3), 189–198.

Frattali, C. (1992). Clinical forum: Functional assessment of communication—Merging public policy with clinical views. *Aphasiology, 6*(1), 63–83.

Fugl-Meyer, A.R., Jääskö, L., Leyman, I., Olsson, S., & Steglind, S. (1975). The poststroke hemiplegic patient. I. A method for evaluation of physical performance. *Scandinavian Journal of Rehabilitation Medicine, 7*(1), 13–31.

Gilson, B.S., Gilson. J.S., & Bergner, M. (1975). The Sickness Impact Profile: Development of an outcome measure of health care. *American Journal of Public Health, 65*(12), 1304–1310.

Granger, C.V., Hamilton, B.B., Keith, R.A., Zielezny, M., & Sherwin, F.S. (1986). Advances in functional assessment for medical rehabilitation. *Topics in Geriatric Rehabilitation, 1*, 59–74.

Granger, C.V., Ottenbacher, K.J., Baker, J.G., & Sehgal, A. (1995). Reliability of a brief outpatient functional outcome assessment measure. *American Journal of Physical Medicine and Rehabilitation, 74*(6), 469–475.

Gresham, G.E., & Labi, M.L.C. (1984). Functional assessment instruments currently available for documenting outcomes in rehabilitation medicine. In C.V. Granger & G.E. Gresham, *Functional assessment in rehabilitation medicine* (pp. 65–85). Baltimore: Williams & Wilkins.

Haley, S.M., Faas, R.M., Coster, W.J., Ludlow, L.H., Haltiwanger, J.T., & Andrellos, P.J. (1989). *Pediatric Evaluation of Disability (PEDI).* Boston: New England Medical Center.

Halstead, L., & Hartley, R.B. (1975). Time Care Profile: An evaluation of a new method of assessing ADL. *Archives of Physical Medicine and Rehabilitation, 56*(3), 110–115.

Hamilton, M. (1960). A rating scale for depression. *Journal of Neurology and Neurosurgical Psychiatry, 23*, 56–62.

Harvey, R.F., & Jellinek, H.M. (1981). Functional assessment performance: A program approach. *Archives of Physical Medicine and Rehabilitation 62*(9), 456–460.

Holland, A. (1980). *Communicative Abilities in Daily Living.* Baltimore: University Park Press.

Jebsen, R.H., Taylor, N., Trieschmann, R.B., Trotter, M.J., & Howard, L.A. (1969). An objective and standardized test of hand function. *Archives of Physical Medicine and Rehabilitation, 50*(6), 311–319.

Jebsen, R.H., Trieschmann, R.B., Mikulic, M.A., Hartley, R.B., McMillan, J.A., & Snook, M.E. (1970). Measurement of time in a standardized test

of patient mobility. *Archives of Physical Medicine and Rehabilitation, 51*(3), 170–175.

Katz, S., Ford, A.B., Moskowitz, R.W., Jackson, B.A., & Jaffe, M.W. (1963). Studies of illness in the aged. *Journal of the American Medical Association, 185*(12), 914–919.

Klein, R.M., & Bell, B. (1982). Self-care skills: Behavior measurements with the Klein-Bell ADL Scale. *Archives of Physical Medicine and Rehabilitation, 63*(7), 335–338.

Labi, M.L.C., & Gresham, G.E. (1984). Some research applications of functional assessment instruments used in rehabilitation medicine. In C.V. Granger & G.E. Gresham, *Functional assessment in rehabilitation medicine* (pp. 86–98). Baltimore: Williams & Wilkins.

Lawton, M.P. (1971). The functional assessment of elderly people. *Journal of the American Geriatric Society, 19*(6), 465–481.

Lawton, M.P., & Brody, E.M. (1969). Assessment of older people: Self maintaining and instrumental activities of daily living. *Gerontologist, 9*(3), 179–186.

Linn, M.W. (1967). A rapid disability rating scale. *Journal of the American Geriatrics Society, 15*(2), 211–214.

Mahoney, F.I., & Barthel, D.W. (1965). Functional evaluation: The Barthel Index. *Maryland State Medical Journal, 14*(1), 61–65.

McCabe, M.A., & Granger, C.V. (1990). Content validity of a pediatric functional independence measure. *Applied Nursing Research, 3*(3), 120–122.

Moinpour, C.M., McCorkle, R., & Sanders, J. (1988). Measuring functional status. In M. Frank-Stromborg (Ed.), *Instruments for clinical nursing research* (pp. 23–45). Norwalk, CT: Appleton & Lange.

Moskowitz, E., & McCann, C.B. (1957). Classification of disability in the chronically ill and aging. *Journal of Chronic Disability, 5*, 342–346.

Radloff, L.S. (1977). The CES–D Scale: A self-report depression scale for research in the general population. *Applied Psychological Measurement, 1*(3), 385–401.

Rankin, J. (1957). Cerebral vascular accidents in patients over the age of 60. II. Prognosis. *Scottish Medical Journal, 2*, 200–215.

Sarno, J.E., Sarno, M.T., & Levita, E. (1973). The Functional Life Scale. *Archives of Physical Medicine and Rehabilitation, 54*(5), 214–220.

Schoening, H.A., Anderegg, L., Bergstrom, D., Fonda, M., Steinke, N., & Ulrich, P. (1965). Numerical scoring of self-care status of patients. *Archives of Physical Medicine and Rehabilitation, 46*(10), 689–697.

Whiteneck, G.G., Charlifue, S.W., Gerhart, K.A., Overholser, J.D., & Richardson, G.N. (1992). Quantifying handicap: A new measure of long-term rehabilitation outcomes. *Archives of Physical Medicine and Rehabilitation, 73*(6), 519–526.

Willer, B., Ottenbacher, K.J., & Coad, M.L. (1994). The Community Integration Questionnaire. *American Journal of Physical Medicine and Rehabilitation, 73*(2), 103–111.

World Health Organization. (1980). *International classification of impairments, disabilities, and handicaps.* Geneva: Author.

Zung, W.W.K. (1965). A Self-rating Depression Scale. *Archives of General Psychiatry, 12*(12), 63–70.

Zung, W.W.K. (1972). The Depression Status Inventory: An adjunct to the self-rating depression scale. *Journal of Clinical Psychology, 28*(4), 539–543.

CHAPTER 5

Relationship among Measures of Disease, General Health, and Functional Status

Marietta P. Stanton, Glen E. Gresham, and Sharon S. Dittmar

BEHAVIORAL OBJECTIVES

After completing this chapter, the reader will be able to
- describe characteristics of general health, disease-specific, and functional assessment measures.
- discuss similarities and differences between general health measures and functional assessment measures.

- explain the uses of general health measures and functional assessment measures.
- identify the value and future uses of health status measures in rehabilitation.

There is ongoing discussion in the health care system concerning measurement of health care outcomes. This discussion has been prompted by several factors. Health care consumes a significant portion of the national budget. There is increasing emphasis on health promotion and disease prevention programs based on the assumption that healthy people have less need to access expensive inpatient care.

In the past 15 years, acute care institutions have been increasingly pressured by public and private third-party payers to monitor and contain the escalating costs of inpatient services. This focus has contributed to the further shift of health care delivery from inpatient to outpatient and subacute care settings. Many diagnostic and treatment services that were previously performed in a hospital are now performed in long-term care, outpatient, and home settings.

Patient care, regardless of setting, is now influenced by what will be paid for by government and private sources. At the same time, many health care regulatory agencies have demanded that the quality of care provided throughout the health care continuum not be compromised by these cost containment imperatives. To ensure that the quality of care provided to patients is not compromised, much attention increasingly focuses on the outcomes of care.

The identification of these outcomes provides a means of measuring quality of patient care. Outcomes also provide an indication of the quality of life and level of independence that a client possesses as a result of health care interventions. Relating outcomes to that care imposes a high degree of accountability for the services of health care providers. In the current, more competitive health care system, the financial viability and survival of health care institutions will be affected greatly by achieving good outcomes despite cost constraints.

Consumers have become much more astute about their own basic health care needs. They also demand more accountability for their care when they must access the health care system. Accordingly, health care providers and institutions are continuously investigating ways to document outcomes of the health care services they deliver to patients. Health care professionals also are examining ways to assess or predict quality of life, not only to improve interventions but to promote the use of their services. The net result is the active effort by all parties involved to assess, predict, and maximize health care outcomes. Thus health care providers have been designing, testing, and using instruments that will provide the best data available to verify outcomes.

The emphasis on outcomes, quality of life, and cost containment is also critical in the rehabilitation process. Rehabilitation medicine has developed its own measures to examine specific outcomes of care. Instruments currently being used in rehabilitation and health care fall into three major classifications: general health, disease-specific, and functional status measures. Functional status measures predominate in terms of evaluating outcomes in rehabilitation.

GENERAL HEALTH MEASURES

General health measures have historically been used in community or public health settings to assess large populations. They are currently being used more frequently in hospitals and long-term care facilities to assess individual patient outcomes. A number of health status measures have been designed because employers, insurers, and government purchasers have paid increased attention to the measurement of patient outcomes and health status (Lansky, Butler, & Waller, 1992). At first, these instruments were oriented toward assessing morbidity and mortality. Later, they focused on disease processes and the ability of the patient to perform routine daily activities. Today, more emphasis is placed on measuring the positive aspects of physical, social, and emotional well-being. These instruments have been used to gather large data sets to influence health care policy. It is only recently that general health measures were considered as a way to assess individual clients. An example of a general health measure is the Sickness Impact Profile (Gilson, Gilson, & Bergner, 1975) discussed in Chapter 4 and Appendix A. As the name implies, this instrument was designed initially to measure behavioral changes due to illness. It was developed specifically to measure performance rather than to assess capacity. Another example of a widely used health status instrument is the MOS 36-Item Short-Form Health Survey (SF–36) (Kurtin, Ross-Davies, Meyer, DeGiacomo, & Kantz, 1992; McHorney, Ware, & Raczek, 1993; Ware & Sherbourne, 1992; Ware, 1993).

There are a number of inherent problems in the use of general health measures. Most vary in terms of what they measure as quality of life indicators. They also are different in terms of how constructs associated with general health are analyzed, interpreted, and scored. A few general measures have been tested and used sufficiently to provide good insight into the type of data collected, biometric properties of the instruments, and reliability of resulting data (see Chapter 3).

Keith (1994) indicated that general health measures were most useful in assessing global or long-term health outcomes but were not sensitive in assessing individual clinical or short-term outcomes of treatment. Deyo and Carter (1992) postulate that general health measures may be useful in clinical settings to screen for functional problems, monitor disease progression or therapeutic response, improve physician–patient communication, assess quality of care, or provide case-mix adjustment for comparing other outcomes between patient groups. Murtaugh (1994) has found health status measures valuable for projecting discharge planning needs when patients are admitted to the long-term care setting. Permanyer-Miralda, Alonso, Anto, Alijarde-Guimera, and Soler-Soler (1991) found that patient outcomes improved when self-reported health status measures were used in conjunction with other forms of clinical evaluation.

Health care providers and consumers have changed their orientation from an emphasis on disease to considerations of health, functioning, and well-being. Therefore, general health measures need to reflect the new priorities and document the natural history of the disease, evaluate treatment effectiveness, and improve case management techniques (Greenfield & Nelson, 1992). Some of the problems of general health measures are confusion and inconsistency about definition of health, medical components of health status, what is included in an index, and how these indicators are scored (Feinstein, 1992). Different statistical analyses have been used to assess the same dimension, making comparisons of data derived from different instruments difficult. In addition, clinical changes related to a particular disease process may not be detected by using a general health measure (Deyo, Diehr, & Patrick, 1991). Often, general health status measures are long and complicated, but shorter questionnaires may have psychometric deficiencies (Jenkinson, 1991). When health status scores are used for quality assurance, average scores for groups of patients have to be adjusted for disease severity, comorbid conditions, demographic characteristics, socioeconomic conditions, and baseline status, thus complicating analysis. Further, the sickest patients may be least able to provide valid health status information because of dementia, frailty, or blindness. Illiteracy and the inability to speak English also interfere with instrument completion and accuracy of results (Deyo & Carter, 1992).

Some experts contend that general health measures are not useful for monitoring functional status in rehabilitation. These experts contend that general measures seem most valuable in assessing overall long-term health status changes (Deyo & Carter, 1992).

The advantages of health status measures are that they appear to provide a broader base of information when compared with that elicited by different disease-specific or functional status measures. Many researchers believe these health status measures can provide powerful tools for assessing long-term clinical changes across a wide variety of illnesses and therefore can be valuable in assessing outcomes. Other researchers have found them not only valuable as a measure for assessing clinical outcomes but predictive of discharge planning needs. The major disadvantage to the use of general measures is that there are many psychometric difficulties with their scoring and administration. They need intensive scrutiny to ensure suitability for varying clinical groups and require adjustment of items in most cases, detracting from their usefulness in a busy clinical setting.

In summary, general health measures may be useful in clinical settings to improve the process and outcomes of care, but their use requires more research. Wider application could be promoted by training health care providers about the methods of health status assessment and their validity as well as the available instruments. The use of these measures would also be enhanced if they could be made more responsive to clinical changes. Both administration and computation of results for general health measures must be simplified (Deyo & Carter, 1992; Deyo, Diehr, & Patrick, 1991). According to Keith (1994), these general health measures could provide a conceptual framework that could broaden health care as well as rehabilitation perspectives. He believes health status measures may not be appropriate for clinical management but might be useful as quality of care and outcome indicators in rehabilitation. The rather limited use of general health measures in rehabilitation to date and the limited amount of research comparing general health with functional assessment measures indicate that much more study is required before general health measures are used in lieu of or in conjunction with functional status measures. This subject is addressed in more detail later in this chapter.

DISEASE-SPECIFIC MEASURES

Disease-specific measures are similar to general health measures in that they are used to assess selected aspects of overall health status. They are dissimilar, however, in that they tend to focus on individual outcomes unique to a specific disease entity.

Disease-specific measures have evolved because of the belief that general health measures do not adequately, and in the depth required, assess individual outcomes related to a specific disease process. However, as with general health status measures, there is debate about their usefulness among practitioners.

Hawley and Wolfe (1992) obtained evidence concerning short- and long-term efficacy of clinical (disease-specific) and general health status measures in rheumatoid arthritis. They concluded that the outcomes documented with the disease-specific measure changed little over time and were not useful in assessing the outcomes of the treatment protocol studied. Their other findings, however, suggested that general health measures provided useful information in all phases of assessment and evaluation related to a particular disease process.

Other researchers, in studying patients with asthma, found that general health measures alone were not adequate to assess treatment outcomes with their patients. They recommended the use of both general health and disease-specific instruments where appropriate (Rothman & Revicki, 1993). Weinberger, Samsa, Tierney, Belyea, and Hiner (1992) were not convinced that general health measures had any applicability to a disease-specific process. They used a disease-specific health status measure, the Arthritis Impact Measurement Scales, in conjunction with a standardized health status measure in their research. After repeated testing and comparison of the general health measure with the disease-specific measure, their results indicated that these two different types of measures provided similar information on many parameters.

In summary, the literature suggests that disease-specific measures may be useful when used alone or in conjunction with a general health measure. It is apparent that disease-specific instruments, although supplying much information about the disease process and outcomes, do not yield the breadth of information about overall health status that is possible with a general measure. General health measures, because of their more comprehensive approach to health status, obtain information that is not possible to obtain with disease-specific instruments alone. In terms of assessing outcomes that have an impact on quality of life, general measures seem to provide greater breadth of data. However, it is important to note that although investigators value the potential use of general measures in their specific area of health care, there is obvious debate about the use of general health measures to the exclusion of disease-specific measures. It is obvious that more research must be completed to settle this question.

FUNCTIONAL STATUS MEASURES

Functional assessment originated in rehabilitation. Again, there are a wide variety of instruments available to measure function. A selection is described in Chapter 4 and displayed in Appendix A. Functional status measures can be self-reported or observations of actual performance. Functional status measures do not vary as greatly conceptually and methodologically as general health measures. In general, functional status measures focus on different aspects of individual patient performance usually associated with specific activities. They may incorporate other parameters pertaining to general health status, but they primarily focus on the patient's level of function and degree of independence in performing various activities, especially activities of daily living. They are not disease specific. Functional status measures tend to assess a constellation of activities associated with chronic, long-term, or debilitating conditions that make up an individual's normal levels of physical and psychosocial function.

Functional status instruments give health care providers standardized criteria for assessing patient performance.

Therefore they do suggest a set of potential individual patient outcomes that serve to guide the process and product of rehabilitation. Conceptually, functional status measures are important because the primary goal of medical rehabilitation is to enhance patient function and independence.

Traditionally, these instruments stressed individual patient outcomes. However, they are being used with increasing frequency to collect aggregate data. The resulting data are currently being used to develop and modify various policies and practices affecting rehabilitative care. For instance, functional status instruments have been used to predict rehabilitation outcomes and resource use. In one study, functional status was consistently related to discharge function and length of stay. The results of this investigation strongly support the implementation of resource use models for rehabilitation (Heinemann, Linacre, Wright, Hamilton, & Granger, 1994).

In the search for an appropriate payment system for medical rehabilitation hospitals and units, functional status measures have become an area of interest. Study results indicate that functional status and functional gain are among the best predictors of resource utilization at rehabilitation facilities. The literature indicates that functional status measures could form the basis for payment models to classify and justify service to rehabilitation clients (Wilkerson, Batavia, & DeJong, 1992). Because so much emphasis is placed on cost containment without compromising quality of care, the use of functional status measures to determine payment for services may provide the fairest and most realistic alternatives for rehabilitation clients.

Functional status measures have also been used to study financial barriers to care. Rehabilitation patients with financial barriers to care scored significantly lower on psychological dimensions than those without financial barriers to care (Hubbell, Waitzkin, & Rodriguez, 1990). This finding indicates that financial barriers alone can impede and alter outcomes of the rehabilitation process.

Functional assessments that use a combination of self-report and performance-based measures have been used with accuracy in predicting mortality and institutionalization in older adults (Reuben, Siu, & Kimpau, 1992). These instruments have been used to predict future outcomes in an older group at risk for frequent and numerous health care problems (Siu, Reuben, Ouslander, & Osterweil, 1993).

In summary, there are many advantages to the use of functional status measures, in rehabilitation, as well as in geriatrics and other forms of long-term care. They continue to be valuable for use with individual clients, and aggregate data are being used more often as a foundation for policy formulation.

There are also disadvantages in using functional status measures. The person who is most affected by the rehabilitation process is the consumer of those services. Most functional status measures focus primarily on functional limitations rather than on handicapping environmental and social factors. Most consumers influenced by the independent living movement focus on their ability to live autonomously in the community. They are most concerned with environmental and societal barriers that prevent them from functioning independently (Batavia, 1992). Functional status measures should assess environmental and social factors that inhibit successful rehabilitation outcomes (see Chapters 6 and 7). Consumer input should be used in developing these dimensions of these instruments.

Functional status measures seem to have a distinct advantage over general health measures for rehabilitation at this time. These instruments do not have the wide variance conceptually and methodologically as that seen with general health measures. The parameters used for individual assessment seem more objective in terms of treatment plans because data are more likely to be performance based and directly observed by health care providers. Functional status measures also seem superior to disease-specific measures in that they can be used for assessing outcomes for a wide range of chronic and long-term conditions. Functional assessment instruments also seem to be the most sensitive (of all measures considered) to short- and long-term outcomes associated with rehabilitation and long-term care treatment.

Many functional status measures seem deficient because they ignore the impact of environmental and societal barriers that affect a patient's ultimate level of independence on returning to the community. Functional status instruments tend to focus on treatment outcomes associated with rehabilitation. General measures have a broader perspective and focus on the whole gamut of health status. Therefore general health measures may provide a greater breadth of outcomes and a more comprehensive overview regarding quality of life.

IMPLICATIONS

In spite of many common areas of interest, general health, disease-specific, and functional status measures have developed separately (Keith, 1994). There are, however, methodological issues that may in the future enrich rehabilitation practice and research.

Although there is a different emphasis, the definition of functional status measures appears very similar to the definition of functional status in most general health measures. Rehabilitation, however, focuses on how patients conduct their lives posttreatment, whereas general health measures tend to focus on the overall quality of life before or after illness, disease, or injury. Another divergence between the two types of measures is that functional assessment traditionally is used in the clinical area to guide individual patient management and outcomes of treatment. General measures have traditionally focused on group outcomes.

Because of the issues discussed in the introduction (i.e., accountability, consumerism, competition, and cost containment), patient outcomes have assumed a more important role. Clinical outcomes in rehabilitation have important policy implications. Rehabilitation outcomes, when assessed by functional measures, have critical implications for payment. Therefore functional assessment scores are now being considered to gauge group performance. Accumulated group data from functional status measures can be used to formulate policy just as data resulting from general measures have been used all along.

Functional status measures have focused traditionally on individual performance, whereas general health measures have focused historically on aggregate data for policy formulation. Only recently have general health measures been used to assess an individual's potential outcomes in the clinical situation. The benefit to considering the use of health status measures in rehabilitation is that they incorporate a more general quality of life aspect than is currently present in most functional status instruments. One of the criticisms of the functional status measures is that they tend to focus on limits associated with physical and mental performance, rather than on a broader base associated with quality of life issues such as independent living. In addition, functional status measures, for the most part, do not reflect or project the impact of environmental or societal barriers on independence and quality of life when the patient returns to the community. On the other hand, general health measures may be so broad that they fail to address critical performance outcomes specifically related to the rehabilitation process.

Illnesses or conditions that require long-term physical, speech, or occupational therapy may produce changes in function that take many weeks or months to become evident. However, these changes may not indicate a significant alteration in general health status. A general health measure may lack the sensitivity to detect slight but critically important changes in physical or mental function. General health measures may not serve the purpose of assessing the day-to-day improvements resulting from therapy in the rehabilitation process, nor would they assess slight degrees of deterioration in function that may be a consequence of degenerative health processes. Therefore in terms of assessing short-term individual, clinical outcomes in rehabilitation, a more sensitive form of instrumentation may be required than a general health measure.

Although general health measures have many psychometric and scoring deficiencies, there is an ongoing effort to make these instruments more valid, reliable, and user friendly. There is a growing consensus in rehabilitation that functional status measures must also address the same issues regarding psychometric properties (Keith, 1994).

CONCLUSION

In this chapter, an overview of general health, disease-specific, and functional status measures has been provided. The historical basis for the evolution of these areas was described. The advantages and disadvantages for each type of instrument were discussed by using research examples from the current literature. Finally, a discussion and comparison for use of general health versus functional status measures in the rehabilitation process have been addressed. In summary, both approaches have potential usefulness in rehabilitation as researchers and practitioners move toward a common ground in assessing individual and group outcomes.

REFERENCES

Batavia, A.L. (1992). Assessing the function of functional assessment: A consumer perspective. *Disability and Rehabilitation, 14*(3), 156–160.

Deyo, R.A., & Carter, W.B. (1992). Strategies for improving and expanding the application of health status measures in clinical settings: A researcher–developer viewpoint. *Medical Care, 30*(Suppl. 5), MS176–186; Discussion MS196–209.

Deyo, R.A., Diehr, P., & Patrick, D.L. (1991). Reproducibility and responsiveness of health status measures: Statistics and strategies for evaluation. *Controlled Clinical Trials, 12*(Suppl. 4), 142S–158S.

Feinstein, A.R. (1992). Benefits and obstacles for development of health status assessment measures in clinical settings. *Medical Care, 30*(Suppl. 5), MS50–56.

Gilson, B.S., Gilson, J.S., & Bergner, M. (1975). The Sickness Impact Profile: Development of an outcome measure of health care. *American Journal of Public Health, 65*(12), 1304–1310.

Greenfield, S., & Nelson, E.C. (1992, May). Recent developments and future issues in the use of health status measures in clinical settings. *Medical Care, 30*(Suppl. 5), MS23–41.

Hawley, D.J., & Wolfe, F. (1992). Sensitivity to change of the health assessment questionnaire (HAQ) and other clinical and health status measures in rheumatoid arthritis: Results of short-term clinical trials and observational studies versus long-term observational studies. *Arthritis Care and Research, 5*(3), 130–136.

Heinemann, A.W., Linacre, J.M., Wright, B.D., Hamilton, B.B., & Granger, C. (1994). Prediction of rehabilitation outcomes with disability measures. *Archives of Physical Medicine and Rehabilitation, 75*(2), 133–143.

Hubbell, F.A., Waitzkin, H., & Rodriguez, F.I. (1990). Functional status and financial barriers to medical care among the poor. *Southern Medical Journal, 83*(5), 548–550.

Jenkinson, C. (1991). Why are we weighting? A critical examination of the use of item weights in a health status measure. *Social Science and Medicine, 32*(12), 1413–1416.

Keith, R.A. (1994). Functional status and health status. *Archives of Physical Medicine and Rehabilitation, 75*(4), 478–483.

Kurtin, P., Ross-Davies, A., Meyer, K., DeGiacomo, J., & Kantz, E. (1992). Patient-based health status measures in outpatient dialysis—Early experiences in developing an outcomes assessment program. *Medical Care, 30*(Suppl. 5), 136–149.

Lansky, D., Butler, J.B., & Waller, F I. (1992). Using health status measures in the hospital setting: From acute care to outcomes measurement. *Medical Care, 30*(Suppl. 5), MS57–73.

McHorney, C.A., Ware, J.E., Jr., & Raczek, A.E. (1993). The MOS 36-Item Short-Form Health Survey (SF–36). II. Psychometric and chemical and clinical tests of validity in measuring physical and mental health constructs. *Medical Care, 31*(3), 247–263.

Murtaugh, C.M. (1994). Discharge planning in nursing homes. *Health Services Research, 28*(6), 751–769.

Permanyer-Miralda, G., Alonso, J., Anto, J.M., Alijarde-Guimera, M., & Soler-Soler, J. (1991). Comparison of perceived health status and conventional functional evaluation in stable patients with coronary artery disease. *Journal of Clinical Epidemiology, 44*(8), 779–786.

Reuben, D.B., Siu, A.L., & Kimpau, S. (1992). The predictive validity of self-report and performance-based measures of function and health. *Journal of Gerontology, 47*(4), 106–110.

Rothman, M.L., & Revicki, D.A. (1993). Issues in the measurement of health status in asthma research. *Medical Care, 31*(Suppl. 3), MS82–98.

Siu, A.L., Reuben, D.B., Ouslander, J.G., & Osterweil, D. (1993). Using multidimensional health measures in older persons to identify risk of hospitalization and skilled nursing placement. *Quality of Life Research, 2*(4), 253–261.

Ware, J.E., Jr. (1993). *SF–36 Health Survey: Manual and Interpretation Guide*. Boston: The Health Institute. New England Medical Center.

Ware, J.E., Jr., & Sherbourne, C.D. (1992). The MOS 36-Item Short-Form Health Survey (SF–36). I. Conceptual framework and item selection. *Medical Care, 30*(6). 473–483.

Weinberger, M., Samsa, G.P., Tierney, W.M., Belyea, M.G., & Hiner, S.L. (1992). Generic versus disease-specific health status measures: Comparing the Sickness Impact Profile and the Arthritis Impact Measurement Scales. *Journal of Rheumatology, 19*(4), 543–546.

Wilkerson, D.L., Batavia, A.L., & DeJong, G. (1992). Use of functional status measures for payment of medical rehabilitation services. *Archives of Physical Medicine and Rehabilitation, 73*(2), 111–120.

CHAPTER 6

Environment as a Mediating Factor in Functional Assessment

Edward H. Steinfeld and Gary S. Danford

BEHAVIORAL OBJECTIVES

After completing this chapter, the reader will be able to
- use a theoretical framework to describe the role of environment in disability.
- recognize current accessibility standards and their appropriateness for individuals with specific disabilities.

- understand issues in measurement with specific functional assessment instruments designed to identify and describe the role of environment in disability.
- describe research to test the environmental components of disability.

In this chapter, the physical environment of everyday living is emphasized as part of functional assessment. An analytical framework for understanding and using the environment in rehabilitation practice, as well as techniques of assessment that can be used to operationalize environmental considerations in the functional assessment process, are described.

Any analytical perspective on the issue of environmental considerations in functional assessment is either explicitly or implicitly grounded in theoretical assumptions about the nature of person–environment relationships. Thus a foundation of theory is set first, so that the reader understands the underlying rationale for the model, especially because this type of theory will be unfamiliar to many readers of this book. Then the practical value of an environmental focus for rehabilitation practice and how that focus can improve validity and reliability of functional assessment methods are demonstrated. Once this background is established, key issues of reliability and validity in measurement are discussed. Finally, the authors' work in development of new measures is used as a case study to illustrate the importance of the environmental viewpoint and the way measurement issues can be addressed in development of methods.

THEORETICAL CONSIDERATIONS

In rehabilitation practice, the environment has been conceptualized as a prosthetic support for functional independence. Standards and codes are used to establish how environmental interventions should be designed. The prevailing view is that an environment is either accessible (meets standards) or inaccessible (does not meet standards). This conceptual model has limited usefulness because it leads to prescriptive approaches that do not consider the complexity of person–environment relationships. Moreover, it limits the development of functional assessment methods because only the environment, and not its influence, is the focus of measurement. How a person behaves in a particular situation is not a simple property of either the person or that person's environment; it is a product of the interaction between the two (Cronberg, 1975; Mead, 1934). This view on the nature of person–behavior–environment relationships is the defining characteristic of what has come to be known as a *transactional perspective* (Altman & Rogoff, 1987; Moore, 1976; Stokols, 1981, 1987; Wandersman, Murday, & Wadsworth, 1979). The transactional model can be very useful in practice. In particular, it can be operationalized in functional assessment to provide tools for measuring the impact of environmental design on functional performance.

Virtually all such transactional models of person–behavior–environment relationships are at least partially grounded in Kurt Lewin's classic concept of *life space*, which is defined by the equation B = f(PE) (Lewin, 1951). Simply stated, Lewin conceived of behavior (B) as being a function (f) of the interaction of personality and individual factors (P) and the perceived environment of the individual (E). Contemporary transactional models are typically more complex. These models continue either the Gestalt psychology tradition such as that promoted by Lewin emphasizing mental processes (e.g., perception) or the behaviorist tradition of Watson and Skinner emphasizing outwardly observable behavior. Nevertheless, they generally acknowledge that behavior is a manifestation of the person–environment interaction, rather than determined by either intrapersonal factors or the environment alone. Both theoretical traditions have their value, and both can be incorporated in transactional models.

The *environmental docility hypothesis* is an example of a transactional model. It demonstrates the focus on the person–environment relationship and introduces the concept of *environmental demand*. On the basis of the concept of stress, the model postulates that environment exerts a *press* on the person, either supportive or challenging. The consequences of that environmental press depend on the *competence* of the person encountering that environment (Nahemow & Lawton, 1973). Nahemow and Lawton argue that mismatches between the press of an environment and the functional capabilities that person may possess can lead to situations in which the person's functional independence and performance could be seriously compromised. This may occur not only with conditions of *overload*, in which press exceeds the coping capacity of an individual, but also in conditions of *deprivation*, in which challenges are well below an individual's capacity. These are positions endorsed by most contemporary transactional theories.

A third concept often reflected in transactional models is captured by Bandura's formulation of *reciprocal determinism* (1978). Bandura's model emphasizes the reciprocity that exists among person, behavior, and environment—each influencing the other two and, in return, being influenced by the consequences of its own effects on those of the other two. Transactional models typically take this reciprocity as a given and proceed to focus on defining the dynamic nature of the relationships among person, behavior, and environment. One such contemporary model is *dynamic reciprocal determinism* (Danford, 1983, 1985). This model melds the three aforementioned concepts and then proceeds to define the dynamics of the relationships in terms that can explain widely divergent outcomes in the same setting. It seeks to explain how the environment's influence can seem at one time to be negligible and at another time to be the primary or even sole determinant of the outcomes resulting from a specific situation (see Figure 6–1). That is, the environment may at times heavily influence behavior and at other times have only a negligible influence on it.

A key factor in the dynamic reciprocal determinism model is a monitoring mechanism. It is proposed that the person or group subconsciously *monitors* the ongoing (or anticipated) behavior–environment transaction and typically submits to the influence of the environment. As long as the environmental press does not violate certain *tolerance thresholds* (i.e., does not violate the person's values, expectations, or capabilities) sufficiently to prompt an attempt to *override* or change the situation, the environment effectively determines the outcomes. The consequence is that "most of the time, most people behave in ways that are compatible with or adaptive to the settings they occupy" (Wicker, 1974, p. 599).

Other theories have represented the same ideas with an emphasis on cognitive and social processes. Symbolic interactionists (see Mead, 1934) would call Danford's monitoring process *interpretation*. They argue that as long as the situation matches one's conception of self or a group's shared understanding about how things should be, no action to change the situation would be taken. If the bounds of an appropriate match are broken, however, some sort of action would occur, such as protesting intolerable conditions, moving to a new place that is more appropriate, renovating the existing environment, or constructing a new environment. A new dimension is introduced when the person–environment relationship is viewed in this way. The resultant action could be entirely mental, a change in values and expectations (i.e., psychological adjustment to the situation). An example is the adjustment from stranger to resident documented by Matthews (1979) in retirement communities. The interactionist view also has an important social component in that social interaction heavily defines what is considered appropriate and how an individual or group will respond. In essence, the interactionist view adds the dimension of social construction.

How successful individuals or groups might be in attempting to overcome an inappropriate situation is determined by their *mastery level* (similar to what Moos [1975] calls *capabilities*). Those with low levels of mastery may find that their attempts to change the situation are ineffective or even maladaptive. The behaviorist would argue that the result would be extinction or suppression of the behavior to change because of lack of reinforcement or negative reinforcement, respectively. The interactionist would argue that individuals or groups adjust by changing their perceptions of self and accepting the situation as a reflection of that new identity. An example is the prisoner who stops resisting incarceration and becomes docile and compliant. As the environmental docility hypothesis demonstrates, if the demands of the environment are so great that mastery is impossible—even for individuals or groups with a high level of competency—

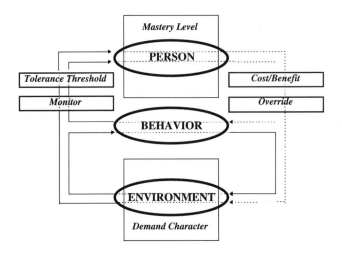

Figure 6–1 Dynamic reciprocal determinism model of person–behavior–environment transactions.

there may be no mental or physical adjustment at all. The individuals or groups may simply succumb to insurmountable stress, as was the case in the recent demise of expert climbers on Mt. Everest, for example. In general, these examples illustrate the importance of separating adaptive behaviors from the person and environment. This separation helps clarify the relationship, as well as aids in analyzing differences between one situation and another.

A term often used to characterize the appropriateness of a particular person–behavior–environment transaction is *congruence* or *fit* (Fisher, Bell, & Baum, 1984). Nahemow and Lawton (1973) defined fit as a sort of equilibrium in which an individual's capabilities are in balance with the press of environment. In their model, equilibrium is not a specific pivot point but, rather, a *zone of adaptation*. Within this zone individuals are sufficiently challenged to ensure continued ability to adapt, yet not so overloaded or deprived that they are under pathological stress. If the dynamic reciprocal determinism model is used, fit would be defined as a relationship that is tolerated by individuals. The individuals conclude that either the benefits to be derived from changing an inappropriate situation are simply not worth the costs in terms of the effort necessary to effect the requisite changes or the changes are not even possible because of the magnitude of the mismatch between individuals' mastery levels and the environment's demand character. In the interactionist conception, fit would be a situation that represents congruence between the desired presentation of self and the reflected self as perceived and affirmed by others. All three conceptions are valid and are not mutually exclusive. In effect, fit can be defined by some objective criterion by an outside observer, the individual, or one's social world.

Obviously, the concept of fit covers a broad range of person–behavior–environment outcomes. It could be achieved by insulating an individual from challenge as mastery level declines, such as when a veteran baseball player is sent to the minor league or a frail older person is relocated to a nursing home. However, it could also be achieved by maintaining a high exposure to challenge and taking a different social role, such as becoming a designated hitter or care recipient in the previous examples. In contemporary rehabilitation practice, with its emphasis on independent living, a common intervention would be to provide environmental support to achieve or maintain competence in the face of stress. However much the professional observer concludes that fit has been achieved, the individual may not and vice versa. The transactional model provides a broader awareness that can assist a practitioner in making informed decisions and understanding the highly variable responses of clients. For example, it can help explain why people may have very different responses to the same modified environment. Some may be willing and able to learn new patterns of living, but others may refuse to deal with even a limited challenge and adapt by restricting their range of movement or social roles. Moreover, it can help explain why some households make modifications to the environment and others do not. Each has a different definition of fit.

ACCESSIBILITY STANDARDS

It might at first seem reasonable to recommend an unquestioning compliance with accessibility standards such as the Americans With Disabilities Act Accessibility Guidelines (*Federal Register*, 1991) as a strategy for ensuring achievement of appropriate person–behavior–environment fit for the person with a disability. The transactional model provides at least three reasons why such a strategy might not yield a desirable outcome (Rubin & Elder, 1980).

First, accessibility standards can be viewed as a socially constructed definition of fit. They do not always represent the latest in knowledge and social values. For example, the inertia of the regulatory process tends to work against timely application of emerging technologies (e.g., building practices, health care delivery services, social customs) with the result that the standards could be not only obsolete but also actually counterproductive. Another example is that accessibility standards are typically written to ensure achievement of minimum levels of facility accessibility. Unquestioning application of such standards in rehabilitation practice could lead to less than optimum responses for an individual's needs.

Second, accessibility standards are largely insensitive to individual differences; that is, they prescribe unvarying responses in the face of varying individual needs. They provide prescriptive guidelines that can compel environmental design changes that may be neither warranted nor beneficial to the individual in question. To the degree that they produce environments that are either too challenging or too supportive their wholesale and indiscriminant application can actually prove deleterious to functional independence and performance.

Third, standards are not based on empirically derived performance models. If empirical data are used as a basis for standards, they usually have been obtained from studies that seek to define boundaries of accessibility, rather than understand the relationship of individual and environment as a dynamic reciprocal system. For example, it is unreasonable to assume that there is one fixed accessible door width for wheelchair users as currently incorporated in all standards. The accessibility of a doorway is a function of an individual's wheelchair width, ability to maneuver, and definition of convenience. The building owner's tolerance for damage to the door frame also plays a role. In addition, standards are often not based on empirical research at all. They are merely reactions to design failures combined with a measure of good intentions with the result that the person–behavior–environment fit afforded by their actual application can sometimes be less than appropriate.

MEASUREMENT ISSUES

There are several important issues that need to be addressed when measuring the fit between individuals and their environments. Some of these issues are related to the administration of assessment measures. Others are related to the quality of the information those measures produce.

The objectives of the measurement will play an important role in determining what measures are most appropriate. For example, an assessment with a goal of determining whether an individual can live in a particular facility requires a measurement technique that will provide information on the overall fit between environment and individual abilities. On the other hand, an assessment with a goal of determining what modifications are needed to facilitate productivity in a workplace requires a more fine-grained measurement technique to identify specific problems that need to be addressed. A related issue is the sensitivity required by the measurement technique. Some methods may identify differences in fit between radically different environments but not between slightly different settings. In addition, the range of difference in performance or perceptions measured may be so slight as to be somewhat meaningless. For example, does it really matter if a person requires five seconds more to toilet in one bathroom compared to another? Cost of administration is a real concern in both research and practice. A measurement technique that is labor intensive to administer and analyze will not be a very useful tool for professionals and researchers operating with limited resources. Moreover, in research such a measurement technique can severely restrict generalizability by limiting the feasible size of samples.

Information quality is determined primarily by the reliability and validity of assessment measures. Few techniques for measuring fit have been systematically tested for reliability. Questions must be asked about whether a particular measure will give the same results on repeated applications in the same setting with the same person. Reliability is particularly affected by instability in the environment and training of the person doing the assessment. Environments can change in very subtle ways that an untrained person may not recognize. For example, light level and background noise can vary slightly but enough to make a difference in performance. Or the placement of any object that must be reached for use in a task (e.g., toothbrush) can make a big difference in performance. Clearly, measures that have proved reliable through systematic testing are preferable, but in practice, it is important that professionals also use them in appropriate ways. This requires training and, in particular, an understanding of how environment can influence results.

Validity in measurement is concerned primarily with whether a particular tool measures what it is supposed to measure. Ideally, a measurement technique should correlate well with related measures. If it does not, this does not necessarily mean that the technique is not valid; it may simply be measuring something very different. For example, self-report and observer ratings may tap entirely different things (e.g., perceptions or performance). In research, multimethod strategies are generally preferred to single measure approaches. They allow triangulation of different perspectives, and they can help uncover differences that may not be apparent by using one method alone. In professional practice, however, the resources, available in time and money, may not be adequate to use multiple methods. It is therefore advisable to ensure that the method selected has been shown to be valid, through rigorous testing and comparison with other measures. It is particularly important that the practitioner understand the different dimensions of person–environment fit and select appropriate techniques accordingly. For example, one would not likely choose a self-report measure if the objective is to assess demonstrated competence in a particular task. On the other hand, one would not likely select an observer rating measure if the objective is to measure an individual's satisfaction with a particular environment.

CASE STUDY IN DEVELOPING MEASURES

In a four-year program of research, we are developing methods to measure the influence of physical environments on functional independence and performance of persons with functional limitations (e.g., mobility impairments, reduced grip strength). These measures examine how environments can enable or disable functional independence and performance.

This outcome measurement capability becomes particularly important when one observes changes in functional independence and performance after an individual is discharged from a rehabilitation program. Such outcome measures can enable one to discern whether a negative change such as a loss in functional independence or performance is attributable to an attenuation in the benefits of the rehabilitation program over time, or whether it is the person's home environment that might be responsible for the change.

The focus of this program of research has been on the development, testing, and refinement of measures to complement the widely used Functional Independence Measure instrument (FIM℠) (Granger, Hamilton, Keith, Zielezny, & Sherwin, 1986). This has been done not only to enable the identification of enabling person–behavior–environment match-ups but also to permit diagnosis of the specific handicapping match-ups. An identification of the latter may begin to provide an explanation for maladaptive or undesirable outcomes such as a person's postrehabilitation decline in functional independence (as measured by the FIM℠) on return to the home environment.

We have developed outcome measures that can accomplish the following:

1. Obtain individuals' self-reports on ease or difficulty of functional performance in selected environments.
2. Examine a person's functional independence and performance in the context of mediating environmental demand character.
3. Diagnose the specific sources of person–environment fit.
4. Assess caregiver burden.

The first measure is a psychophysical Usability Rating Scale (URS℠), which has the person rate perceived ease or difficulty of using specific task environments. The second is the Environmental Functional Independence Measure (Enviro-FIM℠), which scores the person's functional independence in the context of specifically designed physical environments. The third is a Functional Performance Measure (FPM℠), which scores three items: (1) the person's level of effort toward completion of a task, (2) the caregiver's (if applicable) level of assistance provided to the person toward completion of that task, and (3) the demand character of the task environment.

The initial testing and refinement of these outcome measures was conducted by studying the functional independence and performance of persons with disabilities in environments whose demand character varied systematically.

Research Design

Twenty-four women with mobility impairments (i.e., 12 wheelchair users and 12 walking aid users) were selected for the testing and refinement phase of this program. They were asked to simulate the performance of several activities of daily living, such as grooming, toileting, and bathing, in three full-scale simulated bathrooms: (1) challenging, (2) supportive, and (3) intermediate (between challenging and supportive). In these three bathrooms, five sets of design attributes typically addressed in accessibility standards were varied systematically to provide three distinct levels of demand character as contexts for the subjects' performance of those activities and their component tasks:

1. size of open floor area inside the room
2. entry door characteristics
3. lavatory/vanity characteristics
4. toilet characteristics
5. bathtub/shower characteristics

The challenging (i.e., unaccommodating) bathroom configuration (see Figure 6–2) was characterized by the following five design attributes:

1. an open floor area of only 15 square feet
2. a 32-inch entry door equipped with conventional doorknob handles with a swing that swept across the open floor area inside the room
3. an enclosed vanity with small (20 × 20 inch) countertop, traditional dual-knob faucets, and high-mounted (47-inch) mirror/cabinet
4. a 16-inch-high toilet with no attached grab bars or wall grab bars
5. a 15-inch-high bathtub with a fixed position shower head, no wall grab bars, and single knob-handle faucet mounted on center

The supportive (i.e., accommodating) bathroom configuration (see Figure 6–3) was characterized by the following five design attributes:

1. a 25-square-foot open floor area
2. a 34-inch entry door equipped with lever handles with a swing that swept away from the inside of the room
3. an open vanity with even larger (20 × 30 inch) countertop, single lever-handle faucet, and low-mounted (40-inch) mirror/cabinet plus adjustable wall-mounted mirror
4. a higher (18-inch) toilet equipped with both attached grab bars and wall grab bars
5. a roll-in shower stall with an adjustable position hand-held shower, wall grab bars, and single lever-handle faucet mounted off center

Finally, the intermediate (i.e., neither strongly challenging nor supportive) bathroom configuration (see Figure 6–4) was characterized by the following five design attributes:

1. a 20-square-foot open floor area

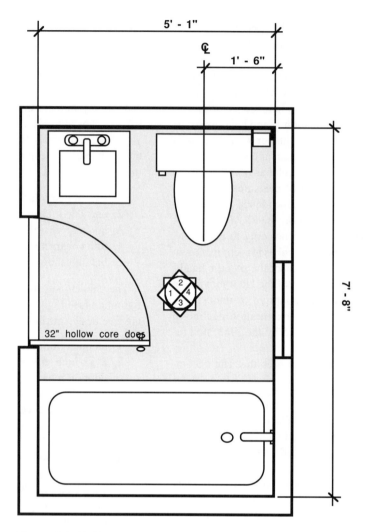

Figure 6–2 Challenging bathroom configuration.

2. a 34-inch entry door equipped with lever handles with a swing that swept across the open floor area inside the room
3. an open vanity with an in-between (20 × 24 inch) countertop, double-lever-handle faucets, and high-mounted (47 inch) mirror/cabinet plus adjustable wall-mounted mirror
4. a 16-inch-high toilet with wall grab bars
5. a 15-inch-high bathtub with fixed position hand-held shower head, wall grab bars, and single lever-handle faucet mounted on center

In addition, the 24 subjects were asked to negotiate their way through 26 distinct door configurations (including entering and exiting door configurations for each of the three bathrooms). These door configurations varied systematically in terms of their

- door width
- direction of door swing
- latch type
- handle type
- latch–side clearance
- force required to open
- interior/exterior projections

The subjects' bathroom and door trials were counterbalanced to control for possible order effect, and standardized instructions were provided for each activity to be performed (e.g., simulating use of the toilet), including each activity's

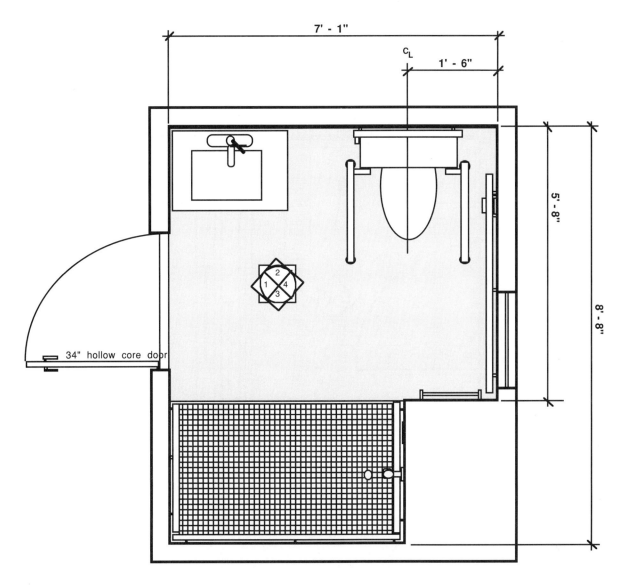

7' - 1"

1' - 6"

C_L

5' - 8"

8' - 8"

34" hollow core door

Figure 6–3 Supportive bathroom configuration.

component tasks (e.g., flushing the toilet). At the end of each activity, each subject was asked to rate how easy or difficult it had been to perform the requested activity in that environment (see URS℠ below). Each subject's performance of each of the requested activities in each environment was also videotaped to permit more detailed analysis at a later time (see Enviro-FIM℠ instrument below).

URS℠

The URS℠ (see Figure 6–5) is an adaptation of a previously developed, tested, and published sequential judgment

scale (Pitrella & Kappler, 1988) that ultimately was simplified to a seven-point bipolar rating scale. The URS℠ was designed to enable examination of individuals' subjective responses to their experiences in designed physical environments. Examination involved a sequential two-step process: (1) making an initial choice among difficult, moderate, and easy characterizations of the activity's performance followed by (2) locating the activity at a specific position on the relevant subsection of the seven-point scale. Subjects' self-reports about the relative ease or difficulty of use of environments were hypothesized to be globally reflective of the environments' influences on functional indepen-

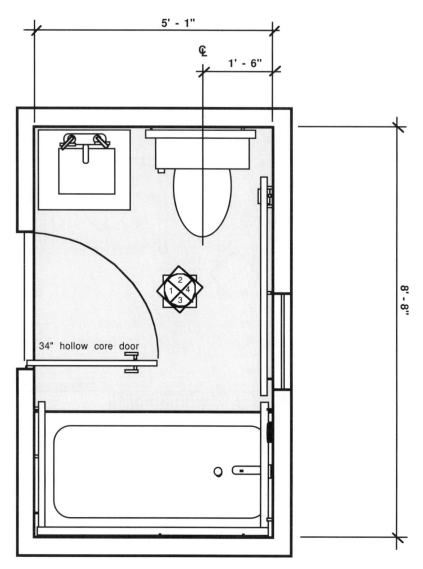

Figure 6–4 Intermediate bathroom configuration.

dence during simulated performance of the requested activities.

Examination of the URS℠ ratings of the three bathrooms by these subjects (see Figure 6–6) supported our hypothesis about these environments' expected enabling or handicapping (or both) influences. Particularly interesting was how the wheelchair users' perceptions suggest that they were more handicapped by certain design features in the intermediate and challenging bathrooms and more enabled by design features of the supportive bathroom, when their reports were compared with those of their walking aid counterparts.

Enviro-FIM℠

The Enviro-FIM℠ instrument (see Figure 6–7) is a derivative of the seven-point FIM℠ instrument. It expands the

FIM℠ instrument's score of six into four scores to create a 10-point measurement scale. In addition, the content of the FIM℠ instrument was expanded to address additional design features in the physical environment (e.g., doors), which were hypothesized to influence individuals' functional independence and performance. The Enviro-FIM℠ instrument was designed to identify, at a global level, possible enabling and handicapping match-ups between physical environments and individuals with disabilities based on those environments' influences on functional independence and performance.

For this aspect of the research program, the performance of the 24 subjects was rated with both the FIM℠, and the Enviro-FIM℠ instruments, and the respective scores for each instrument were evaluated. Examination of the FIM℠

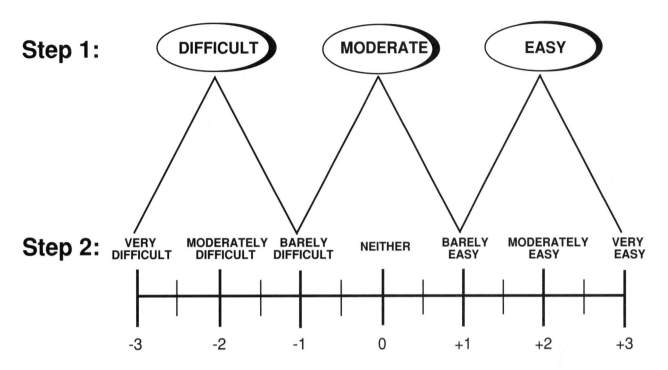

Figure 6–5 Two-step Usability Rating Scale (URS^SM).

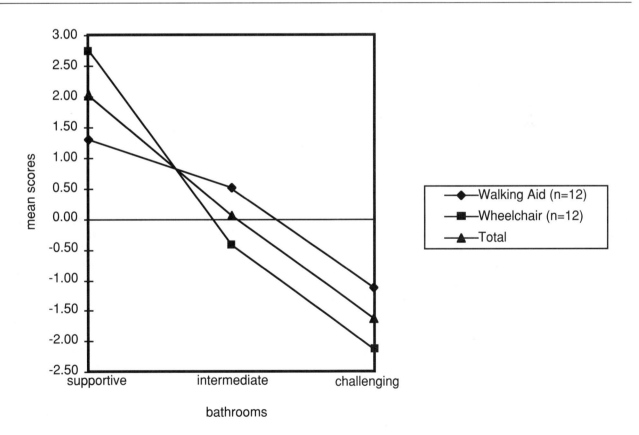

Figure 6–6 Usability Rating Scale (URS^SM) mean scores for supportive, intermediate, and challenging bathrooms.

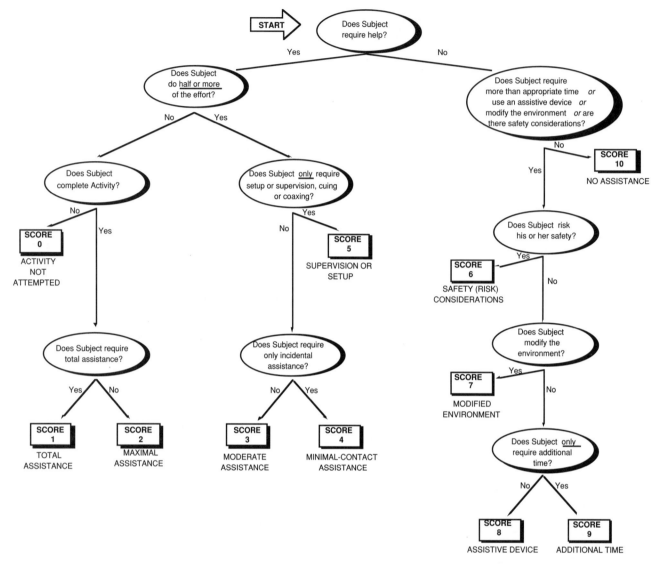

Figure 6–7 Decision tree for Environmental Functional Independence Measure (Enviro-FIM℠).

instrument scores (see Figure 6–8) demonstrated that these scores were not independent of the environmental context in which the subjects performed the requested activities. In comparison with the walking aid users, the wheelchair users' functional independence was more markedly affected by these three environments, particularly the challenging bathroom.

Examination of the Enviro-FIM℠ scores of these same 24 subjects for the three bathrooms (see Figure 6–9) also demonstrated the expected effects of the environments on functional independence of the subjects, again with the wheelchair users being more dramatically affected than the walking aid users by the challenging bathroom's design characteristics.

Comparison of the FIM℠ and Enviro-FIM℠ scores (see Figure 6–10) demonstrates similar effects of the environ-

ments on the subjects' functional independence scores. When the 10-point Enviro-FIM℠ scale is collapsed into a seven-point scale comparable to the FIM℠'s seven-point scale, the two sets of scores fall virtually on top of each other.

Tests of both inter- and intra-rater reliabilities (see Table 6–1) demonstrated relatively high levels of complete agreement with use of the Enviro-FIM℠ instrument. Both reliabilities were only marginally affected by the passage of time (i.e., two weeks of not using the Enviro-FIM℠ instrument).

FPM℠

The third outcome measure, the FPM℠ instrument, uses two eight-point rating scales to score

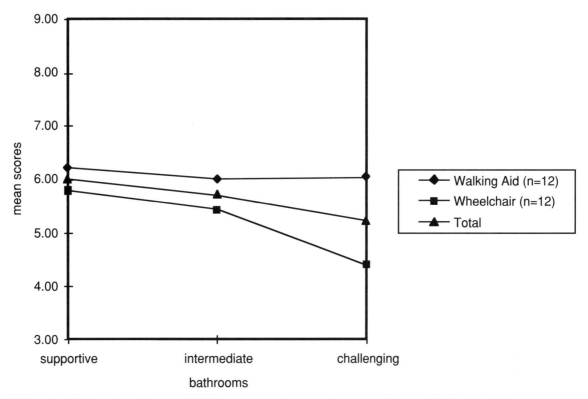

Figure 6–8 Functional Independence Measure (FIMˢᴹ) mean scores in supportive, intermediate, and challenging bathrooms.

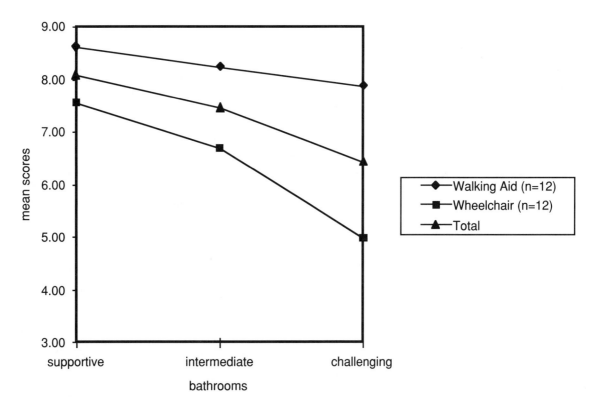

Figure 6–9 Environmental Functional Independence Measure (Enviro-FIMˢᴹ) mean scores in supportive, intermediate, and challenging bathrooms.

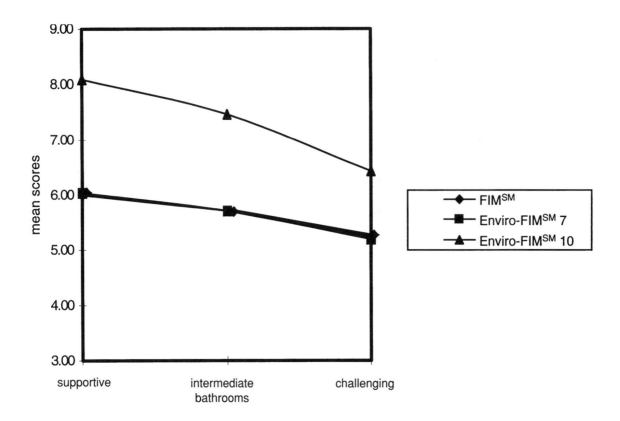

Figure 6–10 Comparison of Functional Independence Measure (FIM^SM) and Environmental Functional Independence Measure (Enviro-FIM^SM) mean scores in supportive, intermediate, and challenging bathrooms.

1. level of effort (X = unknown, 0 = none, and Levels 1–6 of effort) expended by the subject toward task performance
2. level of assistance (X = unknown, 0 = none, and Levels 1–6 of assistance) provided by the caregiver during that task performance in the variously challenging bathroom and door environments tested.

Which of the eight level of effort scores the individual receives (see Figure 6–11) is determined by factors, such as

Table 6–1 Environmental Functional Independence Measure (Enviro-FIM^SM) Reliabilities

Type of Reliability	Enviro-FIM^sm	
	n	% Agreement
Inter-rater (1)	164	96
Inter-rater (2)	164	87
Intra-rater (1)	164	92
Intra-rater (2)	164	89

(1) = Initial trial; (2) = Second trial two weeks later.

- whether successful performance of the task in question is actually required for accomplishment of the activity (e.g., operating the latch for a door that is not equipped with a latch = Level 0), and if so,
- whether any physical effort is required for successful task performance (e.g., closing a door that is equipped with an automatic closer = Level 0), and if so,
- frequency of complaint by the individual as an expression of aggravation, inconvenience, or anxiety during task performance,
- frequency of interruption in the continuity of the individual's task performance,
- amount of time taken for task performance, and
- number of attempts made toward task performance.

Which of the eight level of assistance scores the caregiver receives (see Figure 6–12) is determined by factors, such as

- whether successful task performance is required for accomplishment of the activity (i.e., not required = Level 0), and if so,
- whether any assistance is required for successful task performance (i.e., no assistance required = Level 0) and if so,

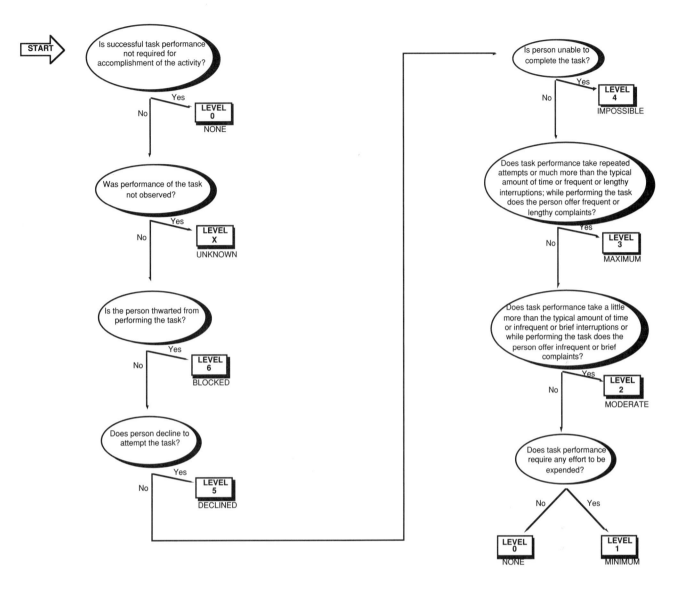

Figure 6–11 Decision tree for Functional Performance Measure (FPM^SM) level of effort.

- whether provided assistance is merely incidental to task performance (e.g., touching or verbal expression intended solely as encouragement or praise = Level 1),
- whether provided assistance directly facilitates the individual's task performance (e.g., instructing, prompting, performing set up, etc. = Level 2), and
- whether assistance provided constitutes direct performance of task for individual by the caregiver (i.e., caregiver performs the task for the person = Level 3).
- Level of Assistance scores 4–6 are directly comparable to the level of effort scores 4–6.

Of the scores obtained from 24 subjects and analyzed using the FPM^SM level of effort and level of assistance scales, the responses from four subjects (i.e., two wheelchair users and two walking aid users) were rescored to permit examina-

tion of both inter- and intra-rater reliabilities. This involved rescoring each of 283 tasks performed by every subject in three bathrooms and all 26 doors—a total of 1,132 level of effort judgments and 1,132 level of assistance judgments.

The intra-rater reliability analysis examined the consistency with which one rater scored the 283 tasks for each of the four subjects. The results (see Table 6–2) showed exact score matches on the eight-point level of effort scale of 97% and exact score matches on the eight-point level of assistance scale of 99%.

Inter-rater reliability analysis examined the agreement between two raters who scored the 283 tasks for each of the four subjects. These results showed exact score matches on the eight-point level of effort scale of 84% and exact score matches on the eight-point level of assistance scale of 96%. Of the 16% exact score level of effort mismatches, only

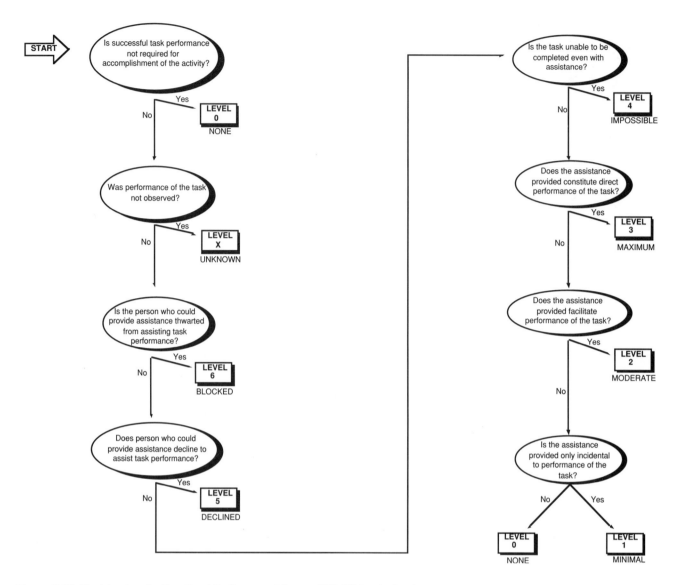

Figure 6–12 Decision tree for Functional Performance Measure (FPM^SM) level of assistance.

1.5% differed by more than one point on the eight-point scale (a remarkable finding given this was achieved without benefit of a formal training program or a written user manual detailing all coding conventions during this testing and development phase).

Level of effort scores for the 24 subjects in the three bathrooms (excluding the bathrooms' door trial components, which were analyzed separately) are shown in Figure 6–13. The walking aid users expended a relatively constant level of effort across the three environments. In contrast, the wheelchair users expended a progressively increasing level of effort as they moved from supportive to intermediate to challenging bathrooms.

Examination of the level of assistance scores (see Figure 6–14) for the 24 subjects in the three bathrooms (again, ex-

cluding the bathrooms' door trials) shows the walking aid users received negligible assistance in any of the bathrooms. In contrast, the wheelchair users received a progressively increasing level of assistance as they moved from supportive to intermediate to challenging bathrooms.

If average level of effort and level of assistance scores for all 24 subjects in all three bathrooms are plotted (see Figure 6–15), the effects of environment are clearly evident. Environment affects not only effort required from the individual but also assistance required from the caregiver as the subject moved from supportive to intermediate to challenging bathrooms.

If mean level of effort scores for all grooming, toileting, and bathing tasks performed by all 24 subjects are plotted against the subjects' comparable FIM^SM subscales' scores

Table 6–2 Functional Performance Measure (FPM^{SM}) Reliabilities

Type of Reliability	Level of Effort		Level of Assistance	
	n	% Agreement	n	% Agreement
Inter-rater (1)	1132	84	1132	96
Intra-rater	1132	97	1132	99

(1) = Level of effort scale inter-rater agreement variance: 1 point off = 14.5%; > 1 point off = 1.5%.

(i.e., grooming, toilet transfer, tub transfer, and bathing) in the challenging bathroom (see Figure 6–16), a remarkably strong relationship exists between the two. As expected, the lower the subject's FIM^{SM} score the higher the level of effort typically required to perform the tasks. In turn, the higher the subject's FIM^{SM} score the lower the level of effort typically required to perform the tasks.

Utility of Measures

The initial motivation for development, testing, and refinement of the URS^{SM}, Enviro-FIM^{SM}, and FPM^{SM} instruments was to use them as complements to the FIM^{SM} instru-

ment, tapping into information about environmental influences on the individual's functional independence and performance that the FIM^{SM} instrument does not address.

The URS^{SM} measure enables one to examine subjects' perceptions of the relative ease or difficulty of performing certain activities-of-daily-living associated with the FIM^{SM} instrument in different physical environmental contexts. Thus how perceptions of ease or difficulty can be influenced by both individuals' functional capabilities and previous experiences and expectations can be demonstrated. The URS^{SM} measure also enjoys the advantages of most such survey instruments; that is, low cost of administration compared with that of the FIM^{SM} instrument. In addition, when used to assess

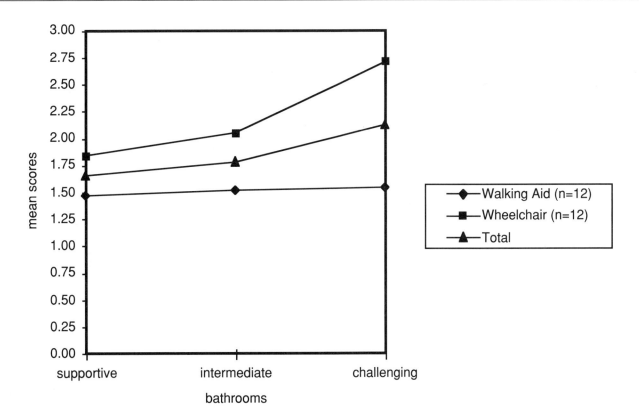

Figure 6–13 Functional Performance Measure (FPM^{SM}) level of effort mean scores in supportive, intermediate, and challenging bathrooms. *Y* axis effort score: 0 = no effort, 1 = minimum effort, 2 = moderate effort, and 3 = maximum effort.

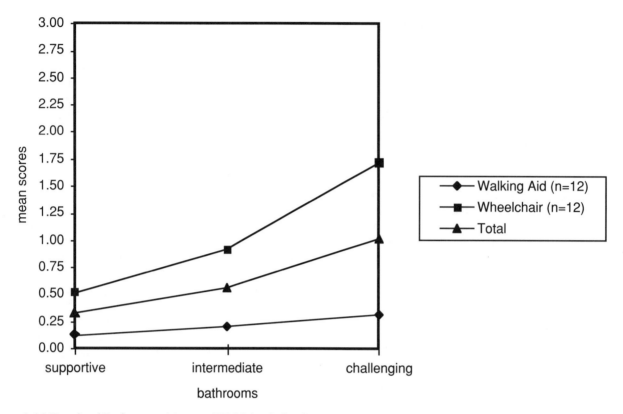

Figure 6–14 Functional Performance Measure (FPM℠) level of assistance mean scores in supportive, intermediate, and challenging bathrooms.

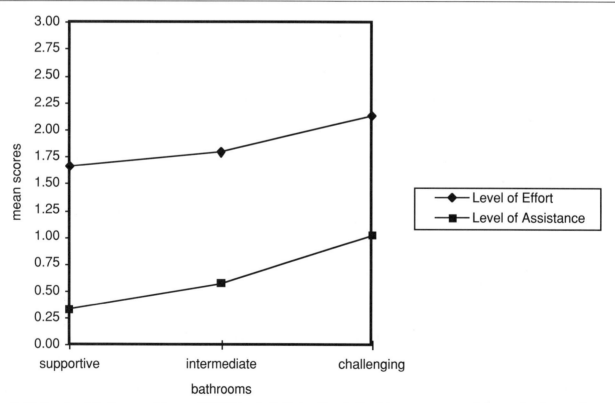

Figure 6–15 Functional Performance Measure (FPM℠) level of effort and level of assistance mean scores in supportive, intermediate, and challenging bathrooms.

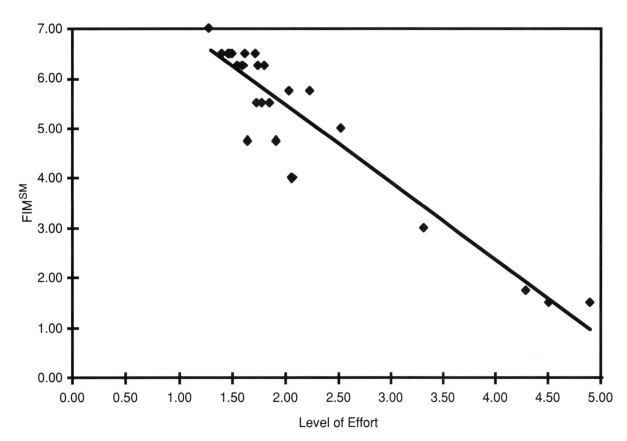

Figure 6–16 Functional Performance Measure (FPM^SM) level of effort mean scores versus Functional Independence Measure (FIM^SM) mean scores.

perceptions of individual subjects, the URS^SM enables measurement of individual differences that may be significant correlates of subsequent functional independence and performance.

The Enviro-FIM^SM instrument provides a means for evaluating design artifacts in terms of their overall impact on functional independence of an individual or a group (e.g., assessing effects of alternative door configurations on functional independence of wheelchair users). The Enviro-FIM^SM instrument also enables a global assessment of fit between subjects and designed physical environments. This outcome measure provides a means for determining whether a mismatch exists between an environment's demand character and a subject's mastery level.

The FPM^SM provides direct measurement of caregiver burden through its level of assistance scale and, thereby, a means of assessing how that burden is affected by changes in specific environments' demand character. The FPM^SM also permits the identification of specific design characteristics in physical environments responsible for problematic activity performance by either individuals or groups. Consequently, the FPM^SM can be used to identify needed design changes in specific task environments that will improve subsequent task

(and therefore activity) performance. That is, it will enable the fine tuning of designed environments to facilitate specific outcome changes in functional independence and performance of either individuals or groups.

A quick demonstration of how these measures are used to these ends can be helpful. Table 6–3 shows average URS^SM and Enviro-FIM^SM scores for door use in each of the three bathrooms. Door configuration characteristics encountered while entering and exiting the supportive bathroom (i.e., doors D1S2 and D4S1, respectively) are clearly perceived as being easy to use by the 24 subjects. The mean Enviro-FIM^SM scores also substantiate this. In contrast, the door configuration characteristics encountered while entering and exiting the challenging bathroom (i.e., doors D9CI1 and D12CI2, respectively) are just as clearly perceived as being more difficult to use by these same 24 subjects (actually moving into the negative half of the bipolar URS^SM). Again, Enviro-FIM^SM scores substantiate this finding with overall mean scores for functional independence during door use that are barely above the level (even with the walking aid users' much higher scores included) where help would typically be required. Clearly, the wheelchair users are being handicapped by the demand character present in these door configurations.

Table 6–3 Utility of Usability Rating Scale (URSˢᴹ) and Environmental Functional Independence Measure (Enviro-FIMˢᴹ) for Identifying Problems

Door	Approach & Swing	Demand	Enviro-FIMˢᴹ	URSˢᴹ
D1S2	Enter & Out	supportive	7.83	2.38
D4S1	Exit & Out	supportive	8.08	2.83
D5I1	Enter & In	intermediate	7.04	0.88
D8I2	Exit & In	intermediate	7.67	1.19
D9CI1	Enter & In	challenging	6.04	−0.40
D12CI2	Exit & In	challenging	6.04	−0.04

Enviro-FIMˢᴹ: 1 to 10, 10 = complete independence; URSˢᴹ: −3 to +3, +3 = very easy.

The FPMˢᴹ average level of effort and level of assistance scores on just the first of those two door configurations for the challenging bathroom (i.e., door D9CI1: entering the difficult bathroom) for wheelchair users versus walking aid users are shown in Table 6–4. Examination quickly reveals the specific door use activity tasks that cause the problems indicated by the URSˢᴹ and Enviro-FIMˢᴹ scores. Maneuvering to close the door and then actually closing the door after entering the room are tasks that the wheelchair users (but not the walking aid users) found virtually impossible to perform. (Recall that a level of effort score of 3 means maximum effort was required, and a level of effort score of 4 means that task performance was impossible even with maximum effort.)

By next examining the design characteristics of the challenging bathroom (return to Figure 6–2) relevant to entering this bathroom through the door, it becomes readily apparent that two specific design characteristics have combined to handicap the wheelchair users. The open floor space inside the bathroom is only 15 square feet, and when opened the door's interior projection of 32 inches sweeps into the bathroom and across large portions of that 15 square feet. This combination leaves insufficient space for the wheelchair to maneuver to get out of the way, so that the door can be closed once the person is inside the room.

CONCLUSIONS

It has been argued that consideration of environment in functional assessment has three implications for the methods of measurement used. First, contemporary transactional models of person–behavior–environment relations view environment as a means toward achieving a fit between an individual and a level of environmental demand or challenge. Environment, then, is a mediating variable in the relationship between individual abilities and outcomes. Therefore, assessment measures must take its influence into account. Second, the experience of a particular environment may be evaluated differently by the individual versus an objective observer. Thus, measurement of fit must include some way to assess perceptions as well as outwardly observable behavior. Third, the appropriate fit between environment and person is socially constructed (e.g., independent living, assisted

Table 6–4 Utility of Functional Performance Measure (FPMˢᴹ) Level of Effort and Level of Assistance Scores for Identifying Causes of Problems

Door No. D9DI1 Task	Level of Effort			Level of Assistance		
	Wheelchair	Walking Aid	Total	Wheelchair	Walking Aid	Total
Approach	1.33	1.25	1.29	0.00	0.00	0.00
Opening Maneuver	1.00	1.42	1.21	0.00	0.00	0.00
Latch Use	1.58	1.25	1.42	0.25	0.00	0.13
Opening	2.42	1.83	2.13	0.00	0.00	0.00
Through Passage	2.17	1.83	2.00	0.00	0.00	0.00
Closing Maneuver	3.67	1.86	2.77	2.25	0.00	1.13
Closing	4.25	1.86	3.06	2.58	0.29	1.44

Level of effort: 0 to 6, 0 = no effort required; Level of assistance: 0 to 6, 0 = no assistance required.

living, accessible). Thus social perceptions play a major role in evaluating environments.

The physical environment cannot be ignored in the measurement of functional ability because it is an integral part of all behavior. Measures that ignore its influence will not provide a complete assessment of an individual's performance. The experiment described earlier demonstrated that the widely used FIM℠ instrument gives different results in different environments. Thus the influence of environment can bias assessments even when the measures are not designed to address the mediating role of environment. It is important to recognize this influence and measure function within the relevant environment. For example, the most accurate assessment of whether a person can function independently should be made within the environment in which he or she is expected to live. On the other hand, if an individual is not functioning independently in one environment, it is possible that he or she may be able to function independently in another of a different design. The Enviro-FIM℠ instrument was developed to incorporate the environment as a variable in functional assessment. It provides data consistent with those obtained with the FIM℠ instrument, but it is more sensitive to environmental influences.

The individual's perception of demand may differ from an objective assessment. It is particularly important to consider the individual's frame of reference. A difficult environment for one person may be perceived as easy for another, even though each observed performance is identical. There are many possible reasons for this, including differences in self-concept, perceived social norms, expectations, motivation, or experience. Regardless of the reason, it is not sufficient to make objective measurements of fit. It is also necessary to obtain subjective responses. Even though it may seem that a person can function independently in a particular setting, the quality of that experience should be a concern in rehabilitation. As studies of technology abandonment have shown, individuals' evaluation of appropriateness is often divergent from that of the rehabilitation professional. In this summary of our research program, we have demonstrated that it is possible to develop a reliable and sensitive subjective measure (the URS℠) that can be used very easily in practice.

Although measures such as the FIM℠ and Enviro-FIM℠ instruments are very useful for obtaining a global measure of function, they are not sufficiently detailed to identify the needed interventions for improving environments. The FPM℠ is a different type of measure that allows very fine-grained analysis of person–environment fit. However, the FPM℠ requires the use of a videotaped record for accuracy. It is useful for research on design and in clinical practice for evaluating alternatives for home and workplace modifications. It is also useful for measuring caregiver burden and identifying environmental design interventions that could relieve it.

The inclusion of environment as a variable in functional assessment introduces three unique reliability problems.

Reliable assessments require multiple trials, but most environments are tiring and can be dangerous to use. Thus when developing measures, it is critical to design experiments that do not create artifacts due to fatigue. The second problem is that new environments are novel and unfamiliar, especially innovative designs. Most people carry out activities of daily living within the same environments everyday. The novelty of new settings such as those used in our experiments can introduce learning effects because users have to adapt habitual routines. Thus it is important to control for those effects in some way. Third, the influence of any particular environment sometimes is and sometimes is not the sum of all its parts. On the one hand, each individual does not use each setting in exactly the same way. For example, one person may use a grab bar to transfer and another may not. So the impact of having a grab bar will be different for each of these two individuals. On the other hand, for some the impact of each feature in a setting may be weak but incremental. It is the total picture that matters for such a person.

In our work, we used a number of methods to control for these problems. Most important, we used counterbalanced trials to counter fatigue and learning effects. In addition, we carefully designed and selected the experimental settings to reflect changes in every identified feature. From the data we have collected with the FPM℠, we can now examine which of those features are the critical ones and develop simplified procedures and settings. These same threats to reliability occur in clinical practice. When studying the fit between environment and person, clinicians need to develop methods for administering assessments that will not be biased by these very same issues. For example, one trial of using a bathroom in a new apartment is not sufficient for assessing its appropriateness.

There is a need for much more research on issues of functional assessment with the environment in mind. One important area of research is to study the predictive ability of assessment methods. It should be possible to develop methods that will predict performance in a particular setting by measuring selected functional abilities and the demand character of the setting itself. It is believed that multimethod intervention studies would be the best approach for establishing predictive validity since other variables that affect rehabilitation outcome as well need to be studied in relationship to environment (e.g., family assistance available).

Codes and standards have hitherto been used as measures of appropriate fit. However, they have never been subjected to validation by using a transactional model. This new paradigm suggests that, although codes and standards may be useful for determining minimum legal guidelines on the basis of a consensus process, interventions for individuals and the achievement of universal design may be more successful if they are based on performance models that reflect differences in needs and preferences. Such models can help define *reasonable accommodations* in a manner that is based on functional ability rather than arbitrary standards.

Another area for future research is comparison of consumer and professional assessments of fit. Results of such studies would help identify the issues that are most significant to consumers. They may demonstrate that consumer-oriented evaluations are more effective and less expensive than professional-oriented ones.

It has been argued that the environment can play a significant role in functional ability. Therefore, it is important to develop and use methods that can measure its contribution. Clearly there are many complex issues that need to be addressed in methods and practice to ensure that measurement of person–behavior–environment relations will be meaningful and useful. Although the field of rehabilitation has always recognized the importance of environment as a prosthetic supportive context for human activities, the relationship is actually more complex and significant. More attention to this topic will no doubt uncover the complexity of the relationship and identify ways to understand it better.

REFERENCES

Altman, I., & Rogoff, B. (1987). World views in psychology: Trait, interactional, organismic and transactional perspectives. In D. Stokols & I. Altman (Eds.), *Handbook of environmental psychology* (Vol. 1, pp. 7–40). New York: Wiley.

Americans With Disabilities Act Accessibility Guidelines. (1991, July 26) *Federal Register.*

Bandura, A. (1978). The self system in reciprocal determinism. *American Psychologist, 33*(4), 344–358.

Cronberg, T. (1975). Performance requirements for building—A study based on user activities. Sweden: Swedish Council for Building Research.

Danford, S. (1983). Dynamic reciprocal determinism: A synthetic transactional model of person–behavior–environment relations. In D. Amedeo, J. Griffin, & J. Potter (Eds.), *EDRA 19: Proceedings of the Fourteenth International Conference of the Environmental Design Research Association* (pp. 19–28). Lincoln, NE: Environmental Design Research Association.

Danford, S. (1985). The reciprocal roles of settings and behavior. In R. Johnson, D. Bershader, & L. Leifer (Eds.), *Autonomy and the human element in space* (pp. 60–70). Washington, DC: National Aeronautics and Space Administration.

Fisher, J., Bell, P., & Baum, A. (1984). *Environmental psychology.* New York: Holt, Rinehart & Winston.

Granger, C., Hamilton, B., Keith, R., Zielezny, M., & Sherwin, F. (1986). Advances in functional assessment for medical rehabilitation. *Topics in Geriatric Rehabilitation, 1*(3), 59–74.

Lewin, K. (1951). *Field theory in social science.* New York: Harper & Row.

Matthews, S.H. (1979). *The social world of older women.* Beverly Hills, CA: Sage, p. 99.

Mead, G. (1934). *Mind, self and society.* Chicago: University of Chicago.

Moore, G. (1976). Theory and research on the development of environmental knowing. In G. Moore & R. Golledge (Eds.), *Environmental knowing: Theories, research, and methods* (pp. 138–164). Stroudsburg, PA: Dowden, Hutchinson & Ross.

Moos, R. (1975). Synthesizing major perspectives on environmental impact: A social ecological approach. In B. Honikman (Ed.), *Responding to social change* (pp. 211–222). Stroudsburg, PA: Dowden, Hutchinson & Ross.

Nahemow, L., & Lawton, M. (1973). Toward an ecological theory of adaptation and aging. In W. Preiser (Ed.), *Environmental design research* (Vol. 1, pp. 24–32). Stroudsburg, PA: Dowden, Hutchinson & Ross.

Pitrella, F., & Kappler, W. (1988). *Identification and evaluation of scale design principles in the development of the extended range sequential judgment scale.* Wachtberg, Germany: Research Institute for Human Engineering.

Rubin, A., & Elder, J. (1980). *Building for people: Behavioral research approaches and directions.* Washington DC: National Bureau of Standards.

Stokols, D. (1981). Group x place transactions: Some neglected issues in psychological research on setting. In D. Magnusson (Ed.), *Toward a psychology of situations: An interactional perspective* (pp. 393–415). Hillsdale, NJ: Erlbaum.

Stokols, D. (1987). Conceptual strategies of environmental psychology. In D. Stokols & I. Altman (Eds.), *Handbook of environmental psychology* (Vol. 1, pp. 41–70). New York: Wiley.

Wandersman, A., Murday, D., & Wadsworth, J. (1979). The environment–behavior–personal relationship–implications for research. In A. Seidel & S. Danford (Eds.), *Environmental design: Research, theory and application* (pp. 162–174). Washington, DC: Environmental Design Research Association.

Wicker, A. (1974). Processes which mediate behavior–environment congruence. In R. Moos & P. Insel (Eds.), *Issues in social ecology: Human milieus* (pp. 598–615). Palo Alto, CA: National Press Books.

CHAPTER 7

A Functional Approach to Psychological and Psychosocial Factors and Their Assessment in Rehabilitation

Marcia J. Scherer and Laura A. Cushman

BEHAVIORAL OBJECTIVES

After completing this chapter, the reader will be able to
- discuss the psychological ramifications of physical disability.
- describe different ways in which individuals with disabilities cope with and adjust to changes in their lifestyle.

- explain the importance of personality and social support in adaptation to physical disability.
- list measures of social support.
- recognize symptoms of psychological disorders experienced by persons with disability.
- locate psychological tests and measures.

Individuals with disabilities vary as much in *how* they adjust to and cope with physical injury and permanent disability as in the extent to which they *do* adjust and cope. To help a person move from withdrawal and hopelessness to adjustment and coping requires attention to physical, social, developmental, and psychological/personal factors. An illustration of the importance of these factors is provided by Ken, one of the individuals who shares personal experiences with and perspectives of the psychological aspects of rehabilitation in the book *Living in the State of Stuck: How Technology Impacts the Lives of People with Disabilities* (Scherer, 1996a).

PSYCHOLOGICAL RAMIFICATIONS OF DISABILITY

At the age of 31, Ken is working as a counselor for an independent living center. He has a C5-6 level spinal cord injury from a fall at the age of 17. His facial features and expression are gentle, and he has a soft-spoken, calm, and kind demeanor. His responses are thoughtful, insightful, and sincere. He comes across as someone who could take charge and get the job done, but in a quiet, low-key manner. Everything about Ken says he is truly caring and sincere, but there

is also a sadness, a resignation, in his tone that says he evolved to this point after considerable trials.

Ken is very active in his community in advocating civil rights for persons with disabilities and is just one of thousands of individuals with disabilities who have adopted an independent living (IL) philosophy. The *independent living movement* was started by a group of consumers who were determined to exercise choice and maximize opportunity and individual autonomy. Independent living centers throughout the United States continue this philosophy and help consumers achieve self-determination, self-advocacy, and assertiveness in their goals to obtain housing, employment, and health and community services.

Fifteen years after his injury, Ken shared his perspective on the emotional aspects of rehabilitation.[1]

> What's needed is a good middle ground between the attitude expressed in the book, *Options*, where you feel like a failure because you know you'll

---

[1]The book that Ken mentions, *Options* (Corbet, 1989), is one that was circulated on his spinal cord unit back in 1974. It contains case examples of people's lives after their injuries and is meant to be inspiring.

never match up to the guys in that book—who all have a $200,000-a-year job, a wife and kids, a big house and brand new sports car—and the need to have some hope held out to you, which *Options* does to an extreme and which can destroy a lot of people attitudinally. It's one thing to give a ray of hope, everybody needs that; but it's quite another to indicate they can get up and walk again someday.

Initially in rehabilitation you need a ray of hope. It gives you something to work toward. But professionals should be more realistic by telling people that, "This is possible, but not likely for everyone." They should build confidence without building hopes so high that people expect they can be completely normal. As rehab moves along, they should emphasize more and more each person's own capabilities and what is realistic for that person. They also need to get people to see that their disabilities do not need to stand in the way of their achievement. You're going to have failures, but you're also going to have successes. Without trying, you're not going to have either.

I wasn't assertive before my injury and that helped because the more aggressive guys [with a lot of hostility and intolerance] have a tougher time with their injuries.

Some people just need more time than others. There were people up on the floor that hated going to therapy. There was no motivation there whatsoever. So, for them, maybe therapy wasn't the answer at that point. They were the ones that got left by the wayside. The people that would come into their sessions and do what was expected, the staff seemed to concentrate more on them.

Some rehab professionals try to make silk purses out of sow's ears, and that isn't being realistic either. Rehab needs to have the attitude of, "Okay, this is what you have, and this is what you can work with. What can you do to make the best out of what you can work with?" They need to focus mainly on those people that are going day-to-day through life, just like the average able-bodied person goes day-to-day through life.

Ken's perspective was formed after a slow recovery from depression and prolonged rehabilitation, which he likened to Elisabeth Kubler-Ross's (1969) stages of dying:

If someone is stuck in the grieving process . . . six to seven years is the average for real adjustment. It's like an adjustment to a death. The only thing is, for an injury or disability, it's not as easy to adjust as with a death because with a death, the person's no longer there. With a disability, you have a constant reminder. So, sometimes it takes even longer to grieve and adjust. A lot of people turn to alcohol and drugs, which is a way of going through denial. As long as you're smashed or stoned, you can forget about your disability. It alters the mind and you can forget about it. Well, you don't forget about it—you just don't quite care as much.

I asked Ken for his opinion about how common it is for people with spinal cord injuries to use drugs and alcohol to avoid confronting the facts of their disabilities. He continued: "Everybody goes through that stage, I think, of using a lot of alcohol or drugs. It's just a coping mechanism. Some break out of it and some don't. I know people who've stayed smashed their whole lives." Ken summarized his perspective on adjustment for the person with a spinal cord injury as follows: "A lot of it is just time. Rehab can't turn your life around in just a couple of months."

Many people with disabilities need time to develop an awareness of their disabilities and a perspective of themselves, which allows them to admit grief and anger and then get on with their lives. Some need months; others need years. For Ken, it took a major life event to turn himself around:

It was a slow process getting fed up with doing nothing. It was like a long, low-grade depression I didn't even know I had until I came out of it. It was just, I was unmotivated. I knew it even while I was doing it. But even when I was in the stage of depression or whatever, in the rut stage, I saw both the positive and negative sides. I never had a real negative attitude. I was in the stoned part, but I wasn't negative. I always tried to keep an optimistic attitude. I think that's what helped me to get out of the depression and progress through the stages.

One of the things that did it, also, was not something I was glad happened and that was my mother's death. My mother, and all my family, were very overprotective—but especially my mother. After she was gone, there was not so much of a dominant figure, so then I had to kind of learn to find my own way. My father . . . he was a very passive person, a farmer most of his life. He died two years ago and he kind of took things as they came and just went through life. Good or bad, I modeled him in a lot of ways. . . . Even though I went through the depression and stuff, there's not a lot of ways to change things. You change things when you can, but you don't go out and constantly knock your head against a wall to try to beat down the system and this type of thing. You make little changes where you can in a . . . quieter way. And it does work. Once you can achieve smaller goals, you can work up.

Through my years I've seen both sides of it. I mean, I've been in rehab so many times they don't want to see me again! But I've seen everything from really high achievers to suicides, you know, people that are planning suicide. Or a couple of people that I know of that are drinking themselves to death. It's just that different people look at it in somewhat different ways.

Ken represents the views of a professional social worker as well as a consumer who has had to come to terms with a severe physical disability. Even though he went through a period of depression and substance abuse, he became what can be termed a *rehabilitation success*. His reflection on *motivation for rehabilitation* was based on his own experience and his knowledge of the experiences of other persons with disabilities. Much attention in the medical and social science literature has been given to theoretical and empirical speculations on the nature of the factors that differentiate people with disabilities who are "successfully rehabilitated" from those who are not. In an attempt to understand the important factors in consumer achievement of rehabilitation goals, Roessler (1980) looked at characteristics of the goal itself (explicit, proximate, not too difficult), client expectations and personal barriers, environmental and social barriers, support from others, and whether the experience of success or failure accompanied the process of goal achievement. He concluded that a diagnostic analysis of these factors would offer providers insights into potential rehabilitation problems and a means to identify influences on consumers' achievement motivation.

Attribution theory has been a commonly accepted framework for research on rehabilitation success and motivation to achieve success (e.g., Maker, 1979; Nielson, MacDonald, & Cameron, 1984; Plotkin-Israel, 1985). It considers the following characteristics within and external to the person as influencing success: one's ability and effort (within) and task difficulty and luck (external).

NEED SATISFACTION IS WHAT MOTIVATES PEOPLE

Psychological theories of motivation and identity relevant to rehabilitation include Abraham Maslow's hierarchy of needs and Erik Erikson's psychosocial development.

Maslow (1954) developed a hierarchy of five basic levels of needs in the order in which individuals attempt to satisfy them:

1. Physical
   a. Survival
   b. Security
2. Social/affiliation
   a. Belonging
   b. Esteem
3. Intellectual/achievement
   a. Knowledge
   b. Understanding
4. Aesthetic
5. Self-actualization

He maintained that (1) needs must be met at each successive level, beginning with the lowest or physical needs, before one can move on to the next, and (2) frustrated needs result in hostility or anxiety (or both). A young adult who receives a traumatic injury (e.g., spinal cord injury) may have been at the higher level of *achievement* only to have to refocus again on the satisfaction of *physical* needs. Often such adults find themselves having to go through each successive stage again, meeting the needs for *affiliation* with new friends and needs for *achievement* in an entirely new career area than originally planned.

Erikson (1963) developed a life span theory of psychosocial development of the normal/healthy personality. He viewed development as a person's search for identity and conceived of eight stages of conflicts persons need to resolve to develop psychologically. The nature of the resolution achieved influences how the succeeding developmental conflicts are addressed. Erikson's stages of psychosocial development, with a focus on the positive outcomes of each conflict or crisis, are as follows:

1. Infancy: Trust vs. Mistrust
   Satisfaction of basic needs leads to trust in self and others and to hope, optimism
2. Toddler: Autonomy vs. Shame and Doubt
   Expression of self-control leads to autonomy
3. Early childhood: Initiative vs. Guilt
   Basis of purpose, ambition
4. School age: Industry vs. Inferiority
   Success at activities leads to a sense of accomplishment and adequacy
5. Adolescence: Identity vs. Confusion
   An understanding of the self, self-confidence, ability to make choices and to express them
6. Young adulthood: Intimacy vs. Isolation
   To give and receive love
7. Adulthood: Generativity vs. Stagnation
   Desire to nurture, produce, create
8. Old age: Integrity vs. Despair
   Viewing one's life as complete and fulfilled

Erikson's and Maslow's theories lead to possibilities for understanding the roots of depression, anxiety, anger, substance abuse, loneliness, social isolation, and other phenomena described by Ken and often encountered when working with persons who have a new disability. An individual's profile, formulated from Maslow's five needs and Erikson's eight stages of development, will lead to a characterization of that person as someone who is coping or not coping with a disability, as well as that person's personality/identity as being more or less adequate.

WAYS OF COPING DIFFER

Some individuals with disabilities cope with their challenges earlier and better than others. They adjust in various ways over time, evidence developmental growth, and—consistent with the study results of Krause (1992) and Krause and Dawis (1992)—show that psychological factors are important in the understanding of both short- and long-term adjustment.

Although some individuals with disabilities share an unwillingness to be held back from pursuing their independence and goals, others (as Ken discussed) seem to lack motivation for increasing their independence. Many individuals emphasize goals they have and their desire to work around obstacles; others view obstacles as being insurmountable. Some appear to meet challenge head-on; others feel defeated. Some pursue a productive and satisfying life; others withdraw into depression, social isolation, and perhaps substance abuse. Still others deny the realities of their limitations or harbor unrealistic hopes for a cure for their disabilities, focusing on a lifestyle incompatible with their current capabilities.

Coping and Non-Coping

In Beatrice Wright's classic text, *Physical Disability: A Psychological Approach* (1960), considerable attention is devoted to coping and non-coping, which are defined as follows:

> Coping—[Seeing] the difficulties associated with a disability as something that [can] be faced in some way or overcome . . . [focusing] on the adjustable aspects . . . coping with the difficulties rather than managing because of blissful ignorance or pretense. (p. 59)

> Succumbing (non-coping)—[Seeing] difficulties as a quagmire through which there [is] no path. Perhaps one doesn't even seek a path, for one is so consumed with the suffering of the disabled state that one is dragged down by despair. (p. 59)

People who cope emphasize what they can do and seek to satisfy their needs for achievement as well as affiliation; persons who succumb focus on what they cannot do. People who cope pursue opportunities; people who succumb are more passive, downplay their competence, and distrust the opportunities presented to them. Coping behaviors are used to overcome limitations—through further education, development of new skills, and participation in rehabilitation programs. Succumbing is characterized by a resignation to and a concentration on limitations.

Research on coping has frequently used ego defense styles as being indicative of the ways in which individuals typically cope with change and challenge. According to Gladstone (1976), "ego defenses are viewed as those defense mechanisms which reflect the individuals' characteristic way of coping with varied internal as well as external stress" (p. 16). She states further that

> coping behaviors are the outcome of a flexible use of appropriate defenses based on a realistic assessment of the nature of [a] threat. Defensive behaviors are described as rigid and compulsive with a less realistic assessment of reality. Thus, ego defenses employed as countermoves to reduce threat are those typically and automatically resorted to under stress, regardless of the nature of the threat. (p. 22)

In 1969, the National Institute of Mental Health sponsored a conference on coping and adaptation, the proceedings of which list many elements belonging to the construct of coping (Coelho, Hamburg, & Adams, 1974). Among those elements are hope, motivation, social support, information-seeking, and appraisal. One of the contributors to this effort was Richard Lazarus. Lazarus, Averill, and Opton (1974) and Lazarus and Folkman (1984) have studied the cognitive appraisal of threat as a transaction between the individual and the environment and as determining individuals' coping behaviors. They believe that "physiological changes may be used to indicate the success or failure of other coping modes, especially the ego defenses" (Lazarus, Averill, & Opton, 1974, p. 277). Lazarus and colleagues note that in the case of severe injury, the individual may be relatively helpless to cope with the harm (through active defense mechanisms), and direct action on the environment has very little value. However, the possibility of direct action on the self may remain, as when the inevitable harm can somehow be mitigated by learning new skills to counteract a disability. When avenues leading to direct action on the self and the environment are closed (or perceived as closed), the individual relies on intrapsychic coping processes (passive defense mechanisms such as denial and rationalization) (Lazarus et al., 1974).

Lazarus and Folkman (1984) define *coping* as "constantly changing cognitive and behavioral efforts to manage specific external and/or internal demands that are appraised as taxing or exceeding the resources of the person" (p. 141). It varies according to both internal and external resources and constraints at the time. Appraisal is a key component. For example, a person in a relationship with an environment may appraise the events within that setting as threatening; coping processes are then applied. Lazarus and Folkman's coping paradigm takes into account individual values and goals and emotions, and these investigators consider demands originating in both the individual and the environment or setting. A cognitive appraisal of threat arises from a transaction between the individual and the environment, and both the history of such transactions and the appraisal determine the individual's coping behaviors.

Lazarus and colleagues believe coping is a *process*. It should not be confused with *outcome*. There are always coping efforts regardless of the outcome, and even negative coping efforts can have (temporary) beneficial effects when looked at retrospectively. (This was Ken's experience from his perspective.) Denial and self-deception are two examples. Initial denial of the seriousness of one's injury can help ward off a flood of overwhelming emotion; deceiving oneself about the strengths of one's talents or abilities can keep hopes and dreams alive. Continued denial of the seriousness of one's disability, however, can lead to inappropriate behaviors and even actions that can prove detrimental to one's recovery and rehabilitation. Prolonged self-deception can prevent a person from taking action that is more suitable, potentially rewarding, and more likely to result in success.

Recent research on coping by Lazarus and associates includes social support, or the quality and quantity of interactions and communication with others (e.g., O'Brien & DeLongis, 1991). While the work of Lazarus and colleagues has greatly influenced coping research, Michigan State University's Coping Study Group and Rudolf Moos at Stanford University have also made important contributions to developing knowledge of coping processes (Moos, 1974).

Coping Is an Unstable Construct and Influenced by Social Support

Coping involves achieving or maintaining control and an identity. When a person has a new disability, a major disequilibrium occurs on both group (as for a family) and individual levels. Some individuals with recently acquired disabilities who experience a major change in lifestyle may not have had earlier experiences and exposures essential to the development of decision making, responsibility, self-control, and so on. Although crises are difficult to handle, they can be especially so for persons with disabilities who did not

psychologically develop in ways compatible with the management of loss, anxiety, and need frustration.

Coping can vary between the extremes of phenomenal success and marginal coping. Non-coping, too, varies from complete withdrawal, helplessness, and hopelessness to maintenance of marginal functioning that develops over time. As individuals develop and mature, they formulate new strategies for goal achievement. When these strategies work and individuals are successful, it seems they are coping. Should their strategies fail them for a time, individuals may then exhibit non-coping behaviors. Coping and non-coping people display significant differences that vary according to the setting in which they find themselves and the kind and amount of personal, professional, social, and financial resources available to them. Thus the psychological response of coping or non-coping is directly linked to the kind and amount of social support individuals receive.

Self-concept, motivation, and personal aspirations of an individual may be shaped by social interactions that control the availability of positive personal regard, resources, and opportunities. Social support systems have a profound influence on how people with disabilities interpret their experiences and evaluate their options and alternatives. They even affect what options and alternatives are presented initially (Scherer, 1996a).

Dew, Lynch, Ernst, Rosenthal, and Judd (1983) discussed a linear chaining of adjustment to a spinal cord injury as follows: One's personality traits influence the recovery and rehabilitation process, length of hospitalization, and number of rehospitalizations. These factors in turn affect adjustment. Dew et al. (1983) studied 111 veterans with severe spinal cord injuries and found that they exhibited a high rate of rehospitalization. Some had spent as much as 77% of their postinjury lives in the hospital. For many, these recurrent interruptions were accompanied by significant changes in their social support system. Many had experienced divorce since their injuries, as well as various other strains on family relationships and social resources. All affected social resources had to be readjusted, and such alterations can lead to psychological distress. This psychological distress can trigger physical distress and medical complications, which in turn can lead to rehospitalization. The outcome of this chain of events would be further disorganization, disintegration, and deterioration of the social support system. Those who do make some adaptations to their injuries may do so because of replacements within their social support system (e.g., being more receptive to therapists, ministers, or teachers). Preexisting personality characteristics may contribute to circumstances surrounding onset of injury, length of hospitalization, and number of rehospitalizations and in turn lead to lack of adjustment.

Thoits (1982, 1995), however, notes that several serious problems underlie the concept of social support and the methods used to assess it. She observed that there are few researchers who have attempted to "develop valid and reliable indicators of the concept" (p. 146) and that the "neglect of multi-dimensionality seems to be especially problematic for work in this area" (p. 147). For example, she notes that not all social ties are supportive, and when effective support is given, it is important to know under what conditions it was actually given (i.e., what was said or done to attract that positive support). She also advocated looking at potential resources from a wider social milieu (e.g., outside the family constellation). Such resources could include medical and health care providers, teachers, and ministers who would not be involved in a reciprocal or symmetric supportive relationship but who would be social support resources.

There is current interest in the interactions between positive and negative social interactions (e.g., Lepore, 1992). Social support theorists have studied negative social interactions and their influence on emotional functioning, as well as differences between *received* and *perceived* support (e.g., Lakey, Tardiff, & Drew, 1994; Sarason, Sarason, & Pierce, 1990).

The interactive relationship of one's (1) personality characteristics and temperament, (2) social network and perceived and received support (or the lack thereof) from that network, and (3) physical functioning is crucial to the understanding of variable coping, adjustment to disability, and motivation for rehabilitation. The assessment of physical functioning is the subject of other chapters in this book. Here, the assessment of personality/temperament and social support are discussed.

ASSESSMENT OF PERSONALITY AND SOCIAL SUPPORT

Investigating the influence of temperament on perceptions of disability, Mayer and Andrews (1981) interviewed 10 people with spinal cord injuries and found great variation in their responses to their injuries:

> The positive change group perceived their disabilities as a challenge or facilitator of personal growth giving them an opportunity to re-examine their lives and to enhance their spirituality. The no change group also perceived their disabilities as a challenge to be circumvented giving them the opportunity to refocus their goals and to move forward with the same high achievement needs that existed prior to their injury. The negative change group perceived their disabilities as a barrier they could not overcome and had not been able to redefine their goals for life satisfaction. The negative change subjects focused on activities that their disabilities prevented them from enjoying. (p. 137)

Differences in coping and adjustment among individuals often are reflective of preexisting personality characteristics. There are many personality tests that can be used to profile a person's personality, but these must be administered and interpreted by a qualified psychologist. Elliott and Umlauf (1995) reviewed many diverse measures of personality and psychopathology. In addition, a list of resources for obtaining a comprehensive review of the wide range of available personality tests as well as measures in other relevant domains of functioning is provided at the end of this chapter. One test will be described in detail in the following paragraphs.

Measures of Personality

In many personality tests it is assumed that there is underlying psychopathology, and the purpose of these tests is to profile such psychopathology and unhealthy personality *traits*. In the case of most individuals with physical disabilities, undesirable behaviors and affect may be exhibited as transient *states* and reactions to their changed physical status. Thus the most appropriate type of personality test is one in which an underlying *normal* personality is assumed. As discussed in Exhibit 7–1, it is important to discern the differences in measures of traits and states and to time the administration of psychological measures appropriately to obtain a fair and accurate indication of the person's personality and temperament.

The Taylor-Johnson Temperament Analysis (Mosher, 1972) is a 180-item inventory that has been widely used in clinical work since the early 1940s. In this measure a normal personality, not psychopathology, is assumed. It profiles the respondent on nine traits (and their opposites) that correlate with positive rehabilitation outcomes:

1. nervous/composed
2. depressive/light-hearted
3. active–social/quiet
4. expressive–responsive/inhibited
5. sympathetic/indifferent
6. subjective/objective
7. dominant/submissive
8. hostile/tolerant
9. self-disciplined/impulsive

The measure also assesses six trait patterns:

1. anxiety
2. withdrawal
3. hostile–dominant
4. dependent–hostile
5. emotionally inhibited/emotionally repressed
6. socially effective

Exhibit 7–1 Temporal Factors in Assessment

The timing of a test relates closely to the instruments selected, anticipated future assessments, and behaviors or constructs being assessed. Most traditional instruments measure a combination of relatively stable behavior (known as traits) and recent (probably temporary) changes in state (status). Because functional assessment is geared toward current behaviors, it is most similar to so-called state measures. However, it may differ in that the changes being measured may be a result of an injury and may not completely reverse. It is often desirable for a functional instrument to assess very subtle changes, by day or week. Nonetheless, the instrument should still be reliable; that is, it should be stable (result in the same score) over very brief intervals and yield essentially the same findings for different raters. These characteristics are known as test-retest and inter-rater reliability, respectively.

Most traditional psychological tests are not designed to be given repeatedly or on a regular basis over time. Some exceptions are lists of adjectives that describe current mood state or lists of symptoms. When specific behaviors are being monitored by observation, however, second and subsequent assessments are part and parcel of the intervention process. Similarly, when small changes in cognitive functioning need to be measured, tests need to be easily repeatable without significant practice effects, as well as designed to have alternative (comparable)

forms. In rehabilitation settings, patients are often given a task many times for both training and evaluation purposes. However, this can produce overestimates of the person's skills as she or he is "trained to the test" but may be unable to do a related task or a similar task in a different setting.

At the outset, consideration should be given to whether regular (repeated) assessment will be done, what constitutes a meaningful interval in which change can be expected to occur, and how various instruments relate to these needs. There is also a need to consider the temporal factor of what kind of assessment is best suited to the phase of rehabilitation and recovery at hand. Psychological assessments have traditionally been done during inpatient acute rehabilitation and as part of vocational planning. It is not difficult to see, however, that certain types of assessments may be useful at virtually all points along the rehabilitation continuum. For example, a mood assessment may be useful in the outpatient setting for a patient who progressed well as an inpatient and then seemed to "stall" as an outpatient. A behavioral assessment of social skills may provide useful input before the patient returns to work or school; an assessment of family functioning or coping skills may be important to community re-entry or vocational plans. Alternatively, a screening assessment of mood or coping before inpatient rehabilitation may help place the patient's behavior in context.

Source: Copyright © Marcia J. Scherer, PhD.

Raw scores on the Taylor-Johnson Temperament Analysis are converted to either percentiles or sten scores by using norm tables provided in the accompanying manual. There are tables for general population norms and adolescents, as well as separate male and female norms within each. Results are plotted on shaded profiles, which are designed so that the trait percentile or sten scores (scores that have been converted to standard scores with values ranging from 1 to 10) can be evaluated according to their placement within four shaded zones. These zones range from excellent to improvement urgent. Placement of the shaded zones varies for each trait. If all scores are in the darker shaded zones, this suggests good personal and social adjustment.

Mosher, in *The Seventh Mental Measurements Yearbook* (1972) reports that the Taylor-Johnson Temperament Analysis possesses adequate internal consistency and stability over two weeks' time. "The factor analysis of the nine traits revealed that each of the scales measures some trait that is distinct from the trait measured by the other scales" (p. 572).

Mosher also notes that it correlates well with tests designed for similar purposes. Correlations and salient factor loadings with the Minnesota Multiphasic Personality Inventory (MMPI) scales and the scales of the Edwards Personality Factor Questionnaire (16PF) are provided in the Taylor-Johnson Temperament Analysis Manual.

In our example, Ken presents himself as fighting his limitations, but he also reported on the Taylor-Johnson Tempera-

ment Analysis that he is often submissive and "too tolerant." His Taylor-Johnson Temperament Analysis profile indicates his drive and fight are competing with a sense of powerlessness. Additionally, his results suggest a confused identity as well as nervousness, depression, and inhibition, all of which suggest that even many years postinjury his identity (ego) was quite fragile.

The Behavioral Observation of Major Personality States

Increasingly, tests and measures are being considered only one facet of assessment as it has become evident that paper-and-pencil tests inadequately measure many of the most important influences on a person's rehabilitation and quality of life. It is helpful in determining the need for psychological testing and perhaps intervention to conduct some behavioral observations and interviewing. The following summaries of major psychological states commonly seen in medical rehabilitation settings focus on observable behaviors indicative of particular patterns of distress.[2]

---

[2]Criteria based on the American Psychiatric Association's Diagnostic and Statistical Manual of Mental Disorders, fourth edition (DSM-IV, 1994).

1. *Some Features of Anxiety Disorders*:
   - Panic attack—shaking, sweating, nausea, dizziness, palpitations or chest pain, fear of dying or losing control
   - Excessive, unreasonable fear in response to, or in anticipation of, a specific object or situation
   - Disruption of normal routines or daily activities
   - Possible extreme fear of social situations
   - Recognition that the fear is extreme
2. *Descriptive Features of Posttraumatic Stress Disorder*:
   - Severe injury or other threat to survival has occurred
   - Fear and helplessness in response to the event, as well as repeated times of reexperiencing the event (unwanted recollections or dreams)
   - Avoidance of reminders of the event
   - General numbing of emotional responses
   - Hyperarousal or startle reflex (or both)
   - Significant disruption of daily life and functioning
   - Duration of disorder for more than one month
3. *Descriptive Features of Acute Stress Disorder:*
   - Development of features of anxiety disorder within one month after exposure to stressor
   - Subjective sense of detachment, "unreality," or being in a daze; possible amnesia (re: the trauma) or feelings of depersonalization
   - Other features similar to posttraumatic stress disorder, arising up to four weeks posttrauma and lasting two days to four weeks
4. *Some Features of Clinical (Major) Depression*:
   - Significant change from prior functioning, lasting two weeks or more; subjective distress
   - Diminished interest or pleasure in virtually all activities
   - Depressed (or irritable) mood most of the time
   - "Vegetative" disturbances: insomnia or excessive sleep; nonpurposeful appetite and weight change (>5%); daily fatigue; periods of excessive activity or slowness almost every day
   - Feelings of low self-worth
   - Very poor concentration; great difficulty making any decision
   - Recurrent thoughts of death or suicidal ideation
5. *Some Features of Adjustment Disorders*—Predominant features similar to anxiety, depression, a mixture of anxiety/depression, or conduct (major violation of social/legal norms) disorders:
   - Clear relationship of disorder and identifiable stressor, within three months
   - Marked, extreme distress relative to stressor
   - Clear disruption of job or social functioning because of disorder

- Most often resolves within six months, but may persist when stressor is chronic (e.g., disabling medical condition)
- Not a product of bereavement

Measures of Social Support

Like Thoits (discussed earlier), Barrera and Ainlay (1983) note that differences in terminology, conceptual disparities, and a lack of precise definition characterize the social support literature. They conducted a content analysis of existing theories and extracted the major and most frequently recurring themes.

Thoits noted that there are few valid and reliable indicators of the multidimensional concept of social support. Barrera (1981) derived a conceptual typology of social support functions and developed inventories of his own based on the typology. Like Thoits, Barrera (1981) advocated looking at potential resources from a wider social milieu to include those who would not be involved in a reciprocal or symmetric supportive relationship but would be social support resources.

Barrera's Inventory of Socially Supportive Behaviors (ISSB) (1981) is a 40-item questionnaire assessing the frequency of social support experienced during the preceding four-week period of a respondent's life. Item responses are on a five-point Likert-type frequency scale, ranging from not at all to about every day. Items cover six content domains:

1. Material Aid: Providing material aid in the form of money and other physical objects
2. Physical Assistance: Sharing of tasks
3. Intimate Interaction: Interacting in a nondirective manner such that feelings and personal concerns are expressed
4. Guidance: Offering advice and guidance
5. Feedback: Providing individuals with information about themselves
6. Social Participation: Engaging in social interactions for fun, relaxation, and diversion from demanding conditions

Items are summed to obtain domain scores and a total score. Thus the ISSB can be used as a global social support instrument, or it can be used to measure particular types of support.

The ISSB is reported to have very high internal consistency (coefficient alpha = .94 and .93). A test–retest reliability coefficient of .88 has been reported (Barrera & Ainlay, 1983). Additional evidence for the reliability and validity of the ISSB is reported by Novack and Gage (1995). The Arizona Social Support Interview Schedule (Barrera, 1981) investigates sources of support in the domains assessed by the ISSB through a structured interview inquiring into support network size and satisfaction with support. Ken (whose experiences are reported in part in this chapter) reported adequate social support in all realms of the ISSB and Arizona Support Interview Schedule at the time of interview (15 years postinjury).

Need To Focus on Outcomes

A better understanding of how and why individuals cope with their injuries and disabilities and achieve personally satisfying lives is critical for improving the cost and general effectiveness of rehabilitation interventions, as well as for enhancing consumer satisfaction and quality of life (Scherer, 1996b). Research is needed to examine different treatment strategies, different ages at disability onset, disability severity, and the psychological and psychosocial predispositions individuals bring to their participation in rehabilitation.

Definition of Outcomes

Outcomes are the result of an intervention. Examples of outcomes are employability, performance of activities of daily living, and consumer satisfaction or subjective quality of life. The last example encompasses the person's sense of well-being, comfort, happiness, and satisfaction with specific areas of functioning, such as work and in social relationships as well as with finances. *Outcomes assessment* has been defined as "what rehabilitation services *ought to* [emphasis added] achieve for the persons receiving them . . . and how those achievements can be identified and measured (Fuhrer, 1987, p. 1).

In its *1995 Standards Manual and Interpretive Guidelines for Behavioral Health*, the Commission on the Accreditation of Rehabilitation Facilities (1995) discusses outcome-based evaluation and the need for organizations to demonstrate that systems have been established to measure outcomes including effectiveness, efficiency, and satisfaction of the persons served.

Measurement of Outcomes

Outcomes measures are used to demonstrate that particular goals established for a consumer have been identified and achieved. One outcome measure is the difference over time in capability and performance (effectiveness). Thus, many functional assessment measures (with a focus on employability, performance of activities of daily living, etc.) are being viewed as a means of demonstrating outcome achievement. Without the use of functional assessment measures, the determination of rehabilitation effectiveness can be affected by incongruence in views held by consumers and therapists regarding disability, rehabilitation success, and so forth. For example, professionals tend to define independence in terms of physical functioning, whereas consumers

more often equate independence with social and psychological freedoms. Outcomes vary among individuals, and one must obtain consumers' perspectives of the most desired outcomes, as well the perspectives of secondary consumers (e.g., family members, caretakers), payers, vendors, and employers. Once the goals of the intervention are specified, a timeline for goal achievement needs to be established.

For many people, the ultimate in outcome achievement is the subjective sense of well-being and comfort the person has when in the community. Quality of life has come to mean global happiness and satisfaction, as well as satisfaction with specific areas of life functioning such as work, social relationships, and finances. A person's view of his or her quality of life is influenced by psychological factors such as mood and outlook, as well as by physical factors such as pain. In addition, the person's perceptions of a broad array of external factors including available social support, money, and transportation, play into the quality of life equation. Further, all these factors are interrelated. Pain influences mood; in turn, mood influences perceived resources and needs.

When outcome achievement is viewed from a quality of life perspective, one means of assessing that quality of life is to have the individual self-report behavioral adaptation at various points during the rehabilitation process. Then he or she can prioritize desired outcomes and rate his or her progress in achieving these outcomes over time. This system is used in the Assistive Technology Device Predisposition Assessment.[3] In this way, outcomes are measured in terms of changes in, for example, the person's satisfaction in being able to get to where he or she wants to go—whether by walking or some other means—rather than just by the functional capability to do so (Scherer, 1996a). Functional capability, however, is an essential means to quality of life achievement.

Quality of life enhancement is the ultimate outcome for medical rehabilitation professionals. These professionals want individuals to be more capable, more independent, able to exercise more choice, and able to take advantage of a wide range of opportunities. As Ken's example has instructed, people have preferences, personalities, and varying life histories and networks of support that need to be taken into account. These factors may change over relatively short spans of time.

---

[3]The Assistive Technology Device Predisposition Assessment was developed from a study in which differences between assistive technology users and nonusers were assessed. The instrument is used to determine individuals' subjective satisfaction with current functioning in many areas, as well as to examine in which areas they want the most improvement. More information on this measure can be found in Chapter 8. (Scherer, 1996a)

RETRIEVAL OF PSYCHOLOGICAL TESTS AND MEASURES

The book, *Psychological Assessment in Medical Rehabilitation* (Cushman & Scherer, 1995), is a comprehensive resource on measures in the following domains:

- measures of coping and reaction to disability
- functional assessment
- bedside screening of neurocognitive function
- behavioral assessment
- assessment of pain and pain behavior
- assessment of family functioning and social support
- assessment of vocational interests and aptitudes
- measurement of personality and psychopathology after acquired physical disability
- assessing awareness of deficits

In addition, the book includes discussions of the role of nonstandard neuropsychological assessment and testing adaptations, as well as the history and context of psychological assessment in rehabilitation psychology.

Resources for locating tests and measures, reviews of tests, and test publishers are as follows:

Mental Measurements Yearbook (MMY)—published by The Buros Institute for Mental Measurements in Lincoln, Nebraska (The Buros Institute for Mental Measurements, 1992). This publication provides descriptions and reviews of tests, including information on reliability, validity, norming data, and scoring and reporting services, as well as whether foreign language versions are available. It also provides publisher and cost information.

Tests in Print—also published by The Buros Institute for Mental Measurements in Lincoln, Nebraska (The Buros Institute for Mental Measurements, 1994). This publication serves as a master index of more than 3,000 tests in print in psychology and education that are available for purchase. No critical reviews nor psychometric information are provided.

Computer Use in Psychology: A Directory of Software—published by the American Psychological Association, Washington, DC (Stoloff & Couch, 1992). More than 8,000 software products are described, including more than 350 listings from computerized tests or scoring/interpretation aids. Hardware requirements, prices, and publisher contact information are provided.

A wide range of informative materials on tests—published by the Science Directorate of the American Psychological Association (750 First Street, NE, Washington, DC 20002-4242; telephone (202) 336–6000) (APA, 1991), including:

- *Finding Information about Psychological Tests: A Guide for Locating and Using Both Published and Unpublished Tests*
- *Standards for Educational and Psychological Testing*

CONCLUSIONS

People's life situations are influenced by their responses to a disability, not the disability itself. As Ken said, "A lot of it is just time." Also important is the ability to look beyond the physical aspects of rehabilitation to the psychological and psychosocial needs of the person. Ken's example illustrates why the person—and not the disability, nor the payer—will always need to come first in rehabilitation.

REFERENCES

American Psychiatric Association. (1994). *Diagnostic and statistical manual of mental disorders* (4th ed.). Washington, DC: Author.

American Psychological Association Science Directorate. (1991). *Finding information on psychological tests and measures*. Washington, DC: Author.

Barrera, M. (1981). Preliminary development of a scale of social support. *American Journal of Community Psychology, 9*, 435–447.

Barrera, M., & Ainlay, S.L. (1983). The structure of social support: A conceptual and empirical analysis. *Journal of Community Psychology, 11*, 133–143.

The Buros Institute for Mental Measurements. (1992). *Mental measurements yearbook (MMY)* (11th ed.). Lincoln, NE: Author.

The Buros Institute for Mental Measurements. (1994). *Tests in print* (4th ed.). Lincoln, NE: Author.

Coelho, G., Hamburg, D., & Adams, J. (Eds.). (1974). *Coping and adaptation*. New York: Basic Books.

Commission on the Accreditation of Rehabilitation Facilities. (1995). *1995 Standards manual and interpretive guidelines for behavioral health*. Tucson, AZ: Author.

Corbet, B. (1989). *Options: Spinal cord injury and the future* (4th ed.). Silver Spring, MD: National Spinal Cord Injury Association.

Cushman, L.A., & Scherer, M.J. (Eds.) (1995). *Psychological assessment in medical rehabilitation*. Washington, DC: APA Books.

Dew, M.A., Lynch, K., Ernst, J., Rosenthal, R., & Judd, C.M. (1983, August). *A causal analysis of factors affecting adjustment to spinal cord injury*. Paper presented at the convention of the American Psychological Association, Anaheim, CA.

Elliott, T.R., & Umlauf, R.L. (1995). Measurement of personality and psychopathology following acquired physical disability. In L.A. Cushman & M.J. Scherer (Eds.), *Psychological assessment in medical rehabilitation*. Washington, DC: APA Books.

Erikson, E. (1963). *Childhood and society* (2nd ed). New York: Norton.

Fuhrer, M.J. (1987). *Rehabilitation outcomes: Analysis and measurement.* Baltimore: Paul H. Brookes.

Gladstone, L.R. (1976). A study of the relationship between ego defense style preference and experimental pain tolerance and attitudes toward physical disability (Doctoral dissertation, New York University, 1976). *Dissertation Abstracts International, 37,* 4679B.

Krause, J.S. (1992). Life satisfaction after spinal cord injury: A descriptive study. *Rehabilitation Psychology, 37*(1), 61–70.

Krause, J.S., & Dawis, R.V. (1992). Prediction of life satisfaction after spinal cord injury: A four-year longitudinal approach. *Rehabilitation Psychology, 37*(1), 49–60.

Kubler-Ross, E. (1969). *On death and dying.* New York: Macmillan.

Lakey, B., Tardiff, T.A., & Drew, J.B. (1994). Negative social interactions: Assessment and relations to social support, cognition, and psychological distress. *Journal of Social and Clinical Psychology, 13,* 42–62.

Lazarus, R.S., Averill, J.R., & Opton, E.M., Jr. (1974). The psychology of coping: Issues of research and assessment. In G.V. Coelho, D.A. Hamburg, & J.E. Adams (Eds.), *Coping and adaptation* (pp. 275–296). New York: Basic Books.

Lazarus, R.S., & Folkman, S. (1984). *Stress, appraisal, and coping.* New York: Springer.

Lepore, S.J. (1992). Social conflict, social support, and psychological distress: Evidence of cross-domain buffering effects. *Journal of Personality and Social Psychology, 63,* 857–867.

Maker, C.J. (1979). Successful handicapped adults: Their perceptions of significant events, causes, and effects (Doctoral dissertation, University of Virginia, 1979). *Dissertation Abstracts International, 40,* 794A.

Maslow, A.H. (1954). *Motivation and personality.* New York: Harper & Row.

Mayer, T., & Andrews, H.B. (1981). Changes in self concept following a spinal cord injury. *Journal of Applied Rehabilitation Counseling, 12,* 135–137.

Moos, R.H. (1974). Psychological techniques in the assessment of adaptive behavior. In G.V. Coelho, D.A. Hamburg, & J.E. Adams (Eds.), *Coping and adaptation* (pp. 334–399). New York: Basic Books.

Mosher, D.L. (1972). Taylor-Johnson Temperament Analysis. In O. Buros (Ed.), *The seventh mental measurements yearbook* (pp. 959–960). Highland Park, NJ: Gryphon.

Nielson, W.R., MacDonald, M.R., & Cameron, M.G.P. (1984, August). *Self-blame and coping following spinal cord injury.* Paper presented at the meeting of the American Psychological Association, Toronto, Canada.

Novack, T.A., & Gage, R.J. (1995). Assessment of family functioning and social support. In L.A. Cushman & M.J. Scherer (Eds.), *Psychological assessment in medical rehabilitation.* Washington, DC: APA Books.

O'Brien, T., & DeLongis, A. (1991). *A three function model of coping: Emotion-focused, problem-focused, and relationship-focused.* Paper presented at the 99th annual convention of the American Psychological Association, San Francisco.

Plotkin-Israel, I. (1985). *Causal attributions, perceived control and coping among MI patients.* Unpublished manuscript, Boston University.

Roessler, R.T. (1980). A quality of life perspective on rehabilitation counseling. *Rehabilitation Counseling Bulletin, 34*(2), 82–90.

Sarason, B.R., Sarason, I.G., & Pierce, G.R. (1990). Traditional views of social support and their impact on assessment. In B.R. Sarason, I.G. Sarason, & G.R. Pierce (Eds.). *Social support: An interactional view* (pp. 9–25). New York: Wiley.

Scherer, M.J. (1995). Comments on DeRuyter's "Evaluating outcomes in assistive technology." *Assistive Technology, 7.1,* 11–12.

Scherer, M.J. (1996a). *Living in the state of stuck: How technology impacts the lives of people with disabilities* (2nd ed.). Cambridge, MA: Brookline Books.

Scherer, M.J. (1996b). Outcomes of assistive technology use on quality of life. *Disability and Rehabilitation, 18* (9), 439–448.

Stoloff, M.L., & Couch, J.V. (Eds.). (1992). *Computer use in psychology: A directory of software* (3rd ed.). Washington, DC: American Psychological Association.

Thoits, P.A. (1982). Conceptual, methodological, and theoretical problems in studying social support as a buffer against life stress. *Journal of Health and Social Behavior, 23,* 145–159.

Thoits, P.A. (1995). Stress, coping, and social support processes: Where are we? What's next? *Journal of Health and Social Behavior,* [Extra Issue], 53–79.

Wright, B.A. (1960). *Physical disability: A psychological approach.* New York: Harper & Row.

CHAPTER 8

A Functional Approach to Technological Factors and Their Assessment in Rehabilitation

Marcia J. Scherer and Lucy T. Vitaliti

BEHAVIORAL OBJECTIVES

After completing this chapter, the reader will be able to
- describe the significance of assistive devices for improving function in persons with physical disabilities.
- explain the importance of matching persons with disabilities with the most appropriate technologies.

- consider consumer attitudes in the selection and use or nonuse of specific technologies.
- discuss the use of functional assessment and general health measures in determining the impact of assistive technologies on disability and quality of life.

People with physical disabilities often require assistance to function more independently. This assistance may come through changes in the environment or from either another person, such as a family member or paid personal care assistant, or an assistive technology (AT) or device. Without personal assistance and assistive devices made possible by relatively low-cost electronic components and computers, many people with physical disabilities would be leading isolated and dependent lives. Today, because of advances in technology, a person with functional movement of the arms and shoulders and above (C6 or lower spinal cord injuries) can live alone, travel, and work in a competitive job. As recently as the early 1960s, most equipment available to individuals with disabilities was only of a mechanical nature. Wheelchairs were literally chairs on wheels. Artificial limbs were plastic or (earlier) metal and wooden replacements for lost arms or legs.

Assistive technologies or devices are tools for enhancing the independent functioning of people who have physical limitations or disabilities. An *assistive technology device*, as defined in the Technology-Related Assistance of Individuals with Disabilities Act of 1988 (Pub. L. 100-407) is "any item, piece of equipment, or product system, whether acquired commercially off the shelf, modified, or customized, that is

used to increase, maintain, or improve functional capabilities of individuals with disabilities." This definition of assistive devices is used in every piece of legislation directed to people with disabilities that has been passed since 1988, and it is the standard definition used in the field.

Assistive devices range from low-tech aids such as built-up handles on eating utensils to high-tech, computerized communication systems for people with speech disabilities and battery-powered wheelchairs for people with mobility limitations. When people speak of high-tech assistive devices, ATs, or rehabilitation technologies they are usually referring to those with electronic components or that are "computerized." Figure 8–1 depicts categories of ATs according to areas of individuals' physical functioning.

The growth in ATs has been tremendous since the advent of the microcomputer in the late 1970s. Statistics from a nationwide survey revealed that in 1969, 6.2 million people used a total of 7.2 million assistive devices. Today, three times that number use the more than 22,000 products that are now available (Scherer, 1996a).

The number of devices that are computerized or electromechanical has increased dramatically in recent years. For purposes of this discussion, the term *complex device* is reserved for those devices. Devices that have either simple

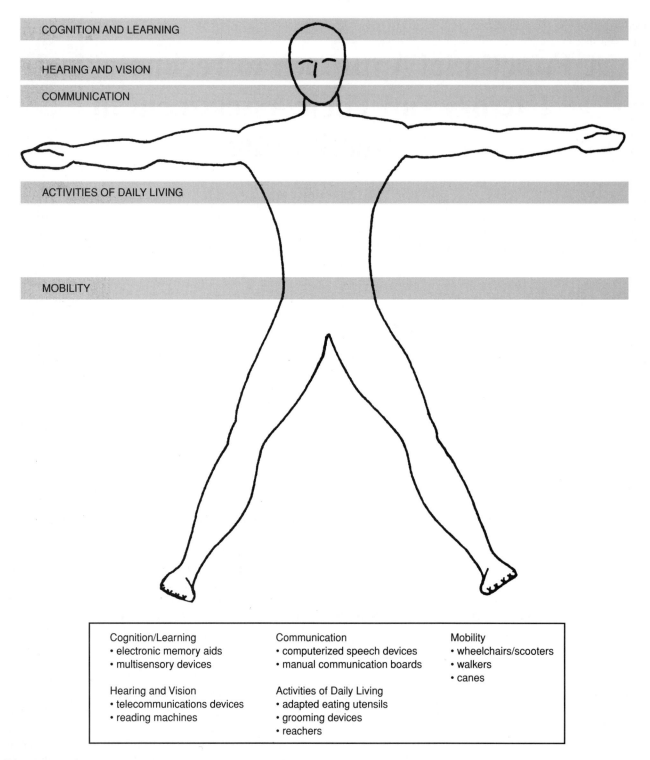

Figure 8–1 Assistive technology functional domains.

mechanical operations or neither mechanical, electrical, nor computerized components are termed *simple devices*. It is important to realize that by law all these devices are ATs and a low-tech device has as much value as a high-tech one for

users who find the device has enhanced their functioning, independence, and quality of life.

It can generally be said that individuals with the most severe disabilities require the most customized and computerized technologies for their enhanced independent functioning. If these technologies were not available, many individuals would not be able to live in the community.

ASSISTIVE DEVICES TO PERFORM ACTIVITIES OF DAILY LIVING FOR PERSONS WITH FUNCTIONAL LIMITATIONS IN FINGERS, HANDS, AND ARMS

The assistive devices used for functional limitations involving fingers, hands, and arms enable independence in fundamental areas, such as grooming, bathing, dressing, eating, and accessing home appliances. Ken (whose commentary was included in Chapter 7) uses a reacher for grabbing items off the floor or that are located up on shelves. Because he has some controllable movement in his arms and hands, Ken uses eating utensils with built-up handles (see Figures 8–2 and 8–3) and a splint that enables him to write independently with a pen or pencil.

Simple devices in this category include nonslip placemats under dinner plates to prevent sliding of the plate, eating utensils that are angled or have a larger surface area for gripping, and sponges to be strapped across the back of the hand for bathing. Other products range from lamps that turn on and off by touching them anywhere on their base to complex environmental control devices that allow several appliances

to be controlled by means of voice or through the use of such objects as a mouthstick. Simple and complex devices are often used together. For example, a mouthstick (a stick held between the teeth that is useful in depressing buttons and dialing phones) is a simple device that provides a means of controlling many complex devices.

Telephones with speaker-phone and abbreviated or quick-dialing capabilities are options that give persons with upper extremity limitations independence in calling and talking with other persons. A person with controllable movement of only the head can independently communicate on the telephone and turn appliances on and off. Regardless of the severity of the disability or need, individuals paralyzed from the neck down as well as those experiencing only weakness in the hands have an array of options available to them. The major differences are that a person with paralysis will generally require the technology to do more and be higher tech than will the person with hand weakness. Table 8–1 is adapted from Scherer (1996a) and illustrates the hierarchy of technologies for increasing limitation.

Just as advances in electronics have made possible products such as environmental control devices, additional advances in materials (plastics, stainless aluminum) have made other devices more lightweight, portable, flexible, and durable. Great strides have been made with technologies for mobility as a result, and within each type of mobility-related device the user can select from a number of options.

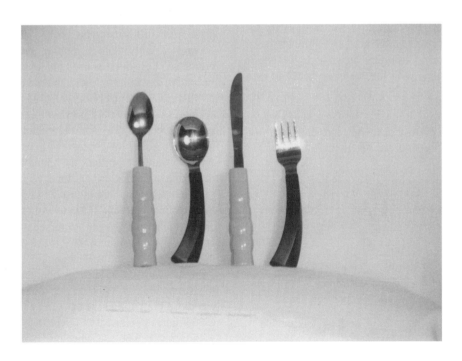

Figure 8–2 Eating utensils with built-up handles. Courtesy of the Center for Assistive Technology, Department of Occupational Therapy, State University of New York, Buffalo, New York.

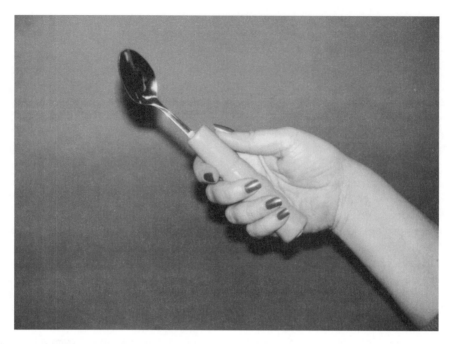

Figure 8–3 Adapted spoon with built-up handle for easier grip. Courtesy of the Center for Assistive Technology, Department of Occupational Therapy, State University of New York, Buffalo, New York.

ASSISTIVE DEVICES FOR MOBILITY FOR PERSONS WITH FUNCTIONAL LIMITATIONS IN BACK, HIPS, AND LEGS

To be mobile is to be able to get around in one's environments, as well as to exercise choice over the environments in which one wishes to be. Products to facilitate mobility include basic canes and crutches. Canes (see Figure 8–4) can be made of wood or metal, as well as have a single foot or three or four feet. A cane with four feet is referred to as a quad cane. Canes are useful for persons with weakness who desire assistance with their balance while walking.

Crutches, too, can be made of wood or metal. Axillary crutches support the person under the arm and require the hand to grip the crutch at hip level. A forearm crutch has a cuff that goes around the arm to assist persons who lack the hand strength for using an axillary crutch. Other names for forearm crutches are Canadian crutches and Lofstrand crutches. These devices need to make up for more functional limitation and thus are more complex in design.

Like canes and crutches, walkers (see Figure 8–5) come in several styles depending on the person's functional needs and preferences. They are wider than a person's body. They have four points of contact with the ground (like a chair does) but are streamlined in appearance so they resemble more of a quilt rack or rack for drying clothes. They provide a wide base of support and may have wheels (helpful on cement or linoleum, but not as useful on carpeting).

Wheelchairs are used by persons who, like Ken, cannot walk unassisted and thus need more assistance with mobility than can be obtained from a walker. Wheelchairs are chairs on wheels, and they are either manual (the wheels are manually propelled or rotated by the user or someone pushes the wheelchair for the user) or battery powered or motorized. (See Figures 8–6 and 8–7.)

Individuals who use wheelchairs need to have additional devices or products to ensure their comfort and safety. These include tilt and recline features of the wheelchair and special support cushions. Optional equipment may involve adding a hydraulic mechanism to raise and lower the wheelchair seat

Table 8–1 Complexity of Devices for Activities of Daily Living According to Extent of Functional Limitation

Extent of Functional Limitation	Complexity of Devices	
	Simple	Complex
Mild	Adapted eating utensils, bath sponge, nonslip placemat	
Moderate		Adapted telephones
Severe		Environmental control device

Source: Reprinted with permission from *Living in the State of Stuck*, 2nd ed., © Brookline Books.

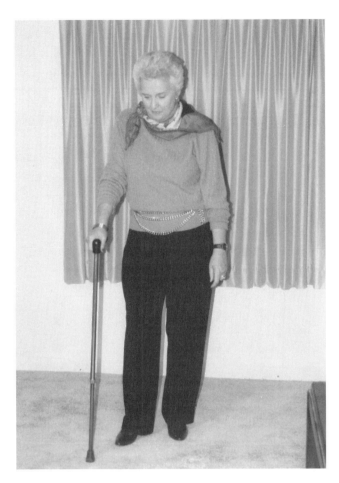

Figure 8–4 Assistive device for mobility—cane. Courtesy of the Center for Assistive Technology, Department of Occupational Therapy, State University of New York, Buffalo, New York.

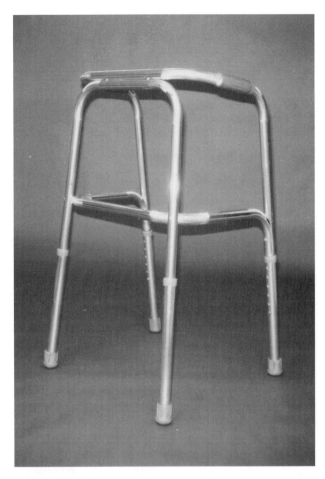

Figure 8–5 Assistive device for mobility—walker. Courtesy of the Center for Assistive Technology, Department of Occupational Therapy, State University of New York, Buffalo, New York.

and accessories, such as wheelchair backpacks, baskets, laptrays, and cup holders. The speed and direction of powered wheelchairs are typically controlled by the user through a joystick, but other means such as a sip-and-puff device (operated by breath) or a voice-activated interface are also used.

Powered wheelchair and powered scooter users (see Figure 8–8) also require ramps for accessing different levels of buildings, lifts for getting into vehicles, and special tie-down and restraint systems when riding in their wheelchairs in buses or vans. A person who uses a powered wheelchair and wishes to drive needs to have a van equipped with hand controls. Users of wheelchairs and scooters have less independent mobility than users of canes, crutches, or walkers, and their assistive technologies are more complex and high-tech in design.

Table 8–2 is adapted from Scherer (1996a) and illustrates the hierarchy of technologies for increasing limitation.

Ken, discussed in Chapter 7, is one of many persons whose limitations in mobility are associated with limitations in functions such as reaching objects in high places or lo-

cated at a distance from the user. Reachers are devices used to grab objects from a distance of approximately three feet from the user. One type is the pistol-grip reacher, which opens and shuts a two-prong gripper on the end by activating a trigger mechanism on the handle.

There are other kinds of assistive devices. In the book, *Evaluating, Selecting, and Using Appropriate Assistive Technology* (Galvin & Scherer, 1996), readers are guided through the system of AT devices and services in the six categories of devices listed below. In addition, a CD-ROM (Co-Net, developed by The Trace Center in Wisconsin) is included with the book. It describes (and in many cases, depicts) the more than 20,000 products in ABLEDATA, a database of assistive devices that is funded by the National Institute of Disability and Rehabilitation Research (NIDRR) and maintained by Macro International. There are

1. *Low-tech aids to daily living and do-it-yourself devices*—Examples of devices in this category help a person bathe, dress, cook, and move about. Specific

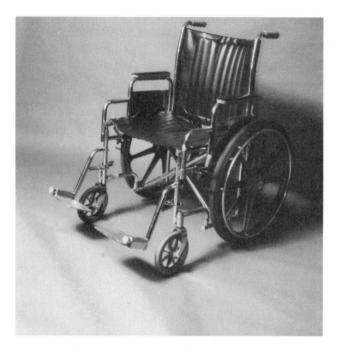

Figure 8–6 Manual wheelchair with footrests. Courtesy of the Center for Assistive Technology, Department of Occupational Therapy, State University of New York, Buffalo, New York.

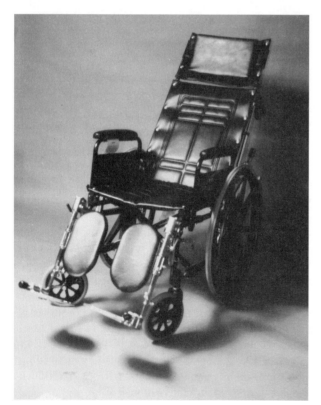

Figure 8–7 Reclining manual wheelchair with footrests. Courtesy of the Center for Assistive Technology, Department of Occupational Therapy, State University of New York, Buffalo, New York.

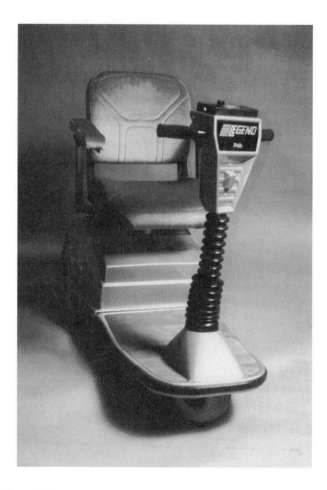

Figure 8–8 Powered scooter. Courtesy of the Center for Assistive Technology, Department of Occupational Therapy, State University of New York, Buffalo, New York.

devices range from long-handled sponges for bathing to hook and loop fasteners instead of buttons on clothing to kettle holders for cooking and canes for walking. Although these devices may not seem to warrant the designation of *technology*, they have been defined as ATs in the Technology-Related Assistance for Individuals with Disabilities Act of 1988. Thus, they can be considered as no-tech ATs, as compared with low-tech (having mechanical parts and mechanisms) and high-tech (having electronic or computerized components and systems) devices.

2. *Seating and mobility aids*—Examples of devices in this category were discussed earlier and include manual and battery-powered wheelchairs, wheelchair cushions and accessories such as desktop-type boards, and backpacks and baskets.

3. *Transportation aids*—Included in this category are aids for adapting vans and cars, including wheelchair

Table 8–2 Complexity of Devices for Mobility According to Extent of Functional Limitation

Extent of Functional Limitation	Complexity of Devices	
	Simple	Complex
Mild	Single foot cane, axillary crutch	
Moderate	Forearm crutches, rolling walkers	Manual wheelchairs with add-on power units
Severe		Powered wheelchairs and scooters

Source: Reprinted with permission from *Living in the State of Stuck*, 2nd ed., © Brookline Books.

lifts, hand controls, and wheelchair carriers. Wheelchair lifts are now on many public buses.

4. *Communication systems and devices*—These items range from manual communication boards to computerized devices with synthesized speech output.

5. *Technologies for blindness and low vision*—Devices in this category are for reading and safe travel. Magnifiers, Braille, or voice output systems for reading and guides for travel are examples.

6. *Technologies for people who are hard-of-hearing or deaf*—Devices in this category are for sound amplification (hearing aids, personal frequency modulation [FM] systems), communication (captioned television, text telephones [TTs] that send printed messages through telephone lines), and alerting/signaling (vibrotactile pagers, flashing timers and alarms). The Americans With Disabilities Act (P.L. 101–336) requires that telecommunication relay services operate 24 hours per day, seven days per week. This enables persons using TTs to communicate with hearing communication partners even though the latter do not have text telephones. A relay operator will speak the text typed by a person with hearing impairment and type the speech of the hearing telephone partner, which appears on the TT of the person with hearing impairment.

Assistive devices are now needed in a variety of contexts and environments. The following are examples of technologies for recreation, play, and work:

• *Recreation and leisure*—Assistive devices have made most sports, recreational, and leisure activities accessible to persons with disabilities, from tethered (attached to a nondisabled skier) sit-skiing to scuba diving, wheelchair basketball, sailing, and card shuffling.

• *Child's play*—Adapted toys and do-it-yourself playthings for children are important assistive devices.

• *Work*—Devices in this group focus on making the worksite accessible to the person with a disability. They include work stations and adapted tools/appliances, as well as desirable modifications in the environment that allow safe and easy movement.

As it became more and more evident that the interest in and need for assistive devices would keep growing, a new field—rehabilitation engineering—was created to design, fabricate, and modify devices while studying and monitoring their general feasibility. Many rehabilitation engineering research centers have been established in the United States through the National Institute on Disability and Rehabilitation Research. Each has its own core area of research, such as augmentative communication, wheelchair mobility, technology and aging, prosthetics and orthotics, and technology evaluation and transfer.

In general, *prosthetic devices* (e.g., artificial limbs) replace or substitute a part of the body (like arms and legs). *Orthotic devices* (e.g., braces) are used to provide support for a weakened part of the body. *Assistive devices* are really just what the term implies: They assist individuals in performing certain functions such as getting around in wheelchairs and in specially designed vans. *Adapted equipment* (e.g., eating utensils with built-up handles) refers to devices designed for the general population that are adapted in ways to be useful for people with disabilities. Some adapted devices are so widely used and accepted that they are not thought of as adapted equipment at all. One example is the large pencils children use when they learn to write. Other technologies frequently encountered in rehabilitation medicine are *biomedical devices*, such as indwelling catheters as well as hemodialysis machines and respiratory ventilators (Campbell-Heider & Knapp, 1993). These technologies are considered invasive because they (or their access) enter a body orifice or go under the skin in the individual.

IMPORTANCE OF MATCHING PERSONS WITH THE MOST APPROPRIATE TECHNOLOGY

Assistive technologies can replace or reduce the amount of assistance required of other persons by enhancing independent functioning and minimizing disability. Although there are federal mandates for comprehensive, consumer-responsive AT and technology-related services, obtaining such devices and services often remains an arduous task for both individual and professional. Thus in this time of reduced resources in many areas, matching a person with the most appropriate AT is essential yet challenging at the individual, system, and funding levels.

ATs May Be Used, Avoided, or Abandoned

Data from the 1990 U.S. Census Bureau's *National Health Survey on Assistive Devices* show that more than 13.1 million people in the United States (more than 5% of the total U.S. population) used ATs in 1990. In 1969, 6.2 million people used a total of 7.2 million assistive devices. In 21 years, the number of persons using ATs doubled because of three key factors: (1) people with disabilities surviving severe trauma and disease and living longer, (2) advances in microelectronics and availability of microcomputers, and (3) legislation regarding persons with disabilities passed since 1988 that has mandated the consideration of AT. There are no data on how these figures compare with the total number of devices prescribed or purchased during this time span, nor are there comparable indicators of this population's predisposition to technology use in general.

It is known that people with disabilities differ in the degrees to which they use ATs, and they have differing views of the extent to which they believe ATs improve the quality of their lives. For example, a survey conducted by the American Association of Retired Persons indicates that many aging individuals who could benefit from ATs avoid them outright, whereas others try them only to abandon them to the basement, closet, or bedside table (Smith, 1996). Depending on the type of AT, nonuse or abandonment can be as low as 8% or as high as 75%. On the average, one-third or more optional ATs are abandoned, most within the first three months of trial (Scherer & Galvin, 1994). No information is available about the number of people who must continue to use devices that they are unhappy with because they cannot abandon these devices without more severe consequences.

Technology abandonment can have a series of repercussions. Although unused and abandoned technologies represent wasted resources, so do people not performing at their functional best. Nonuse of a device may lead to decreases in functional abilities, freedom, and independence, as well as increases in monetary expenses. On a service-delivery level, device abandonment represents ineffective use of limited funds by federal, state, and local government agencies, insurers, and other providers.

The body of research on abandonment of AT devices illustrates the complexity of the interface between a person and a device. A review of that literature indicates that the overarching factor associated with technology abandonment is failure to consider user opinions and preferences in device selection. Other major reasons devices are not used by consumers (in no particular order) include the following:

- changes in consumer functional abilities or activities
- lack of consumer motivation to use the device or do the task
- lack of meaningful training on how to use the device (especially for individuals who are elderly or who have cognitive impairments)
- ineffective device performance
- environmental obstacles to use such as narrow doorways
- lack of access to and information about repair and maintenance
- device unnecessary
- unsatisfactory device aesthetics, weight, size, and other characteristics
- minimal need for device

Most of these issues can be addressed appropriately in a comprehensive selection process (see Exhibit 8–1) that (1) considers the person's ongoing needs and (2) takes a long-term view of an individual's assistive device use, which is first and foremost consumer directed. A better understanding of how and why technology users decide to accept or reject a device is critical to improving the effectiveness of AT interventions and enhancing consumer satisfaction.

Desirability of a Model for Evaluating Needs for AT and Matching Person and Technology

Successful AT use requires adapting the AT to the person's capabilities and temperament, not vice versa. It is also important to adapt the person, family, coworkers, and others to the realities and situations of AT use. This is true with biomedical devices as well as ATs (Campbell-Heider & Knapp, 1993).

One method that is useful in organizing the many influences on a person's predisposition to use a more optional type of AT is the Matching Person and Technology (MPT) Model (Scherer, 1991). This model advocates addressing separately three variables:

Exhibit 8–1 Establishing Quality Pathways to Evaluation, Selection, and Use of Appropriate Assistive Technologies

1. Establish goals/expectations for person.
2. Assess need for simple and complex devices.
3. Match person and technology.
4. Select and fit assistive technology to the person.
5. Train person for assistive technology use.
6. Assess/evaluate outcomes of assistive technology use according to goals/expectations.
7. [Return to #1.]

Source: Reprinted from M.J. Scherer and J.C. Galvin, An Outcomes Perspective of Quality Pathways to the Most Appropriate Technology, in *Evaluating, Selecting, and Using Appropriate Assistive Technology*, J.C. Galvin and M.J. Scherer, eds., pp. 1–26, © 1996, Aspen Publishers, Inc.

Table 8–3 Assistive Technology Influences in the Matching Person and Technology (MPT) Model

		Milieu	*Personality*	*Technology*
U	*Optimal*	Support from family/peers/ employer Realistic expectations of family/employer Setting/environment fully supports and rewards use	Proud to use device Motivated Cooperative Optimistic Good coping skills Patient Self-disciplined Generally positive life experiences Has skills to use device Perceived discrepancy between desired and current situation	Goal achieved with no pain, fatigue, or stress Compatible with/enhances use of other technologies Is safe, reliable, and easy to use and maintain Has desired transportability No better options currently available
S				
E	*Partial/Reluctant*	Pressure for use from family/peers/employer Assistance often not available Setting/environment discourages use or makes use awkward	Embarrassed to use device Unmotivated Impatient/impulsive Unrealistic expectations Low self-esteem Somewhat intimidated by technology Technology partially or occasionally fits with lifestyle Deficits in skills needed for use	Goal not fully achieved or with discomfort/strain Requires a lot of set-up Interferes somewhat with use of other technologies Device inefficient Other options to device use exist
N	*Avoidance*	Lack of support from either family/peers/ employer Unrealistic expectations of others Assistance not available Setting/environment disallows or prevents use	Person does not want device Embarrassed to use device Depressed Unmotivated Uncooperative Withdrawn Intimidated by technology Many changes required in lifestyle Does not have skills for use	Perceived lack of goal achievement or too much strain/ discomfort in use Requires a lot of set-up Perceived or determined to be incompatible with use of other techniques Too expensive Long delay for delivery Other options to device use exist
O				
N				
U	*Abandonment*	Lack of support from either family/peers/ employer Setting/environment discourages or makes use awkward Requires assistance that is not available	Embarrassed to use device Depressed Low self-esteem Hostile/angry Withdrawn Resistant Poor socialization and coping skills Many changes in lifestyle with use Lacks skills to use device and training not available	Goal not achieved and/or discomfort/strain in use Is incompatible with use of other techniques Has been outgrown Difficult to use Device inefficient Repairs/service not timely or affordable Other options to use became available
S				
E				

1. characteristics of the *milieu* (environment and psychosocial setting) in which the AT is used
2. pertinent features of the individual's *personality* and temperament
3. salient characteristics of the assistive *technology* itself.

The influences on AT use delineated in the Matching Person and Technology (MPT) model are shown in Tables 8–3 and 8–4. The information provided in the tables is an attempt to profile a person's predisposition to use a particular AT. It is important to note that predispositions to use can vary over time. For example, Ken had characteristics associated with

Table 8–4 Technology Use Worksheet for Matching Person and Technology (MPT) Model

In which of the following areas does the person (1) use, (2) have past use, and (3) need a technology? Check all that apply, and record the information requested under each area.

Limitations	Technology(ies) Currently Used			Technology(ies) Used in Past			Technology(ies) Needed		
	Name of Technology	Percentage of Day Used	Satisfaction with technology (1 = very dissatisfied, 3 = neutral, 5 = very satisfied)	Percentage of Day Used	Satisfaction with technology (1 = very dissatisfied, 3 = neutral, 5 = very satisfied)	Reason No Longer Using	Needs and Wants But Does Not Have	Needs, But Does Not Want	Reason
___ Communication	1. 2. 3.								
___ Mobility	1. 2. 3.								
___ Vision	1. 2. 3.								
___ Hearing	1. 2. 3.								
___ Employment	1. 2. 3.								
___ Reading/Writing	1. 2. 3.								
___ Household activities	1. 2. 3.								
___ Health maintenance	1. 2. 3.								
___ Recreation	1. 2. 3.								
___ Self-care	1. 2. 3.								

Table 8–4 continued

	Technology(ies) Currently Used			Technology(ies) Used in Past			Technology(ies) Needed		
Limitations	Name of Technology	Percentage of Day Used	Satisfaction with technology (1 = very dissatis- fied, 3 = neutral, 5 = very satisfied)	Percentage of Day Used	Satisfaction with technology (1 = very dissatisfied, 3 = neutral, 5 = very satisfied)	Reason No Longer Using	Needs and Wants But Does Not Have	Needs, But Does Not Want	Reason
__ Employment	1.								
	2.								
	3.								
__ Learning/cognition	1.								
	2.								
	3.								

AT use as far as milieu/environment and technology variables are concerned, but several years after discharge from a rehabilitation program he seemed to be a reluctant user according to the characteristics listed for personality. The personality/temperament influences indicated a need for modification or some intervention for Ken to gain maximum satisfaction and functional gain from the use of his AT. Later, when he no longer described himself as withdrawn and depressed, Ken more closely approximated the profile of an optimal user of AT.

One device with a high rate of abandonment is hearing aids. According to results of a study conducted by Scherer and Frisina (1994), factors associated with nonuse of hearing aids include characteristics of the technology, such as discomfort with ear molds and expense and visibility of the aids. A key characteristic of the person influencing abandonment of hearing aids is the expectation that perfect hearing will be restored. Milieu/environment characteristics affecting hearing aid use include cooperation of significant others in avoiding noisy environments in which it is difficult for the hearing aid user to discriminate a speaker's voice from background noise. The discussion that follows provides more depth on psychological and psychosocial aspects of AT use as measured by the Assistive Technology Device Predisposition Assessment (ATD PA) (Scherer, 1991).

Individual and Psychosocial Incentives and Disincentives to AT Use

Incentives

Users of ATs such as Ken, who see these devices as valuable enablers for their goals, activities, and independence, tend to exhibit common affirming views and experiences. They

- attribute AT use to inner motivation and exhibit an unwillingness to be held back from self-expression as well as pursuit of their goals and independence.
- emphasize new or regained capabilities and try to work around their disabilities, which they view as less important.
- strive actively for social integration in school, the workplace, and their interpersonal relationships.
- have more social support than nonusers—their employers hold jobs for them; their families build ramps and modify the family home and are reluctant to have them return home unaided; and their family relationships are stable. They play a key role in family caretaking.

Disincentives

Nonusers of ATs tend to have opposing views and experiences to those of AT users. They

- exhibit little motivation to overcome their disabilities. Rather, they focus on barriers caused by their own limitations and societal obstacles.
- believe societal integration is unattainable and are socially withdrawn (a situation that they often attribute to a nonaccepting society).
- admit to little life satisfaction and say that they are better off financially by not working or going to school.
- wait for a cure for their disability or for the availability of technologies that are far superior to those currently available.

For many individuals, the role of patient or client requires a submission to professionals, which they resent. They believe that they have lost individuality and freedom of choice and may easily become frustrated and discouraged. To alleviate this frustration and discouragement while a match of potential user to an AT is being sought, the rehabilitation professional should try to include ample choices and not allow training sessions to end in frustration or disappointment.

Individual Characteristics

Once the feasibility of use of a particular AT has been established, the likelihood of its use will often depend on the user's particular expectations and aspirations—both for AT use and functioning in general. Below are individual characteristics that commonly influence use of an AT.

AT use preferred to alternatives—Successful AT use depends on consumers' judgments that they will (1) benefit from use of an AT, (2) achieve a goal with the AT that might not otherwise be possible, and (3) derive more benefit from the AT than from alternatives.

AT use matches consumers' basic lifestyle—Assistive technologies that are forced on individuals and do not fit with their ways of doing things have a low probability of use. For example, an AT that requires discipline, patience, and perseverance, as well as delayed gratification, may not appeal to a young, strong-willed, adventuresome man with a spinal cord injury who takes pride in his free spirit and spontaneity. Alternatively, adults who were born with a disability frequently develop fewer coping skills than those who were injured later in life and experienced normal development. The self-esteem of the former can be threatened by ATs.

User expectations of AT—Research findings have shown that the major reason for abandonment of an AT is the device's failure to meet the user's expectations for that device (Phillips & Zhao, 1993; Scherer & McKee, 1989; Scherer, 1996c). With a collaborative approach to evaluation and selection of a technology, a user's expectations will be more realistic.

User excitement and sense of control—Assistive technology users seem to meet challenges head on and actively try to improve their quality of life. In contrast, nonusers often seem to believe they have little control over their quality of life, and many express little motivation to overcome their disabilities.

User's desire for AT—There can be secondary gains for actually not using a technology. Some nonusers prefer to depend on family members and other individuals. Other nonusers have an aversion to the use of a technology or feel intimidated by it.

Sense of status or self-esteem—The most used ATs are the same as (or similar to) those used by the general population. These devices are often designed to look functional and utilitarian to satisfy funding sources but leave users feeling self-conscious and stigmatized. Moreover, a peer culture may exert a strong influence on the acceptability of an AT, such as among members of the deaf community in which hearing aid users are viewed as rejecting the deaf culture.

Independence from others' assistance—Assistive technologies that require a lot of help and effort from others to set up, maintain, or use probably will not be used to the extent desirable. An example is the case of computerized communication systems, which require a lot of listener cooperation (such as standing by patiently to read a digital display or waiting for a printout.)

Requirements of the AT Compared with Resources of the Consumer

After it has been determined how closely the characteristics of the AT match the preferences of the potential user, the selected technology or user's resources may require modification to optimize the match. The following characteristics are assessed on the ATD PA (described in detail later in this chapter).

Physical demands—Answers to several key questions can maximize an AT–consumer match when physical demands of the AT are considered with the user's physical capabilities. For example: Can the technology be made lighter or smaller or can the user be given assistance in moving it? Can the technology be incorporated into the frame of a wheelchair? Can it be appropriately used in one place? If the weight and size of the technology do not match the user's strength, a different AT must be chosen.

Physical/sensory requirements—One of the most obvious and most crucial device characteristics that must match the capabilities of the user is that of the physical/sensory requirement. For example, an AT that requires hearing cannot be used by a deaf person without modification. In such cases, modification can be made easily by adding a flashing light to a warning buzzer. In some cases, however, the AT must simply be judged inappropriate for the individual.

Expense—When the cost of the technology is beyond a person's resources, funds must be found or the technology is clearly not practical. The situation is less clear when the technology strains the user's resources but can still be purchased. If this situation occurs, the most appropriate AT must be chosen and the potential for optimal use must be high.

Support services/training—It is important that the requirements for support or training match the resources and skills of the user. If these needs and skills do not match and neither can be feasibly modified, the technology is probably not a good choice for that user.

Service delivery—Whether the device can be procured and delivered in a timely fashion before the user's condition changes is key. If delivery will be delayed, it should be ascertained whether use of the device on a trial basis or loan is feasible.

Cognitive demands—Many computerized devices require that the user be able to grasp complex information and have special training. This base level of cognitive abilities is necessary for rewarding use by the consumer. If this level is not assured or demonstrably present, it may be possible to simplify the cognitive demands placed on the user by modifying the technology (e.g., through use of picture instructions or special software).

In addition to the above listed considerations, potential users of ATs can respond to questionnaires, providing valuable information for AT–consumer fit (see Exhibit 8–2).

DESCRIPTIONS OF AVAILABLE MEASURES FOR DETERMINING IMPACT OF ATs ON DISABILITY AND QUALITY OF LIFE

As emphasized in several chapters of this book, many assessment measures and instruments are available to the rehabilitation professional for determining and optimizing consumer needs and capabilities. This section brings together and addresses measures that are integral to the impact of ATs in disability and quality of life of an individual. Some (e.g., the Matching Person and Technology [MPT] Model [Scherer, 1991]) were introduced briefly earlier in this chapter; others were highlighted in Chapters 4 and 5 and are discussed in more depth in Appendix A.

Matching Person and Technology (MPT) Model

The Matching Person and Technology (MPT) Model consists of checklist-type assessment instruments to record consumer goals and preferences, views of the benefits to be gained from a technology, and changes in self-perceived outcome achievement over time.

Exhibit 8–2 Which Is the Most Appropriate Assistive Technology for Me?

Functional Abilities, Goals, and Tasks
What is my disability? Is it stable or changing?
Do I have the physical and mental abilities to use the device?
Have I identified my needs clearly?
Can I change my activities so that I can do them without a device?
Is there a device that can help me meet my needs?
Will I need assistance to use the device?
Will an assistant need to use the device?

Personal Characteristics, Abilities, and Preferences
What technology do I currently use?
How do I currently manage my daily activities?
Is it important to me to do things as independently as possible?
Does technology help me be more independent or dependent?
Am I comfortable using technology?
Will this device contribute significantly to my quality of life?

Environment
Where will I use the equipment? At home, work, community, all of those?

Is the environment architecturally accessible?
Is transportation available?
Can my environment support the technology?
Are people available to assist if needed?
Could the environment disrupt device performance, i.e., electronic interference?
How would the device affect other people in my environment?
Will I have the training and support I need to use the device?

Device
What kind of device do I prefer?
Does the device reflect my lifestyle, age, personality, values?
Have I considered all the devices available?
How well does the device work?
How much will it cost to buy and maintain?
Will it be easy to use and maintain?
How long is it likely to last?
Will I be able to try it before I buy it?

Source: Reprinted from M.J. Scherer and J.C. Galvin, An Outcomes Perspective of Quality Pathways to the Most Appropriate Technology, in *Evaluating, Selecting, and Using Appropriate Assistive Technology,* J.C. Galvin and M.J. Scherer, eds., pp. 1–26, © 1996, Aspen Publishers, Inc.

One pair of instruments, the ATD PA, was developed in connection with an assessment of differences between AT users and nonusers (Scherer, 1986). The ATD PA elicits subjective information regarding individuals' satisfaction with current functioning. Areas in which the most improvement in functioning or consumer–AT fit is desired can be ascertained from the report. The consumer version has two forms: (1) questions given *per consumer* on temperament, psychosocial resources, and views of disability and (2) questions *per technology* on the consumer's views of and expectations for that particular technology.

Table 8–5 provides a portion of the consumer version of the ATD PA. Companion professional forms are similarly constructed, so that criss-cross comparisons of professional and consumer views can be made. The items emerged from the actual experiences of technology users and nonusers, so they have content validity. Additional psychometric evidence indicates that they are quality assessments (Brown, 1996; Crewe & Dijkers, 1995; Cushman & Scherer, 1996).

OT FACT

The OT FACT is a computerized functional assessment instrument that solicits practitioner or consumer judgments on the perceived level of functional performance (Smith, 1993, 1995). The instrument contains five domains of function: role integration, activities of performance, integrated skills of performance, components of performance, and environment performance. The entire question set includes more than 900 trichotomous-scaled computer branching questions. Efficiency is managed by using global screening questions that request detail only in needed areas. In addition, the question set can be customized by users to minimize the overall depth of the assessment.

The OT FACT specifically addresses the area of AT by allowing consumer or practitioner scoring, producing performance scores with and without the use of AT for side-by-side comparison, and prompting the scorer to identify the specific technologies used. Optimizing reliability and validity has been key to the design of OT FACT, which led to the computerized dynamic questioning approach used. As a dynamic question set, however, reliability and validity determination has challenged traditional instrument test procedures. Thus a multidirectional set of classical and more modern reliability and validity measures have been and are continuing to be administered to document the effectiveness of the computerized question structure on which OT FACT is based.

Functional Independence Measure

The Functional Independence Measure (FIM^{SM}) is an 18-item, seven-level ordinal scale developed to provide uniform measurement of disability and rehabilitation. It can be completed in approximately 20 to 30 minutes. (The FIM^{SM} is described more fully in Appendix A.)

CHART: Craig Handicap Assessment and Reporting Technique

The CHART is designed to measure societal limitation in persons in the community with spinal cord injuries. It also may have promise for persons with other diagnoses.

The CHART assesses physical independence, mobility, occupation, social integration, and economic self-sufficiency. Psychometric properties, reliability, and validity have been shown to be adequate. (CHART is described more fully in Appendix A.)

MOS 36-Item Short-Form Health Survey (SF-36)

The SF-36 was developed initially by the RAND Corporation as a measure of patient perception of wellness to predict future health care use. It has eight health concepts: physical functioning, bodily pain, role limitations due to physical health problems, role limitations due to personal or emotional problems, emotional well-being, social functioning, energy/fatigue, and general health perceptions. The SF-36 and subsequent versions have gained widespread acceptance as a good measure of predicting ongoing and future health care utilization. (See also Chapter 5.)

Other Measures

With these (and all other) forms of measurement, the consumer is the most important component of the assessment of both rehabilitation process and outcomes. By demonstrating the changes in a consumer's life, positive or negative, an assessment can serve as an indicator of the effects of an AT intervention (Batavia, 1992).

Regardless of the means used to assess potential quality of the match of person and AT, it is crucial for professionals to ensure that

1. they as professionals have the support they need to become knowledgeable about a variety of technologies and relevant resources.
2. consumer needs, not particular features of an AT or its availability, drive the matching process.
3. different perspectives of professional and consumer become evident so they can be addressed.
4. a variety of interventions, from no tech to simple tech to complex tech, are considered.

5. trial periods with the interventions in situations of actual use are arranged.
6. desirable interventions are selected with the necessary support systems established to ensure their success.
7. specific objective criteria by which to judge the intervention's usefulness to the consumer, along with a timeline, are identified.

OUTCOMES MEASURES AND AT SERVICE DELIVERY: VARIOUS MEANS TO AN END

Professionals working with ATs need to demonstrate that what they do makes a difference in the lives of persons with disabilities. Insurance companies and other payers are increasingly asking for documentation of value related to the costs of AT services. Other demands for documentation focus on functional status, consumer satisfaction, and quality of life. Providers and suppliers of ATs must know how to assess and document outcomes of an intervention at both program and consumer levels (Scherer, 1996b; Smith, 1996).

The Rehabilitation Engineering and Assistive Technology Society of North America (RESNA) is committed to developing a means of assuring consumers, payers, and a variety of service providers that AT devices and services offered are effective. A key aspect of this quality assurance effort is educating its membership on outcome measurement. Outcomes measures are used to demonstrate that particular goals established for a consumer have been identified and then achieved. Outcome data will become increasingly essential for justifying to payers (and others) the need for AT evaluation, provision, and training.

Definition of Outcomes

Outcomes can be the result of an intervention. Examples of outcomes are employability, performance of activities of daily living, and consumer satisfaction or subjective quality of life. The last example encompasses the person's sense of well-being, comfort, happiness, and satisfaction with specific areas of functioning, such as work and in social relationships as well as with finances.

Measurement of Consumer Outcomes

To determine the most appropriate measure for outcome of an AT intervention, the objectives and goals of the intervention must be identified (Smith, 1996). Outcomes vary among individuals, and one must obtain consumers' perspectives of the most desired outcomes as well as the perspectives of secondary consumers (e.g., family members, caretakers, payers, vendors, and employers). Exhibit 8–3, adapted from DeRuyter (1996), lists the kinds of stakeholders that need to be taken into account, and Exhibit 8–4 provides a comparison of what different stakeholders value and accept as outcomes data.

Table 8–5 Assistive Technology Device Predisposition Assessment—Consumer Version

On one side of the consumer form are questions given *per consumer*. They address characteristics of the person's temperament, psychosocial arena, and view of disability. The following are sample portions of the assessment in each of these areas.

ATD PA Consumer Form Item 3: View of Disability

How are your current capabilities in the following areas? Circle the best response for each:

	Poor		Average		Good
a. Vision	1	2	3	4	5
b. Hearing	1	2	3	4	5
c. Speech	1	2	3	4	5
d. Upper extremity control	1	2	3	4	5
e. Lower extremity control	1	2	3	4	5
f. Mobility	1	2	3	4	5
g. Dexterity	1	2	3	4	5

Put a [–] beside any of the above that you believe are or will be deteriorating over time. Then put a [+] beside any you believe are or will be improving over time.

ATD PA Consumer Form Item 4: View of Disability/Quality of Life

How satisfied are you with what you have achieved in the following areas? Please circle the best response for each:

	Not Satisfied		Satisfied		Very Satisfied
a. Independent living skills	1	2	3	4	5
b. Physical comfort and well-being	1	2	3	4	5
c. Overall health	1	2	3	4	5
d. Ability to go where desired	1	2	3	4	5
e. Emotional well-being	1	2	3	4	5

Put a [+] beside the one(s) you most want to improve over time.

ATD PA Consumer Form Sample Items Regarding Temperament

Check all statements below that apply to you a majority of the time:

❑ curious and excited about new things
❑ cooperative
❑ have many things I want to accomplish
❑ discouraged
❑ often depressed

The other side of the ATD PA consumer form addresses characteristics of a technology being proposed for that person's use.

These questions need to be completed *on each technology* being matched with the consumer. Sample items are the following:

ATD PA items regarding characteristics of the particular technology:
  1. Can you use this device with little or no assistance from others?
  5. How much do you believe you will benefit from using this device?
  9. How much will this device require changes in how you usually go about doing this?
  10. How will you feel about using this device?

	Embarrassed			Proud
a. Around your family	1	2	3	4	5
b. Around your friends	1	2	3	4	5

The primary purpose of the ATD PA is to flag potential mismatches between person and technology in the hopes that early identification of mismatches will:

  (a) reduce technology nonuse or inappropriate use
  (b) identify needed technology modifications, and
  (c) eliminate frustration that occurs with a poor match of person and technology

Source: Copyright © Marcia J. Scherer, PhD.

Exhibit 8–3 Stakeholders Other Than Consumers in the Measurement of Outcomes

Policymakers	State and federal agencies
	Program administrators/Boards of directors
Providers	Practitioners
	Technology consultants
	Clinical/community support
	Teachers
Payers	Medicaid
	Medicare
	Developmental disabilities agencies
	Insurance carriers

Source: Adapted from DeRuyter (1996).

Once the goals of the intervention are specified, a timeline for goal achievement needs to be established. The timeline will indicate points when it is most appropriate to assess outcomes.

In measuring or recording data for outcome measures, care must be taken to avoid losing important information throughout the process. Issues surrounding data collection must include, but not be limited to, answers to the following 11 questions.

1. Where are the data to go?
2. Who is the audience for which data are being collected?
3. What should the data measure?
4. How can data collection systems be developed and designed so that programs can work collaboratively to collect these data within their states, regions, and nations?
5. Which practitioners need these data and information?
6. Which payers need these data and information?
7. Is the means of data collection scientifically reliable and valid?
8. How are data disseminated to consumer groups?
9. Which adults or seniors with disabilities can provide these data?
10. How can data be obtained from a variety of settings and contexts?
11. How can the various stakeholders document the use of sundry AT in normal activities?

Outcomes sought by each stakeholder (unique to their roles and relative AT service provided) are described as follows.

Policymaker (e.g., program administrator)—Ensure strategies are in place to maintain user's independence in cost-effective ways. Key foci include

- minimal involvement of provider
- aggregated information
- efficient communication

Provider (e.g., practitioners, occupational therapist, physical therapist, speech-language pathologist)—Assist consumer in becoming independent in functional activities; that is,

- assist with technology support
- provide and facilitate stimulating environment(s)
- advocate for money and services to upgrade care and technologies

Provider (e.g., technology consultants, clinical/community support, teachers)—Promote successful use of equipment; that is,

- eliminate barriers
- organize resources (technology and training)
- ensure social interaction needs are met

Payer (e.g., Medicaid)—Reduce costs; that is,

- pay now for services to save later
- decrease use of support staff
- ensure successful outcome to conserve money

Measurement of Outcomes from a Variety of Dimensions of a Person's Life

Outcomes are derived from a variety of dimensions of a person's life. In addition to outcomes regarding functional status, cost, consumer satisfaction, and quality of life, it is also important to assess these outcomes according to the most appropriate environments/settings in which they occur (educational setting, place of employment, community, etc.).

Functional Status

The measurement of a person's functional status using AT can be addressed in a general framework of broad areas of function for participation in all aspects of life. Functional categories or domains may comprise the following:

Self-care
1. dressing
2. grooming
3. feeding
4. toileting
5. bathing
6. eating

Mobility
1. transfer
2. locomotion
3. transportation

Exhibit 8–4 Stakeholder Perspectives

Stakeholder	Clinical Results	Functional Status	Quality of Life	Consumer Satisfaction	Cost Factors
Administrator	No	Yes	No	Yes	Yes
Consumer	No	Yes	Yes	Yes	No
Clinician	Yes	Yes	Yes	Yes	No
Payer	Yes	Yes	No	Yes	Yes

Communication
1. comprehension
2. expression

Social skills
1. environmental control
2. cognition and problem solving
3. leisure and recreation
4. intimacy/sexuality
5. participation in education/learning or vocation/working (or both)

Providers may find the following questions helpful, realizing that a general approach is taken to allow for application to specific technologies:

1. What does function mean? Is it an issue of control? (see Chapter 1)
2. Do service providers need to intervene?
3. Do service providers need to create a new AT?

The pragmatics of AT dictate that there are needs directly and specifically tethered to reimbursement. Solutions are often sought and found before the problems are fully defined. It should also be remembered that the AT should not be the place to start; it is the *tool* by which the outcome is reached. Other important questions to ask include

- What functions make a difference?
- What needs to happen?
- What are the consumer's and other stakeholders' desired functional outcomes?
- How do these functional outcomes relate to minimal and optional functional performance?
- Are consumers better off after receiving the AT services and devices?

Functional ability must be measured in different contexts. It must also be measured over time to demonstrate change in ability level of an individual. All stakeholders should attempt to keep the measure simple and straightforward and identify targeted goals and what the consumer wants to achieve in terms of function. For example, walking may be a *rehabilitation goal*, but not the *individual's goal*.

With a basic and observed definition that function is the ability to perform or to have performed tasks in a manner that works, the following questions can be considered:

- Is the consumer able to perform, or have performed, daily tasks in a manner that is efficient and acceptable to him or her?
- Are expectations appropriate for the individual's current stage of life?
- Does the technology augment the individual's life, so that he or she is able to do what peers can do?
- Have capacities as well as limitations been assessed?

To know whether a person *can* do something is important, but to know whether he or she *actually does* it is equally important.

Cost

Cost must be considered whenever outcomes are discussed. It can be looked at from many perspectives. As an example, from a provider perspective if there is not proper cost accounting, services may be eliminated despite what the consumer needs and wants.

Currently, in certain circumstances costs seem to be driving policy decisions. Thus providers must be aware of the need to demonstrate that what they do is both cost effective (value of outcomes compared with expenditures) and cost efficient (appropriate use of resources) (Warren, 1993).

The following four recommendations provide a starting point for addressing the need to demonstrate both cost effectiveness and cost efficiency:

1. Measure both costs and benefits (e.g., durability, staying power) over time.
2. Consider long-term and secondary benefits (e.g., employability down the road).
3. Identify and quantify benefits of the person's functioning with and without the use of an AT.
4. Examine the impact of an AT on need for personal assistance.

Assistive technology alone does not increase a person's functioning. It is important to quantify as many benefits from

ATs as possible to ensure their continued development and availability. *Note*: More detailed information and suggested resources on cost outcomes with AT devices and services can be obtained from RESNA (RESNA, 1700 N. Moore Street, Suite 1540, Arlington, VA 22209-1903. Telephone: 703/524-6686; Fax no: 703/524-6630; TTY: 703/524-6639.)

Consumer Satisfaction

Users of ATs have an important role in developing measures that will accurately reflect the status or effect (or both) of the AT in their lives. With the assumption that the consumer was served by a competent professional, questions can be asked to generate the outcomes protocol that would address consumer satisfaction by goal definition. Those desired goals must be met. In addition, the process, program, and system for delivery of the technology and services must be evaluated. The process of bringing about consumer satisfaction includes consensus by all stakeholders that the consumer is the key to the process. Measurement of satisfaction derives from the appropriate and specific set of goals that all stakeholders have defined.

The process of addressing and documenting consumer satisfaction should include the following eight (and often repetitive) steps:

1. Identify the consumer's needs.
2. Establish a set of desired outcomes as defined by the entire rehabilitation team as well as all other stakeholders.
3. Develop the action plan for achieving the desired outcomes.
4. Establish that the user, family members of the user, members of the team, and stakeholders are satisfied with the action plan.
5. Implement the action plan.
6. Measure whether the user, his or her family members, team members, and stakeholders are satisfied with the implementation process.
7. Measure whether the user, his or her family members, team members, and stakeholders are satisfied with achieving the desired outcome.
8. Establish new desired outcomes as appropriate.

Ongoing follow-up of consumer satisfaction is critical to ensure positive outcomes. Follow-up questions can include, but should not be limited to, the following:

- Did you feel that your input was wanted and needed?
- Did you feel that you got what you needed? If not, is what you received appropriate?
- If you are dissatisfied, why? What do you recommend be done about it now?

All follow-up directed toward measuring satisfaction of the consumer with the intervention should include the following two concepts:

1. Treat consumers and family with respect.
2. Use open-ended questions to maintain ongoing communication with the consumer (i.e., What was good? What do we keep? What do we change?)

In addressing the first of these two suggested concepts, targeted questions can be used to address specific areas of service:

- Were you treated by someone whom you feel is competent?
- Were you made aware of your rights and options with regard to assistive technology?
- Were your needs met in a timely manner?
- Did you feel more in control of your life as a result of assistive technology service provision?
- Is there anything you can discuss about the process (e.g., what you would like to see changed)?

As recommended in the second concept, open-ended questions can be used when querying consumers regarding their satisfaction level. The following questions may help in discussing with the consumer the AT intervention and its success or failure across dimensions:

- Do you feel the intervention met your desired needs?
- Did the assistive technology meet expectations?
- If the intervention has not yet addressed your needs, are you confident it will in the future?
- Have your needs changed? (If so, the action plan needs to be reexamined.)
- Were your needs met in a timely manner?
- Was your request for information met appropriately?

Quality of Life

There are many definitions for quality of life. The World Health Organization (1947) defined *quality of life* as the achievement of a state of complete physical, mental, and social well-being, not just the absence of disease, impairment, or disability. According to contributors to the book *Quality of Life for Persons with Disabilities* (Goode, 1994), quality of life is the discrepancy between achieved and unmet needs and desires (as in Maslow's [1954] hierarchy of needs), an index of an individual's relationship with his or her environment, and one's sense of contentment and fulfillment. All definitions share the perspective that the construct *quality of life* is subjective and dynamic and that it has personal meaning for each individual according to his or her values, preferences, and goals within one or more environments. As such, it has many aspects for each person, and consumers may need assistance in defining their particular view of a high quality of life and the role they have for assistive technology in achieving it

(Scherer, 1996c). For some individuals who have not had any AT intervention, even the wrong intervention may seem wonderful and result in the consumer's subsequent satisfactory report. All stakeholders must ask and maintain an awareness of the subjectivity of this construct, as well as try not to impose their definition of a high quality of life on consumers.

To optimize the accuracy as well as fairness and objectivity of the measurement of quality of life, a blend of objective and subjective measures (known as mixed methods research/evaluation) is necessary.

CONCLUSIONS

The appropriate match of person and technology, as well as the demonstration of that appropriateness both in the short-term and over time, requires that the practitioner become knowledgeable about assessment tools and methods according to several different models.

The rehabilitation practitioner is a crucial resource for the continued assessment of an individual's functioning, enhancement of the person's ability to recognize and use support, and provision of links to opportunities for skill building. In addition, the practitioner can provide a valuable service by identifying potential mismatches of AT and individual. In turn, the frequency of nonuse or inappropriate use of ATs can be reduced and the disappointment and frustration that often accompany less than ideal use can be minimized. Assistive technologies are meant to be helpful and enhance functioning, and the practitioner needs to be involved at multiple levels in making this occur.

REFERENCES

Batavia, A. (1992). Assessing the function of functional assessment: A consumer perspective. *Disability and Rehabilitation 14*(3), 156–160.

Brown, D.L. (1996). Personal implications of functional electrical stimulation standing for older adolescents with spinal cord injuries. *Technology and Disability, 5*(3,4), 295–311.

Campbell-Heider, N., & Knapp, T.R. (1993). Toward a hierarchy of adaptation to biomedical technology. *Critical Care Nursing Quarterly, 16*(3), 42–50.

Crewe, N.M., & Dijkers, M. (1995). Functional assessment. In L.A. Cushman & M.J. Scherer (Eds), *Psychological assessment in physical rehabilitation* (pp. 101–144). Washington, DC: APA Books.

Cushman, L.A., & Scherer, M.J. (1995). *Psychological assessment in medical rehabilitation.* Washington, DC: APA Books.

Cushman, L.A., & Scherer, M.J. (1996). Measuring the relationship of assistive technology use, functional status over time, and consumer-therapist perceptions of ATs. *Assistive Technology, 8*(2), 103–109.

DeRuyter, F. (June, 1996). *Outcomes management in assistive technology.* Paper presented at the annual meeting of the Rehabilitation Engineering and Assistive Technology Society of North America (RESNA), Salt Lake City, UT.

Galvin, J.C, & Scherer, M.J. (Eds.). (1996). *Evaluating, selecting, and using appropriate assistive technology* (pp. 9, 15). Gaithersburg, MD: Aspen Publishers.

Goode, D. (Ed.). (1994). *Quality of life for persons with disabilities.* Cambridge, MA: Brookline Books.

Maslow, A.H. (1954). *Motivation and personality.* New York: Harper & Row.

Phillips, B., & Zhao, H. (1993). Predictors of assistive technology abandonment. *Assistive Technology, 5*, 36–45.

P.L. 101-336. (1990). The Americans with Disabilities Act.

Scherer, M.J. (1986). Values in the creation, prescription, and use of technological aids and assistive devices for people with physical disabilities (Doctoral dissertation, University of Rochester, 1986, and final report to the National Science Foundation). *Dissertation Abstracts International, 48*(01), 49. (University Microfilms No. ADG87–08247)

Scherer, M.J. (1991). Matching Person and Technology (MPT) Model and accompanying assessment instruments. Rochester, NY: Author.

Scherer, M.J. (1996a). *Living in the state of stuck: How technology impacts the lives of people with disabilities* (2nd ed.). Cambridge, MA: Brookline Books.

Scherer, M.J. (1996b). Introduction to outcomes measurement. *Technology and Disability, 5*(4), 283–284.

Scherer, M.J. (1996c). Outcomes of assistive technology use on quality of life. *Disability and Rehabilitation, 18*(9), 439–448.

Scherer, M.J., & Frisina, D.R. (1994). Applying the Matching People and Technologies Model to individuals with hearing loss: What people say they want and need from assistive technologies. *Technology and Disability, 3*(1), 62–68.

Scherer, M.J., & Galvin, J.C. (1994). Matching people with technology. *Rehabilitation Management, 7*(2), 128–130.

Scherer, M.J., & McKee, B.G. (1989). But will the assistive technology device be used? *Proceeding of the 12th Annual Conference: Technology for the Next Decade* (pp. 356–357). Washington, DC: RESNA.

Smith, R.O. (1993). Assessing the impact of assistive technology using OT FACT version 2.0. *Proceedings of RESNA '93*, Arlington, VA: Rehabilitation Engineering and Assistive Technology Society of North America.

Smith, R.O. (1995). *OT FACT software system for integrating and reporting occupational therapy functional assessment, v2.0. [computer software and manual].* Rockville, MD: American Occupational Therapy Association.

Smith, R.O. (1996). Measuring the outcomes of assistive technology: Challenge and innovation. *Assistive Technology, 8*(2), 71–81.

Technology-Related Assistance of Individuals with Disabilities Act of 1988, Pub. L. No. 100–407.

U.S. Census Bureau. (1990). *National health interview survey on assistive devices (NHIS–AD).* Washington, DC: Author.

Warren, C.G. (1993). Cost effectiveness and efficiency in assistive technology service delivery. *Assistive Technology, 5*, 61–65.

World Health Organization. (1947). *Constitution of the World Health Organization.* New York: Author.

Description and Display of Selected Functional Assessment and Outcome Measures in Physical Rehabilitation

CATEGORIES OF FUNCTIONAL ASSESSMENT INSTRUMENTS TO MEASURE DISABILITY:

A. Comprehensive Functional Assessment Instruments
B. Activities of Daily Living (ADL) Instruments
C. Outpatient Functional Status Monitoring Instrument
D. Cognitive Function and Affect Measures
E. Functional Communication Instruments
F. Tests of Sensorimotor Function
G. Test of Hand Function
H. Medical Diagnosis–Specific Functional Assessment Instruments
I. Functional Assessment Instruments Used with Specific Age Groups

CATEGORIES OF FUNCTIONAL ASSESSMENT INSTRUMENTS TO MEASURE SOCIETAL LIMITATION:

J. Family Functioning
K. Vocational Function
L. Community Integration
M. Quality of Life

Appendix A

Table of Contents

CATEGORIES OF FUNCTIONAL ASSESSMENT INSTRUMENTS TO MEASURE DISABILITY

A. Comprehensive Functional Assessment Instruments

Edinburgh Rehabilitation Status Scale

The Edinburgh Rehabilitation Status Scale (ERSS) (Affleck, Aitken, Hunter, McGuire, & Roy, 1988) (see Exhibit A–1) is a global "measure of medicosocial dysfunction" that contains four subscales: (1) independence/dependence, (2) activity/inactivity, (3) social integration/isolation, and (4) effect of symptoms on lifestyles (p. 230). "Each subscale has eight grades, 0–7," covering all grades of severity (with higher numbers indicating greater severity) (p. 230). The time scale for observation is seven days unless otherwise stated (see rater's manual). It was originally applied to a group of 150 rehabilitation patients with multiple diagnoses. Sensitivity to change was documented, and further study showed correlations of –0.76 and 0.87 with the Barthel Index (Mahoney & Barthel, 1965) and the PULSES Profile (Moskowitz & McCann, 1957), respectively. Reliability studies produced correlations of 0.65 to 0.97.

Mattison, Aitken, and Prescott (1991) studied the interrelationships of the ERSS, Barthel Index, and PULSES Profile by assessing simultaneously 364 outpatients with physical disabilities. Using Spearman rank-order correlation coefficients, Mattison and colleagues found strong overall correlations among the three sets of scores (0.59 to –0.69) with more variable correlations within some sets of subscores. They concluded that all three instruments were indeed measuring physical disability, albeit with some variability in component items. Mattison, Aitken, and Prescott (1992) extended this work to a study of 129 outpatients with neurological impairments and physical disabilities. Forty-six percent of the subjects also had mental retardation. Results of the study revealed that the ERSS was superior to the Barthel Index and the PULSES Profile in differentiating the subsets with and without mental retardation in a population who all had physical disability.

In another study conducted in New Zealand, the ERSS was compared with the Functional Independence Measure (FIM^{SM}) (Granger, Hamilton, Keith, Zielezny, & Sherwin, 1986) to predict hours of care needed by 75 persons with disabilities and neurological impairments. Results showed that both ERSS and FIM^{SM} scores "correlate well with hours of care required but their association with hours of supervision is poor" (Disler, Roy, & Smith, 1993, p. 139).

A rater's manual, information checklist, and record sheet are available from the Rehabilitation Studies Unit, Princess Margaret Rose Hospital, Edinburgh, Scotland EH10 7ED.

REFERENCES

Affleck, J.W., Aitken, R.C., Hunter, J.A., McGuire, R.J., & Roy, C.W. (1988). Rehabilitation status: A measure of medicosocial dysfunction. *The Lancet, 1*, 230–233.

Disler, P.B., Roy, C.W., & Smith, B.P. (1993). Predicting hours of care needed. *Archives of Physical Medicine and Rehabilitation, 74*(2), 139–143.

Granger, C.V., Hamilton, B.B., Keith, R.A., Zielezny, M., & Sherwin, F.S. (1986). Advances in functional assessment for medical rehabilitation. *Topics in Geriatric Rehabilitation, 1*, 59–74.

Mahoney, F.J., & Barthel, D.W. (1965). Functional evaluation: The Barthel Index. *Maryland State Medical Journal, 14*(1), 61–65.

Mattison, P.G., Aitken, R.C.B., & Prescott, R. (1991). Rehabilitation status—the relationship between the Edinburgh Rehabilitation Status Scale (ERSS), Barthel Index, and PULSES profile. *International Disability Studies, 13*(1), 9–11.

Mattison, P.G., Aitken, R.C.B., & Prescott, R.J. (1992). Rehabilitation status in multiple handicap. *Archives of Physical Medicine and Rehabilitation, 73*(10), 926–929.

Moskowitz, E., & McCann, C.B. (1957). Classification of disability in the chronically ill and aging. *Journal of Chronic Diseases, 5*(3), 342–346.

Exhibit A–1 Edinburgh Rehabilitation Status Scale

The Four Subscales

I. *SUPP: SUPPORT SUBSCALE*

Subscale orientation: This subscale describes the *frequency and extent to which the patient relies on others* for self-care, economic arrangements (e.g., rent, money management), and administration of any medicine or treatment required. The patient's ability to dress, toilet, and feed himself or herself will be taken into account. Help may be supplied by relatives or friends or by regular visits from professionals, such as nurses and home helps. There may be attendance at a day hospital or center, or the patient may live in residential care where assistance is provided.

0 = Independent. Has a living place and is economically stable. May have aids or appliances or has successfully used an adapted house. Not requiring help from spouse, relatives, or friends. Gets medical attention and any necessary treatment from his or her general practitioner. Responsible for own medication and self-care irrespective of the standard achieved.

1 = Intermittently dependent. Usually independent but has required outpatient consultation or occasionally has had help within the time scale—irregularly or at patient's initiative.

2 = Intermediate grade.

3 = Supported by staff, relatives, or friends. Needs help of others with aids or in other ways. Lives in own home or in lodgings or supported accommodation with the understanding that he or she can cope with some domestic and economic responsibilities. Regular visits from professionals (e.g., nurse, occupational therapist, home help) and/or other arranged contacts may be needed. Day hospital or day center may be used. Relatives may provide an unusual amount of support, but this will be at long time intervals (i.e., the patient is unsupported for several hours at a time). When alone, he or she will be able to make a hot drink and answer the door and telephone. (See Practice Note.)

4 = Intermediate grade.

5 = Monitored out of hospital. Provided with essential supervision (i.e., for toilet, moving around the house). This may be in a residential home with non-nursing personnel or at home with a relative or other person who carries the overall domestic responsibilities and perhaps shares such monitoring with staff, where, for example, the patient attends a day center.

6 = Intermediate grade (e.g., in hospital ward but makes major contribution to self-care).

7 = In hospital or at home having full nursing monitoring and care.

Practice Note

The scores should describe the degree of support accepted from others and the extent to which the patient fails to cope or requires to be monitored. They should indicate what actually happens (i.e., the services accepted), not assumed potential capacities.

II. *INACT: INACTIVITY (OCCUPATION AND LEISURE) SUBSCALES*

Subscale orientation: This subscale assesses the *ability to initiate, sustain, and effectively perform* the activities involved in occupations, domesticity, and leisure—physical and intellectual. If the patient or client is not employed, his or her other initiatives will be considered. There is no emphasis on paid employment, nor on the person's type of employment. All, including housewives and retired persons, will be rated on their effective purposeful activity over the whole day. The consequences of some syndromes are expressed in failure to undertake activities, whereas others result in ineffectiveness. This may occur because of difficulties with mobility or dexterity or as a result of weakness, lethargy, or psychological factors.

Leisure activities, insofar as they keep the individual occupied, should be considered in relation to this subscale, whereas other aspects come under the social integration subscale.

0 = Within the time scale has consistently undertaken, effectively and without difficulty, the physical and mental tasks involved in occupational, domestic, and leisure purposes.

1 = Intermittently inactive or occasionally ineffective. Usually active but occasionally within the time scale has needed or taken time off work or failed to maintain nonwork activities (e.g., self-care), which are usually accomplished and/or pastimes or interests.

2 = Intermediate grade.

3 = Modified activity. Effectiveness is impaired. Levels of activities have been modified by making them less responsible or reduced in time or at a more leisurely pace. May have a sympathetic employer, special arrangements, or sheltered employment. Household work and leisure activities similarly modified. (See Practice Note.)

4 = Intermediate grade.

5 = Limited activities. Inefficient or needs to have arrangements made or needs encouragement to sustain tasks or routine activities. Leisure activities similarly restricted.

6 = Intermediate grade.

7 = Very restricted or very ineffective. Unoccupied or essentially inactive. Cannot sustain purposeful activities.

Practice Note

Where a patient's levels of activity in employment, domestic work, and leisure differ, the score given should reflect the total amount of purposeful effective activity within the time scale.

continues

2

Exhibit A–1 continued

III. *ISOL: SOCIAL INTEGRATION/ISOLATION SUBSCALE*
Subscale orientation: This is a social behavioral subscale *for involvement in roles, relationships, a social network, and communications*. The degree and frequency of participation and sharing are rated. This will be done by assessing the frequency and ease of social functioning (e.g., in conversation), cooperation in routine contacts and tasks, and the use of leisure.

Social or psychological problems associated with impairment or coincidental with them and that increase isolation or alienation, will be considered (e.g., after disfigurement or with conspicuous impairment). Avoidance of new relationships may be noted to restrict the individual to relatives and old friends who may be less emotionally demanding.

Some patients achieve a degree of social integration by talking to visitors, telephoning, or exchanging letters.

0 = Within the time scale period, he or she has interacted frequently, competently, and appropriately with a varied range of people. When in hospital this level is not usually possible.
1 = Occasional difficulties. Intermittent problems in social integration. In certain situations fails to participate; or fails to produce the appropriate social response; or may avoid or reject or be rejected from some sustained or intimate relationships.
2 = Intermediate grade.
3 = Noticeably limited participation. Impairments limit social integration or impose disadvantages by restricting contacts or making personal relationships difficult. Participation may be restricted to family and old friends and people in certain special situations (e.g., tradesmen or day care acquaintances and staff). Psychological impairments may show a failure to deal adequately with everyday social encounters, avoidance of new contacts, or very superficial participation. (See Practice Notes.)
4 = Intermediate grade (e.g., little spontaneous participation or any passive participation in social situations).
5 = Severely restricted contacts and relationships. Has dealt with certain few individuals only (e.g., close family and professional staff) *or* may be uncommunicative, unresponsive, intermittently disruptive, or otherwise socially incompetent.
6 = Intermediate grade.
7 = Very isolated and/or almost constantly alienated.

Practice Notes

1. Frequency of contacts and competence/incompetence is rated excluding any assumed potential that might occur by other opportunities.
2. Premorbid difficulties or levels of functioning should not influence the score, which should rate the current level.
3. Contacts by telephoning or letter writing may merit a better grade.

IV. *EFFSYM: EFFECTS OF CURRENT SYMPTOMS SUBSCALE*
Subscale orientation: This is an assessment of the extent to which the *severity and constancy of symptoms and impairments affect the individual's lifestyle*. The frequency and severity of the symptoms/signs, difficulties and distress that occur, and extent to which they determine the life pattern are noted. The effects are rated from the patient's subjective experiences, the clinical observations, and behavior that is noticeable to the patient's friends and acquaintances. Drug side effects may be of relevance.

0 = Symptom free within the time scale. This level is given even if a simple drug regimen is required to maintain it.
1 = Occasional or mild symptoms. Medications may be onerous and/or aids or appliances, though unobtrusive, may impinge on freedom.
2 = Intermediate grade (e.g., as in "3" below but symptoms only intermittent).
3 = Noticeable but moderate effects of symptoms/signs within the time scale. Clinical assessment reveals moderate effects of dysfunction (e.g., appreciable difficulty with mobility or dexterity, pain, dyspnea, or some psychological impairments or problems). Evidence of patient role is noticeable to friends and acquaintances (e.g., symptoms, aids). However, the patient's daily routine is accomplished without much difficulty, though work or leisure may be interrupted by treatment, need to adjust appliances, and so forth. (See Practice Notes.)
4 = Intermediate grade (e.g., moderate symptom effects but difficulty in maintaining a functioning routine *or* severe symptoms/signs but routine continues well, such as managing efficiently in a wheelchair).
5 = Obviously severe symptoms (including behavioral problems). The symptom effects are constant or nearly so, and they will often be disturbing or distressing to the patient and his or her caretakers. These effects will be seen by others as they will obviously interfere with the patient's lifestyle. In spite of this she or he manages to cooperate in an agreed regimen, probably with difficulty.
6 = Intermediate grade.
7 = Incapacitated. Life pattern is determined almost entirely by symptoms and/or medical or nursing needs.

Practice Notes

1. Current symptoms only are assessed whether or not they are associated with the original diagnosis.
2. It is important to avoid halo effects of behavior already scored and/or diagnosis already given (e.g., dependency is not necessarily at the same level as symptomatology).
3. Prognosis, which implies potential, must be disregarded when making the assessment.
4. Note special reference to wheelchair users in Grade 4.

Source: Courtesy of R.C. Aitken, Rehabilitation Studies Unit, Princess Margaret Rose Hospital, Edinburgh, Scotland.

Functional Independence Measure

The Functional Independence Measure (FIM^SM) (see Exhibit A–2) was designed to meet a longstanding need for a minimum uniform data set that would document the severity of patient disability and the outcomes of medical rehabilitation (Granger, Hamilton, Keith, Zielesky, & Sherwin, 1986; Granger & Gresham, 1993). A task force appointed by the American Academy of Physical Medicine and Rehabilitation and the American Congress of Rehabilitation Medicine developed the minimum data set with grant support from the National Institute on Disability and Rehabilitation Research (*Guide for the Uniform Data Set for Medical Rehabilitation [Adult FIM^SM]*, 1993; *Questions and Answers about the Functional Independence Measure [Adult FIM^SM]*, 1993). The FIM^SM—the outgrowth of this project—measures progress or lack of change in patients in rehabilitation programs.

The FIM^SM is a measure usable by any trained health care professional regardless of discipline and has been judged acceptable by clinicians in the medical rehabilitation field (*Guide for the Uniform Data Set for Medical Rehabilitation [Adult FIM^SM]*, 1993; *Questions and Answers about the Functional Independence Measure [Adult FIM^SM]*, 1993). The instrument is currently used in more than 700 facilities in the United States and throughout the world. A guide for use has been developed to explain the underlying principles, describe coding of the data set, and define levels of function and their scores. The appendixes to the guide offer sample cases, follow-up instructions and a sample follow-up interview, *International Classification of Diseases, Ninth Edition, Clinical Modification (ICD-9-CM)* coding policy, answer sheets for sample case studies, references, impairment group codes, and blank coding sheets (*Guide for the Uniform Data Set for Medical Rehabilitation [Adult FIM^SM]*, 1993; *Questions and Answers about the Functional Independence Measure [Adult FIM^SM]*, 1993; U.S. Dept. HHS, 1994). The United States UDSMR^SM database contains more than 1 million patient records.

Nature of Items. The task force reviewed 36 published and unpublished functional assessment instruments and selected the most common and useful functional assessment items. The most appropriate rating scale was also chosen (*Guide for the Uniform Data Set for Medical Rehabilitation [Adult FIM^SM]*, 1993; *Questions and Answers about the Functional Independence Measure [Adult FIM^SM]*, 1993). This comprehensive instrument captures data on self-care, sphincter management, transfers, locomotion, communication, and social cognition.

Scaling Categories, Including Biometric Properties. A seven-point scale is used to measure gradations in independent and dependent behaviors. The scale is divided according to a *no helper* category (levels six and seven) where no

other person is required to help with the activity and a *helper* category (levels one through five) where the client needs minimal to total assistance from another person to accomplish the activity. Scores range from a high of 126 to a low of 18, where high scores indicate higher levels of independence. It is unweighted (i.e., each item is scored by the same method). Scaling is ordinal and consists of the following: 1 = total assist, 2 = maximal assist, 3 = moderate assist, 4 = minimal assist, 5 = supervision (or setup), 6 = modified independence, and 7 = complete independence. Definitions for each level of dependence/independence are given according to functional label (i.e., eating, grooming).

In addition, client demographic characteristics, diagnoses, impairment groups, length of hospital inpatient stay, and hospital charges are recorded (*Guide for the Uniform Data Set for Medical Rehabilitation [Adult FIM^SM]*, 1993; *Questions and Answers about the Functional Independence Measure [Adult FIM^SM]*, 1993).

Standardization. Results of some studies have demonstrated that the FIM^SM and the Patient Evaluation Conference System probably measure the same motor skills (Silverstein, Fisher, Kilgore, Harley, & Harvey, 1992). Further studies are needed to establish which functional assessment instruments, if any, are measuring the same dimensions of performance.

Validity. The FIM^SM has been tested for validity in more than 50 facilities across the United States and found to have face validity. Pilot, trial, and implementation studies since 1984 have assisted the developers in establishing face validity (Granger, Cotter, Hamilton, & Fiedler, 1993; Granger & Hamilton, 1992, 1993, 1994; Granger, Hamilton, Fiedler, & Hens, 1990; Hamilton, Laughlin, Fiedler, & Granger, 1994; Linacre, Heinemann, Wright, Granger, & Hamilton, 1994; Ottenbacher & Fiedler, 1995; Segal, Ditunno, & Staas, 1993).

Reliability. Reliability has also been determined. Interrater reliability was studied in New South Wales in 1990 and found to be .97 among a multidisciplinary staff who had been involved in training. On individual items, there was a high correlation ($r = .85$) on ADL items, and a range of .721 to .846 was found on the five items addressing communication and social cognition (Lee, 1992).

Sensitivity. The FIM^SM is not sensitive enough to measure change in disability among some patient populations (e.g., patients with high-level spinal cord injury [C4-5 and C5-6], chronic pain sufferers, and some patients with traumatic brain dysfunction). This limitation has led to the development of the Functional Assessment Measure to expand the 18-item FIM^SM by 12 items (Ditunno, 1992; Hall, 1992; Hall & Johnston, 1994). Validity has been established (Hall, Hamilton, Gordon, & Zasler, 1993). When determining the validity of the FIM^SM subscales for communication and social cognition, the findings of Davidoff, Roth, Haughton, and

Ardner (1990) suggest that these subscales should not, and were not intended to, substitute for comprehensive neuropsychological assessment in persons with spinal cord injury and cognitive dysfunction.

Sensibility. The FIM℠ is a practical instrument to use. Time required to complete an assessment is approximately 20 minutes. The items are displayed on one page, and scores can be recorded easily and observed at three or more different points in time: admission, discharge, and follow-up. Keypunch of data can be accomplished easily; comparisons among and between programs also can be made. Interobserver reliability can be established through uniform training of personnel. This training is available, and credentialing in use of the FIM℠ can be arranged through the Uniform Data System office at the State University of New York, University at Buffalo, Center for Functional Assessment Research (232 Parker Hall, Buffalo, NY 14214, Telephone: 716-829-2076).

Intended Use. The FIM℠ is constructed to assess severity of disability in a uniform and reliable manner. Documentation consists of observing and recording what a person *actually* does, not what he or she ought to be able to do. Data can be used by clinicians to measure individual functional progress over time, administrators to evaluate rehabilitation programs, and researchers to study functional attributes in relation to outcomes of rehabilitation programs. Data have been used to determine the amount of care needed to achieve and maintain a certain quality of life. When used to identify rehabilitation needs of individuals with stroke, Oczkowski and Barreca (1993) found that "1) impairment variables alone are insufficient as prognostic indicators of outcome; 2) absolute admission FIM score, not the change in the FIM score is the best predictor of outcome disability and place of discharge; and 3) subgroups of stroke survivors with differing rehabilitation needs can be identified" (p. 1291). The FIM℠ allowed these investigators to classify persons with stroke according to their needs.

Strengths. The FIM℠ is short, easy to administer, and valid, and it can be administered by any credentialed member of the rehabilitation team. One of the unique characteristics of the FIM℠ is the ability to measure areas of communication and social cognition.

Limitations. Although designed to be scored by any rehabilitation team member, some disciplines may have more difficulty than others in assessing particular items on the FIM℠. For instance, a nurse is more likely to assess sphincter management, whereas a speech-language pathologist is more likely to determine communication status and a physical therapist more likely to assess mobility. Therefore assessment is commonly divided among nurses and therapists. Adamovich (1992) found that nurses assigned significantly higher scores than did speech-language pathologists when rating communication of patients with left hemisphere damage. The FIM℠ is a minimum data set. Thus it does not incorporate all activities that would be possible or that might need to be measured for specific clinical purposes or individuals with special problems.

Examples of Use as Cited in Literature. The FIM℠ has been used extensively in the United States and Australia. As a result, both benefits and criticisms of the FIM℠ have been noted. Forty-one occupational therapy (OT) departments in Australia were surveyed with a return of responses from 36 (88% response rate). Because the use of the FIM℠ is considered a threat to the professional domain of the OT, in addition to the fact that it can be administered by any trained health professional and it focuses on activities of daily living, it is interesting to note that the use of the FIM℠ in OT departments quadrupled within three years. Therapists, however, were not totally happy with the FIM℠ or with various modifications of the Barthel Index, especially in the areas of communication and social cognition as well as ordinal scale design. Some OTs also criticized the lack of measurement of performance of activities of daily living in the community (Marosszeky, 1993)

The following are examples of findings from other studies:

1. Outcome can be predicted. Patients with functional scores greater than 100 could be discharged home regardless of impairment depending on type of living arrangement or social support. For patients whose admission scores were less than 65, the presence of a spouse was critical to discharge (Lee, Durkin, & Winsor, 1992).

2. Number of hours of care needed by a person with a disability cannot be predicted. Findings suggested that neither the FIM℠ nor the Edinburgh Rehabilitation Status Scale were good measures to determine the number of hours of supervision needed by subjects who are cognitively impaired (Affleck, Aitken, Hunter, McGuire, & Roy, 1988).

3. Patients with stroke can be identified according to discharge groups. Statistically significant differences in FIM℠ scores were found between groups of patients with stroke discharged home alone, home with relatives, to hostel or special accommodation, and to nursing home. Thus it was concluded that the FIM℠ may be useful for determining discharge destination for persons with stroke (Hunter, Rawicki, & deGraaf, 1992).

4. A FIM℠/Function Related Groups case mix classification system for medical rehabilitation—using four predictor variables, including diagnosis leading to disability, admission scores for motor and cognitive functional status subscales as measured by the FIM℠, patient age, and 53 Function Related Groups—may

represent a solution for classifying medical rehabilitation patients for payment, facility planning, and research investigating rehabilitation variables, such as outcome, quality, and cost (Stineman, Escarce, Goin, Hamilton, Granger, & Williams, 1994).

5. Categories of supervision were identified when combinations of functional assessment item, subscale, domain, and full-scale scores were used in a population of persons after traumatic brain injury. The purpose of the study was to predict (1) need for assistance of specific physical care tasks according to minutes of another person's help per day in the home and (2) subject's level of satisfaction with life in general. The latter prediction was made with the Brief Symptom Inventory. Categories of supervision identified were constant (all the time), periodic (daily or weekly), or not at all (Granger, Divan, & Fiedler, 1995).

Comments. The recent development and widespread use of the FIM[SM] indicates that this instrument may become the gold standard as a screening instrument on admission to medical rehabilitation and the outcome measure on discharge. Further research is needed to establish standardization of measures, as well as validity, reliability, and sensitivity for specific patient populations, before the FIM[SM] is adopted as *the measure* for reimbursement and program evaluation. Research conducted by the Rehabilitation Research and Training Center on Functional Assessment and Evaluation of Rehabilitation Outcomes at the University at Buffalo will add to the body of knowledge necessary to base health care decisions on this measure. The instrument is similar to the Barthel Index in practicality but has the added advantages of eliciting more information and giving specific definitions of measurement domains. The application of Rasch analysis to FIM[SM] scores is discussed in Chapter 3.

REFERENCES

Adamovich, B. (1992). Pitfalls in functional assessment: A comparison of FIM[SM] ratings by speech-language pathologists and nurses. *NeuroRehabilitation, 2*(4), 42–51.

Affleck, J.W., Aitken, R.C., Hunter, J.A., McGuire, R.J., & Roy, C.W. (1988). Rehabilitation status: A measure of medicosocial dysfunction. *The Lancet, 1,* 230–233.

Davidoff, G.N., Roth, E.J., Haughton, J.S., & Ardner, M.S. (1990). Cognitive dysfunction in spinal cord injury patients: Sensitivity of the Functional Independence Measure subscales vs neuropsychologic assessment. *Archives of Physical Medicine and Rehabilitation, 71*(5), 326–329.

Ditunno, J. Jr. (1992). Functional assessment measures in CNS trauma. *Journal of Neurotrauma, 9* (suppl 1), S301–S305.

Granger, C.V., Cotter, A.C., Hamilton, B.B., & Fiedler, R.C. (1993). Functional assessment scales: A study of persons after stroke. *Archives of Physical Medicine and Rehabilitation, 74*(2), 133–138.

Granger, C.V., Divan, N., & Fiedler, R.C. (1995). Functional assessment scales: A study of persons after traumatic brain injury. *American Journal of Physical Medicine and Rehabilitation, 74*(2), 107–113.

Granger, C.V., & Gresham, G.E. (1993). Functional assessment in rehabilitation medicine: Introduction and brief background. *Physical Medicine and Rehabilitation Clinics of North America, 4*(3), 417–423.

Granger, C.V., & Hamilton, B.B. (1992). UDS report: The uniform data system for medical rehabilitation report of first admissions for 1990. *American Journal of Physical Medicine and Rehabilitation, 71*(2), 108–113.

Granger, C.V., & Hamilton, B.B. (1993). The uniform data system for medical rehabilitation report of first admissions for 1991. *American Journal of Physical Medicine and Rehabilitation, 72*(1), 33–38.

Granger, C.V., & Hamilton, B.B. (1994). The uniform data system for medical rehabilitation report of first admissions for 1992. *American Journal of Physical Medicine and Rehabilitation, 73*(1), 51–55.

Granger, C.V., Hamilton, B.B., Fiedler, R.C., & Hens, M.M. (1990). Functional assessment scales: A study of persons with multiple sclerosis. *Archives of Physical Medicine and Rehabilitation, 71*(11), 870–875.

Granger, C.V., Hamilton, B.B., Keith, R.A., Zielesky, M., & Sherwin, F.S. (1986). Advances in functional assessment for medical rehabilitation. *Topics in Geriatric Rehabilitation, 1 (3),* 59–74.

Guide for the uniform data set for medical rehabilitation (Adult FIM[SM]), version 4.0 (1993). Buffalo: State University of New York.

Hall, K.M. (1992). Overview of functional assessment scales in brain injury rehabilitation. *NeuroRehabilitation, 2,* 98–113.

Hall, K.M., Hamilton, B.B., Gordon, W.A., & Zasler, N.A. (1993). Characteristics and comparisons of functional assessment indices: Disability Rating Scale, Functional Independence Measure, and Functional Assessment Measure. *Journal of Head Trauma Rehabilitation, 8*(2), 60–74.

Hall, K.M., & Johnston, M.V. (1994). Outcomes evaluation in traumatic brain injury rehabilitation. Part II. Measurement tools for a nationwide data system. *Archives of Physical Medicine and Rehabilitation, 75*(12-S), SC10–18.

Hamilton, B.B., Laughlin, J.A., Fiedler, R.C., & Granger, C.V. (1994). Inter-rater reliability of the 7-level functional independence measure (FIM[SM]). *Scandinavian Journal of Rehabilitation Medicine, 26*(3), 115–119.

Hunter, R.A., Rawicki, H.B., deGraaf, S. (1992). Functional Independence Measurement in Stroke Patients. Assessment of Use as Predictor of Discharge Destination. In *Programs and Abstracts of the Twelfth Annual Scientific Meeting of the Australasian College of Rehabilitation Medicine* (p. 49), Melbourne, Australia.

Lee, L. (1992). Measuring to Manage in the Real World: Non-acute Case Mix Experience in the Illawarra. In *Programs and Abstracts of the Twelfth Annual Scientific Meeting of the Australasian College of Rehabilitation Medicine* (p. 33), Melbourne, Australia.

Lee, R., Durkin, J.T., & Winsor, A. (1992). The Functional Independence Measure (FIM^SM) To Predict Rehabilitation Outcome in an Inpatient Rehabilitation Unit. In *Programs and Abstracts of the Twelfth Annual Scientific Meeting of the Australasian College of Rehabilitation Medicine* (p. 79), Melbourne, Australia.

Linacre, J.M., Heinemann, A.W., Wright, B.D., Granger, C.V., & Hamilton, B.B. (1994). The structure and stability of the Functional Independence Measure. *Archives of Physical Medicine and Rehabilitation, 75*(2), 127–132.

Marosszeky, J.E. (1993). The uniform data system from an international perspective. *Physical Medicine and Rehabilitation Clinics of North America, 4*(3), 571-586.

Oczkowski, W.J., & Barreca, S. (1993). The Functional Independence Measure: Its use to identify rehabilitation needs in stroke survivors. *Archives of Physical Medicine and Rehabilitation, 74*(12), 1291–1300.

Ottenbacher, K.J., & Fiedler, R.C. (1995). The uniform data system for medical rehabilitation report of first admissions for 1993. *American Journal of Physical Medicine and Rehabilitation, 74*(1), 62–66.

Questions and answers about the Functional Independence Measure (Adult FIM^SM), version 4.0 (1993). Buffalo: State University of New York.

Segal, M.E., Ditunno, J.F., & Staas, W.E. (1993). Interinstitutional agreement of individual Functional Independence Measure (FIM^SM) items measured at two sites on one sample of SCI patients. *Paraplegia, 31*(10), 622–631.

Silverstein, B.S., Fisher, W.P., Kilgore, K.M., Harley, J.P., & Harvey, R.F. (1992). Applying psychometric criteria to functional assessment in medical rehabilitation. II. Defining interval measures. *Archives of Physical Medicine and Rehabilitation, 73*(6), 507–518.

Stineman, M.G., Escarce, J.J., Goin, J.E., Hamilton, B.B., Granger, C.V., & Williams, S.V. (1994). A case-mix classification system for medical rehabilitation. *Medical Care, 32*(4), 366–379.

U.S. Department of Health and Human Services, Publication No. 89-1260, HHS-PHS. Health Care Financing Administration, 1994. *The International Classification of Diseases, Ninth Revision, Clinical Modification* (ICD-9-CM). Rockville, MD: Author.

Exhibit A–2 Functional Independence Measure

FIM℠ Instrument

L E V E L S	7 Complete Independence (Timely, Safely) 6 Modified Independence (Device)	**NO HELPER**

	Modified Dependence
	  5 Supervision
	  4 Minimal Assist (Subject = 75% +)
	  3 Moderate Assist (Subject = 50% +)
	
	Complete Dependence
	  2 Maximal Assist (Subject = 25% +)
	  1 Total Assist (Subject = 0% +)
		HELPER

	ADMIT	DISCHARGE	FOLLOW-UP
Self-Care			
A. Eating			
B. Grooming			
C. Bathing			
D. Dressing—Upper Body			
E. Dressing—Lower Body			
F. Toileting			
Sphincter Control			
G. Bladder Management			
H. Bowel Management			
Transfers			
I. Bed, Chair, Wheelchair			
J. Toilet			
K. Tub, Shower			
Locomotion	Walk / Wheelchair / Both	Walk / Wheelchair / Both	Walk / Wheelchair / Both
L. Walk/Wheelchair			
M. Stairs			
Motor Subtotal Score			
Communication	Auditory / Visual / Both / Vocal / Nonvocal / Both	Auditory / Visual / Both / Vocal / Nonvocal / Both	Auditory / Visual / Both / Vocal / Nonvocal / Both
N. Comprehension			
O. Expression			
Social Cognition			
P. Social Interaction			
Q. Problem Solving			
R. Memory			
Cognitive Subtotal Score			
Total FIM			

Note: Leave no blanks; enter 1 if patient not testable due to risk.

Source: Reprinted with permission from Uniform Data System for Medical Rehabilitation, a division of U B Foundation Activities, Inc. *Guide for the Uniform Data Set for Medical Rehabilitation (Adult FIM℠) Version 4.0.* © 1993, State University of New York, Buffalo, New York.

The Functional Life Scale and Its Adaptations (LORS, LORS–II, LORS–IIB, LADS, LORS–III)

The Functional Life Scale (FLS) (Sarno, Sarno, & Levita, 1973) (see Table A-1) was designed to "provide a quantitative measure of an individual's ability to participate in all of the basic activities which are customary for the majority of human beings" (p. 214). It consists of 44 items in five categories: 14 on cognition; 7, activities of daily living; 8, activities in the home; 9, outside activities; and 6, social interaction (including vocational status). The original article in which the authors presented and described this instrument (Sarno et al., 1973) reproduces the entire scale and scoring format. Actual performance, not capacity, is measured. The FLS requires a community, not a hospital setting, in which to be used because of the broad range of functional domains. It can be administered by a trained interviewer/rater (who need not be a physician).

Each of the 44 items on the FLS is rated, where appropriate, for "self-initiation, frequency, speed and overall efficiency" (Sarno et al., 1973, p. 216) on a continuum of zero to four. Subscores are important because the same overall score can be achieved by different combinations of subscores. Reliability and internal consistency were established by 11 observers on 25 patients with a variety of disabilities. Videotaped interviews were used, and nonparametric statistics showed highly significant correlations. Concurrent validity was tested by comparison with independent expert-clinician assessments.

The FLS was used in a controlled trial of drug treatment for Alzheimer's disease (Wilcock et al., 1993). Because of its exemplary standardization, the FLS has been listed in several reviews (Fleming, 1991; Gresham & Labi, 1984; Kelley, Kawamoto, & Rubenstein, 1991; Unsworth, 1993).

The Level of Rehabilitation Scale (LORS) (Carey & Posavac, 1978) was adapted from the FLS as an instrument for use in physical medicine and rehabilitation program evaluation (i.e., a measure for functional improvement between admission and discharge, maintenance of functional gains, relative contributions of rehabilitation interventions and spontaneous recovery, and as a basic research instrument). After reviewing a number of previous evaluation approaches, Cary and Posavac (1978) chose the FLS as the basis for the LORS. The five content subscales were retained, but the four dimensions of performance were dropped.

The format of the LORS is given in the original article in which the instrument is first presented and described (Carey & Posavac, 1978). Inter-rater reliability was established, and a pilot evaluation study of 69 patients with stroke, admitted to inpatient rehabilitation, was done. The results showed improvement between admission and discharge, an inability to differentiate the effect of rehabilitation interventions from spontaneous recovery, and maintenance of functional gains at the 4½-month follow-up. Numerous inferences regarding program evaluation were possible from the results obtained.

The LORS was used in two major clinical studies of stroke patients (Schmidt et al., 1986; Wood-Dauphinee, Williams, & Shapiro, 1990), as well as in a study of chronicity and family/patient interaction in a Japanese schizophrenic population (Nojima, 1989). In addition, the LORS was included in several reviews of rehabilitation program evaluation methodologies (Gonnella, 1992; Gresham & Labi, 1984).

In 1982, a revision of the LORS was published (Carey & Posavac, 1982). Termed the LORS–II, the subscales used were for the three major domains of activities of daily living, mobility, and communication. Comparison studies, with program evaluation guidelines of the Commission for the Accreditation of Rehabilitation Facilities, were carried out. The LORS–II was used in a major study of functional gains made by 6,194 rehabilitation patients in 22 facilities in 1985 and 1986 (Carey, Seibert, & Posavac, 1988). Subsequent revisions of the LORS (e.g., LORS–II, LORS–IIB) and their use in the LORS American Data System (LADS) are discussed in detail by Gonnella in her comprehensive chapter on rehabilitation program evaluation (Gonnella, 1992). She also describes the Rehabilitation Outpatient Evaluation Scales component of the LADS System. Carey and colleagues have also written extensively about the development of this system (Carey, 1990; Carey & Posavac, 1982; Carey & Seibert, 1988). Currently, the LORS–III is part of the Formations' Outcome System and is no longer used as such. The Formations' Outcome System is available from Formations in Health Care, Inc., 1144 West Wrightwood Ave., Chicago, IL 60614.

REFERENCES

Carey, R. (1990). Advances in rehabilitation program evaluation. In M. Eisenberg (Ed.), *Advances in clinical rehabilitation: Vol. III* (Section V). New York: Springer.

Carey, R.G., & Posavac, E.J. (1978). Program evaluation of a physical medicine and rehabilitation unit: A new approach. *Archives of Physical Medicine and Rehabilitation, 59*(7), 330–337.

Carey, R.G., & Posavac, E.J. (1982). Rehabilitation program evaluation using a revised level of rehabilitation scale (LORS-II). *Archives of Physical Medicine and Rehabilitation, 63*(8), 367–370.

Carey, R.G., & Seibert, J.H. (1988). Integrating program evaluation, quality assurance, and marketing for inpatient rehabilitation. *Rehabilitation Nursing, 13*(2), 66–70.

Carey, R.G., Seibert, J.H., & Posavac, E. J. (1988). Who makes the most progress in inpatient rehabilitation? An analysis of functional gain. *Archives of Physical Medicine and Rehabilitation, 69*(5), 337-343.

Fleming, J. (1991). Overview of functional health status measures in nursing. In H. Hibbard (Ed.), *Proceedings of primary care research: Theory and methods* (AHCPR91-0011, pp. 67–72). Rockville, MD: U.S. Department of Health and Human Services, Public Health Service.

Gonnella, C. (1992). Program evaluation. In G.F. Fletcher, J.D. Banja, B.B. Jann, & S.L. Wolf (Eds.), *Rehabilitation medicine: Contemporary clinical perspectives* (pp. 243–268). Philadelphia: Lea & Febiger.

Gresham, G.E., & Labi, M.L.C. (1984). Functional assessment instruments currently available for documenting outcomes in rehabilitation medicine. In C.V. Granger & G.E. Gresham (Eds.), *Functional assessment in rehabilitation medicine* (pp. 76–77). Baltimore: Williams & Wilkins.

Kelley, F.A., Kawamoto, T.T., & Rubenstein, L.Z. (1991). Assessment of the geriatric patient. In J.M. Kiernat (Ed.), *Occupational therapy and the older adult: A clinical manual* (pp. 76–98). Gaithersburg, MD: Aspen Publishers.

Nojima, S. (1989). *Chronicity and family/patient interaction in a Japanese schizophrenic patient population.* Unpublished doctoral dissertation, University of California, San Francisco.

Sarno, J.E., Sarno, M.T., & Levita, E. (1973). The Functional Life Scale. *Archives of Physical Medicine and Rehabilitation, 54*(5), 214–220.

Schmidt, S.M., Herman, L.M., Koenig, P., Leuze, M., Monahan, M.K., & Stubbers, R.W. (1986). Status of stroke patients: A community assessment. *Archives of Physical Medicine and Rehabilitation, 67*(2), 99–102.

Unsworth, C. A. (1993). The concept of function. *British Journal of Occupational Therapy, 56*(8), 287-292.

Wilcock, G.K., Surmon, D.J., Scott, M., Boyle, M., Mulligan, K., Neubauer, K.A., O'Neill, D., & Royston, V.H. (1993). An evaluation of the efficacy and safety of tetrahydroaminoacridine (THA) without lecithin in the treatment of Alzheimer's disease. *Age & Ageing, 22*(5), 316–324.

Wood-Dauphinee, S.L., Williams, J.I., & Shapiro, S.H. (1990). Examining outcome measures in a clinical study of stroke. *Stroke, 21*(5), 731–739.

Table A–1 Functional Life Scale*

	Not Applicable (NA)	Self-initiation	Frequency	Speed	Overall Efficiency	Total
COGNITION						
1. Is oriented for time (e.g., hour, day, week).	X	X	X	X		
2. Uses "yes" and "no" appropriately.	X	X	X	X		
3. Understands speech (e.g., simple commands, directions, television).	X	X	X	X		
4. Calculates change (money).	X	X	X	X		
5. Does higher calculation (balance checkbook, etc.).	X	X	X	X		
6. Uses appropriate gestures in lieu of speech (not applicable for patients without speech impairment).						
7. Uses speech for communication.	X					
8. Reads (e.g., street signs, ability to follow written instructions, books).	X					
9. Writes (e.g., signs name, writes or types letters) (include motor disability).	X					
10. Social behavior is appropriate.	X	X	X	X		
11. Able to shift from one task to another with relative ease and speed.	X	X	X	X		
12. Aware of self (e.g., of mistakes, inappropriate behavior, poor judgment, etc.).	X	X	X	X		
13. Attempts to correct own errors (e.g., of judgment, mistakes).	X	X	X	X		
14. Has good memory (e.g., names of people, recent events).	X	X	X	X		
ACTIVITIES OF DAILY LIVING						
15. Able to get about (with or without brace, wheelchair, etc.).	X		X			
16. Does transfers.	X		X			
17. Feeds self.	X		X			
18. Uses toilet.	X		X			
19. Grooms self (e.g., wash, brush teeth, shave).	X					
20. Dresses self.	X		X			
21. Bathes self (including getting in and out of tub or stall).	X					
HOME ACTIVITIES						
22. Prepares simple food or drink (e.g., snacks, light breakfast).						
23. Performs light housekeeping chores (e.g., meals, dishes, dusting).						
24. Performs heavy housekeeping chores (e.g., floor or window washing).						
25. Performs odd jobs in or around house (e.g., gardening, electrical, auto, mending, sewing).	X					
26. Engages in solo pleasure activities (e.g., puzzles, painting, reading, stamps).			X	X		

*X = not scored.

continues

Table A–1 continued

Item	Not Applicable (NA)	Self-initiation	Frequency	Speed	Overall Efficiency	Total
HOME ACTIVITIES (continued)						
27. Uses telephone (e.g., dialing, handling; do not rate speech proficiency).	X					
28. Uses television set (e.g., changing channel).			X			
29. Uses record player or tape recorder.			X			
OUTSIDE ACTIVITIES						
30. Engages in simple pleasure activities (e.g., walk, car rides).	X			X	X	
31. Goes shopping for food.					X	
32. Does general shopping (e.g., clothes, gifts).	X				X	
33. Performs errands (e.g., post office, cleaner, bank, pick up newspaper).	X					
34. Attends spectator events (e.g., theater, concert, sports, movies).	X			X	X	
35. Uses public transportation accompanied (mass transportation).				X		
36. Uses public transportation alone (rate NA if item 35 is 0).				X		
37. Takes longer trips accompanied (plane, train, boat, car).				X	X	
38. Takes longer trips alone (rate NA if item 37 is 0).				X	X	
SOCIAL INTERACTION						
39. Participates in games with other people (e.g., cards, chess, checkers).				X		
40. Participates in home social activities (e.g., family gathering, party, dancing).				X	X	
41. Attends social functions outside of home (e.g., home of friend, dining at restaurant, dance).				X	X	
42. Participates in organizational activities (e.g., religious, union, service club, professional).				X	X	
43. Goes to work or school at comparable premorbid level (not housekeeping at home) (*Do not rate* if item 44 is to be rated.)				X		
44. Goes to work or school at lower than premorbid level (*Do not rate* if item 43 has been rated) (Multiply item 43 or 44 by 2.)				X		

Table A–1 continued

Scoring Sheet

	Total Score	Maximum Score	NA	Adjusted Maximum (Maximum – NA)	Total Score Adjusted Maximum	Proportion
Cognition		104				
ADL		92				
Home activities		112				
Outside activities		96				
Social interaction		60				
Overall score		464				
Self-initiation score		136				
Frequency score		104				
Speed score		84				
Overall efficiency score		140				

Source: Courtesy of Institute of Rehabilitation Medicine, New York, New York.

Patient Evaluation Conference System

The Patient Evaluation Conference System (PECS©) (see Exhibit A–3) was first published by Harvey and Jellinek in 1981. It is an interdisciplinary system in which rehabilitation patients are graded in each of 76 distinct functional performance areas. Items used include physical, medical, psychological, social, and vocational variables (examples emphasized are feeding, dressing, ambulation, denial of physical disability, and ability to live independently). Separate preconference worksheets are available for each rehabilitation discipline.

The PECS© scoring system "utilizes a 0 to 7 scale which reflects 1 as the most dependent and 7 as the most independent. . . . Zero is the value which reflects either an unmeasured or unmeasurable function. The scaling also reflects the key change from dependent with minimal assistance at 4, to independent with self-help aids at 5" (Harvey & Jellinek, 1981, p. 457). Harvey and Jellinek's first published series was composed of data from the evaluation of 125 rehabilitation patients. They believed the system met their goals of sensitivity; tracking ability; breadth of component variables; consistency in rating; and clarity and ease of understanding by rehabilitation professionals, reviewing bodies, and agencies. Their approach to the management of aggregate data was done "by determining the percentage of patients as a group or by diagnostic category who reached independent function" (Harvey & Jellinek, 1981, p. 460).

In 1984, the PECS© was used as an outcome measure for 30 patients with closed head injury (Rao, Jellinek, Harvey, & Flynn, 1984). Results of the study documented the value of computerized axial tomography in predicting functional outcomes in this group of patients. Before this study, a shortened version of the PECS© had been used similarly in a long-term follow-up study of individuals with brain injury. The findings showed significant negative relationships of levels of distress to function in various PECS© variables (Jellinek, Torkelson, & Harvey, 1982). Other work during the 1980s successfully used the PECS© as the functional outcome measure for studies on stroke as well as traumatic brain injury (Chaudhuri, Harvey, Sulton, & Lambert, 1988; Korner-Bitensky, Mayo, Cabot, Becker, & Coopersmith, 1989; Parke, Penn, Savoy, & Corcos, 1989; Rao, Jellinek, Harberg, & Fryback, 1988).

Such use of the PECS© continued during the 1990s, including use with pediatric patients (Clydesdale, Fahs, Kilgore, & Splaingard, 1990); prediction of stroke outcome (Korner-Bitensky, Mayo, & Poznanski, 1990); the effectiveness of a training program (Cronin-Stubbs, Swanson, Dean-Baar, Sheldon, & Duchene, 1992); and return to work (Rao & Kilgore, 1992). In addition, a new series of analyses was conducted to elucidate the precise biometric properties of the PECS©. Harvey et al. (1992) applied discriminate analysis using Rasch ability estimates to document the construct validity of the PECS©. Harvey and colleagues had previously explored undimensionality (Silverstein, Kilgore, Fisher, Harley, & Harvey, 1991) and performed a Rasch analysis to ascertain the degree to which interval measure requirements are met by the PECS© (Silverstein, Fisher, Kilgore, Harley, & Harvey, 1992). Further applications of Rasch analysis to the PECS© were published in 1993 (Kilgore, Fisher, Silverstein, Harley, & Harvey, 1993).

The PECS© has been adapted concurrently to computer software and selected as one of the three leading systems for rehabilitation program evaluation (Gonnella, 1992), along with the Uniform Data System (using the Functional Independence Measure [see Chapter 1]) and the LORS American Data System.

REFERENCES

Chaudhuri, G., Harvey, R.F., Sulton, L.D., & Lambert, R.W. (1988). Computerized tomography head scans as predictors of functional outcome of stroke patients. *Archives of Physical Medicine and Rehabilitation, 69*(7), 496–498.

Clydesdale, T.T., Fahs, I.J., Kilgore, K.M., & Splaingard, M.L. (1990). Social dimensions to functional gain in pediatric patients. *Archives of Physical Medicine and Rehabilitation, 71*(7), 469–472.

Cronin-Stubbs, D., Swanson, B., Dean-Baar, S., Sheldon, J.A., & Duchene, P. (1992). The effects of a training program on nurses' functional performance assessments. *Applied Nursing Research, 5*(1), 38–43.

Gonnella, C. (1992). Program evaluation. In G.F. Fletcher, J.D. Banja, B.B. Jann, & S.L. Wolf (Eds.), *Rehabilitation medicine: Contemporary clinical perspectives* (pp. 253–265). London: Lea & Febiger.

Harvey, R.F., & Jellinek, H.M. (1981). Functional performance assessment: A program approach. *Archives of Physical Medicine and Rehabilitation, 62*(9), 456–460.

Harvey, R.F., Silverstein, B., Venzon, M. A., Kilgore, K.M., Fisher, W.P., Steiner, M., & Harley, J.P. (1992). Applying psychometric criteria to functional assessment in medical rehabilitation. III. Construct validity and predicting level of care. *Archives of Physical Medicine and Rehabilitation, 73*(10), 887–892.

Jellinek, H.M., Torkelson, R.M., & Harvey, R.F. (1982). Functional abilities and distress levels in brain injured patients at long-term follow-up. *Archives of Physical Medicine and Rehabilitation, 63*(4), 160–162.

Kilgore, K.M., Fisher, W.P., Silverstein, B., Harley, J.P., & Harvey, R.F. (1993). Application of Rasch analysis to the patient evaluation and conference system. In C.V. Granger & G.E. Gresham (Eds.), *New developments in functional assessment* (pp. 493–515). Philadelphia: W.B. Saunders.

Korner-Bitensky, N., Mayo, N., Cabot, R., Becker, R., & Coopersmith, H. (1989). Motor and functional recovery after stroke: Accuracy of physical therapists' predictions. *Archives of Physical Medicine and Rehabilitation, 70*(2), 95–99.

Korner-Bitensky, N., Mayo, N.E., & Poznanski, S.G. (1990). Occupational therapists' accuracy in predicting sensory, perceptual-cognitive and functional recovery post stroke. *Occupational Therapy Journal of Research, 10*(4), 237–250.

Parke, B., Penn, R.D., Savoy, S.M., & Corcos, D. (1989). Functional outcome after delivery of intrathecal baclofen. *Archives of Physical Medicine and Rehabilitation, 70*(1), 30–32.

Rao, N., Jellinek, H.M., Harberg, J.K., & Fryback, D.G. (1988). The art of medicine: Subjective measures as predictors of outcome in stroke and traumatic brain injury. *Archives of Physical Medicine and Rehabilitation, 69*(3, Part 1), 179–182.

Rao, N., Jellinek, H.M., Harvey, R.F., & Flynn M.M. (1984). Computerized tomography head scans as predictors of rehabilitation outcome. *Archives of Physical Medicine and Rehabilitation, 65*(1), 18–20.

Rao, N., & Kilgore, K.M. (1992). Predicting return to work in traumatic brain injury using assessment scales. *Archives of Physical Medicine and Rehabilitation, 73*(10), 911–916.

Silverstein, B., Fisher, W.P., Kilgore, K.M., Harley, J.P. & Harvey, R.F. (1992). Applying psychometric criteria to functional assessment in medical rehabilitation. Part II. Defining interval measures. *Archives of Physical Medicine and Rehabilitation, 73*(6), 507–518.

Silverstein, B., Kilgore, K.M., Fisher, W.P., Harley, J.P., & Harvey, R.F. (1991). Applying psychometric criteria to functional assessment in medical rehabilitation. Part I. Exploring undimensionality. *Archives of Physical Medicine and Rehabilitation, 72*(9), 631–637.

Exhibit A–3 Patient Evaluation Conference System

Sample PECS© Items

1. LifeScale™: Impairment Severity

   Discipline: MED (usually completed by rehabilitation physicians)

   There are two methods for assessing the MED items: a qualitative set of descriptors (also used for the Narrative Report) and Rehabilitation Medicine checklist which is a "symptom checklist."

   MED1 Motor Loss

   0 Not assessed
   1 Severe: all 4 extremities and trunk
   2 Moderate: all 4 extremities
   3 Moderate: 2 extremities and trunk
   4 Moderate: 1 or 2 extremities
   5 Mild: independent functional ability in best extremity
   6 Mild: independent functional ability in 2 or more best extremities
   7 Normal function

2. LifeScale™: Applied: Self-Care

   Discipline: NSG (usually completed by Nursing)

   NSG1 Effectiveness of Bowel Program
   Regulation of bowel elimination and prevention of complications includes any of the following: regulation of food and fluid intake; high fiber diet for bowel management; medications for softening, bulk formation, stimulation or prevention of diarrhea; digital stimulation; and, colostomy care.

   0 Not assessed.
   1 Ineffective program: effective less than 25% of the time.
   2 Effective 25%-49% of the time with beginning response to program. Dependent: requires physical assistance for any or all parts of bowel program.
   3 Effective 50%-74% of the time. May require occasional modifications to maintain regularity, prevent constipation, diarrhea, etc. Dependent: requires physical assistance for any or all parts of the bowel program.
   4 Effective 75%-100% of the time. Dependent: requires physical assistance for any or all parts of the bowel program.
   5 Effective 50%-74% of the time. Independent: occasional lapse in effectiveness due to non-adherence to program or need for program modification.
   6 Effective 75%-100% of the time. Independent: regular adherence to program.
   7 Within normal limits–self maintenance and prevention; no aids, special dietary consideration, or medications needed.

3. LifeScale™: Motor Skills
   Discipline: PHY (usually completed by Physical Therapy)

PHY1 Transfer

Moving to and from wheelchair to mat table and bed from both directions. Set up for transfer and management of wheelchair parts necessary for safe transfer are included.

0 Not assessed.
1 Maximal assistance: patient attempts to participate or provide some physical assistance in carrying out the activity, but requires significant physical and verbal assistance to complete the activity. Patient is able to assist with up to 25% of the activity.
2 Moderate assistance: patient attempts to participate or provide some physical assistance in carrying out the activity, but requires physical and verbal assistance to complete the activity. Patient is able to assist with 25%-75% of the activity.
3 Minimal assistance: patient is able to participate fully in the activity, but requires intermittent physical assistance and/or contact guard. Patient is able to assist with 75% or more of the activity.
4 Standby assistance: patient performs the activity without physical/hands on assist. May require verbal cuing, prior demonstration or supervision to complete the activity safely.
5 Limited independent: patient is independent in the activity but requires an assistive device or environmental modification.
6 Functional independent: patient is independent in the activity but demonstrates an altered quality of movement or requires an unreasonable amount of time.
7 Within normal limits: patient is independent in the activity with reaction time and quality of movement appropriate for age.

Discipline: ADL (usually completed by Occupational Therapist)

ADL1 Performance in Feeding—Ability to use utensils, cut and eat food, pour and drink liquids, use condiments, and pass food at the table.

0 Not assessed
1 Functional and manual assistance and assistive device: caregiver required to assemble/gather equipment, apply device(s); manual assistance needed to complete task.
2 Functional with manual assistance: caregiver required to complete (e.g., cut food, put pants over feet, apply toothpaste, transfer to bed/toilet).
3 Functional with supervision and assistive device: caregiver required to provide verbal cues as patient uses assistive device(s) (e.g., use of dressing aids, transfer to tub seat, use peeling board).
4 Functional with supervision: caregiver required to provide verbal cues to initiate dressing, direct sequence of activity, keep patient on task.

continues

Exhibit A–3 continued

5 Functional with assistive device: patient able to complete task with assistive device (e.g., mobile with wheelchair, dress with dressing stick, peel vegetables stabilized on spike board, write with writing device).

6 Functional: no caregiver needed, but patient needs increased time to complete task.

7 Within normal limits: normal function.

4. LifeScale™: Cognition

Discipline: COM (usually completed by Speech Therapist)

COM1 Ability To Comprehend Verbal Language
Understands information presented verbally.

0 Not assessed.

1 Brain Injury: no purposeful response to auditory stimuli.
   Stroke: no purposeful response to auditory stimuli.

2 Brain Injury: maximum cuing required to attend to environmental and concrete single-step auditory stimuli; inconsistent responses characterized by latency and variable accuracy.
   Stroke: maximum cuing required. Inconsistently responds to auditory stimuli.

3 Brain Injury: responses indicate comprehension of brief personal and contextual based stimuli; reliability decreases for comprehension of abstract stimuli which requires increased structure and repetition; inconsistent carryover from minute to minute.
   Stroke: needs repetition and cuing for comprehension of personally and contextually based stimuli, comprehension of non-contextual stimuli is inconsistent.

4 Brain Injury: relies upon the speaker to provide necessary repetition and clarification for comprehension of non-contextually bound stimuli such as multistep commands, conversation on familiar topics.
   Stroke: may need repetition and clarification for comprehension of non-contextually bound stimuli such as simple commands, short phrases and brief conversation on familiar topics.

5 Brain Injury: patient comprehends auditory stimuli associated with activities of daily living. Patient demonstrates emerging responsibility for clarification and repetition to enhance auditory comprehension. Breakdown may occur with decreased structure and increased length and complexity.
   Stroke: patient's auditory comprehension is functional for activities of daily living; however, breakdown occurs with increased length and complexity.

6 Brain Injury: patient is independent in utilizing compensatory techniques to maximize recall and new learning for comprehension in his [or her] premorbid environments. Sustained concentration to auditory stimuli may be affected by distractions and/or mental fatigue.

Stroke: comprehension of verbal language is functional for conversation. Minimal difficulty occurs with lengthy or complex auditory stimuli which may be associated with premorbid level of functioning.

7 Brain Injury: comprehension of verbal language is functional for all situations at the patient's premorbid level of functioning.
   Stroke: comprehension of verbal language is functional for all situations at the patient's premorbid level of functioning.

5. LifeScale™: Community Reintegration

Discipline: PSY (usually completed by Psychologist)

PSY1 Distress/Comfort
Decreasing comfort (and increasing distress) is indicated by the intensity of muscular tension, somatic complaints, pain complaints, expressed fears, social withdrawal, reports of feeling "blue, down in the dumps, frustrated, lonely, nervous," disturbed sleep, difficulty concentrating, lack of animation in gestures and facial expression, crying, anger, irritability. Overall score on the SCL-90 is a psychometric measure of distress which contributes to this assessment. Although many of these variables are also correlated with clinical depression (as measured by the Beck Depression Inventory), the cognitive distortions (e.g., overgeneralization, arbitrary inference) associated with clinical depression are absent or not consistently displayed by distressed persons who are not depressed. A distressed person usually focuses his [or] her distress in one or two modalities of expression, whereas a depressed person displays significant and sustained disturbance in behavior affect cognition.

0 Not assessed.

1 Extreme psychological distress: may be expressed through extreme muscle tension, somatic complaints, phobias, severe affect problems (anxiety, depression, anger, quiet), or social withdrawing, resulting in poor reality contact and inability to participate in rehab program.

2 Severe psychological distress: expressed through severe muscle tension or somatic complaints, phobias, severe affect problems (anxiety, depression, anger, guilt) or social withdrawal and patient's participation in rehab program is affected, but reality contact is not impaired.

3 Marked psychological distress: may be expressed through a marked level of muscle tension or somatic complaints; there are objective indications of abnormal affect which the patient is unable to control and participation in the rehab program is affected.

4 Moderate psychological distress: may be expressed through a moderate level of muscle tension or somatic complaints; there are objective indications of abnormal affect: although patient can control negative behavior, participation in the rehab program is affected.

continues

Exhibit A–3 continued

5 Mild or intermittent psychological distress: patient may have some muscle tensions, somatic complaints, or subjective feelings of distress (feeling blue, worried, lonely, nervous, or irritable), but not to a degree where these are noticeable to an observer nor do they interfere with patient's rehab program.

6 Minimal psychological distress: patient is experiencing and reports mild feelings of distress, but they are not noticeable to an observer.

7 Patient is psychologically comfortable the vast majority of the time.

6. LifeScale™: Pain

Discipline: PAI (usually completed by Pain Team consensus)

PAI1 Behavior

Verbal and non-verbal complaints; moans, gasps, facial grimaces, distorted standing posture, impaired mobility (limping), body language (clutching or rubbing pain site), abnormal movement and position shifts. Also includes a lack of appropriate requests for help.

0 Not assessed.

1 Extreme pain behavior: verbal and non-verbal pain behavior is extreme and interferes with social appropriateness and ADL task functioning.

2 Marked: verbal and/or non-verbal pain behavior often interferes with social appropriateness and ADL task functioning.

3 Moderate pain behavior: verbal and/or non-verbal pain behavior occasionally interferes with social appropriateness and ADL task functioning.

4 Mild: limited verbal or non-verbal pain behavior, but patient cannot effectively communicate his [or her] physical limitations or ask for help even when appropriate.

5 Occasional pain behavior, but patient is demonstrating an attempt to modify.

6 Minimal pain behavior: patient rarely exhibits verbal or non-verbal pain behaviors. Patient effectively communicates his physical limitations, but seldom asks for help even if appropriate.

7 No pain behaviors. Patient effectively communicates his [or her] physical limitations and can ask for help when appropriate.

Source: Copyright © Dr. Richard F. Harvey, Rehabilitation Foundation, Inc., Wheaton, Illinois.

PULSES Profile

PULSES Profile (Moskowitz & McCann, 1957) is a scored profile of six categories, each of which has four subcategories (see Exhibit A–4). The name PULSES represents the initial letters of each of the six categories. The measure was originally developed by the authors to provide an overall representation of the physical function of a given patient, to supplement the traditional medical diagnoses that do not contain this needed information. It was methodologically based on the Pulhems Profile method developed by the Canadian Army and subsequently adopted by the U.S. Army during World War II (Moskowitz & McCann, 1957).

The authors first used the PULSES to screen 115 residents of the Westchester County Home (Moskowitz & McCann, 1957). They concluded that the disability evaluation information generated a necessary supplement to the medical diagnoses and believed it would also be useful in establishing individual rehabilitation goals and documenting functional change (either improvement or deterioration) as the process of rehabilitation proceeded.

Gresham and Labi (1984) summarized a number of important studies that had been accomplished by using the PULSES Profile. Moskowitz, Fuhn, Peters, and Kearley (1959) were able to document the subsequent functional outcomes of the 115 residents studied originally. Results of another study showed the functional disability course (over one year) of 163 nursing home residents (Moskowitz, Goldman, Randall, Fox, & Brumfield, 1960), as well as of 518 persons from a stroke registry (followed for three years) (Moskowitz, Lightbody, & Freitag, 1972). In their summary, Gresham and Labi (1984) concluded that the PULSES "is an effective means of monitoring service requirements . . . the effects of rehabilitation efforts . . . and able to detect cases of unexpected functional deterioration where more intensive evaluation and intervention were needed" (p. 67).

Other investigators, including Reynolds, Abramson, and Young (1959), have used the PULSES Profile to assess rehabilitation potential of patients in institutions for treatment of chronic disease as well as in studies of cerebral palsy (Goldkamp, 1984), vocational status (Goldberg, Bernad, & Granger, 1980; Goldberg, Hannon, & Granger, 1977), and amputees (O'Toole, Goldberg, & Ryan, 1985). By far the most dramatic, however, was the modification and use of the PULSES Profile along with the Barthel Index (Granger, Greer, Liset, Coulombe, & O'Brien, 1975). Granger et al. (1975) made criteria modifications and added a scoring system. Then Granger and colleagues conducted a series of studies on stroke and overall rehabilitation outcomes, which culminated in a landmark paper (Granger, Albrecht, & Hamilton, 1979) documenting in a 10-center study that functional status of medical rehabilitation patients does improve during active rehabilitation and that this improvement is sustained for at least two years.

REFERENCES

Goldberg, R.T., Bernad, M., & Granger, C.V. (1980). Vocational status: Prediction by the Barthel Index and PULSES Profile. *Archives of Physical Medicine and Rehabilitation, 61*(12), 580–583.

Goldberg, R.T., Hannon, H., & Granger, C. (1977). Vocational and functional assessments of clients reopened for service. *Scandinavian Journal of Rehabilitation Medicine, 9*(2), 85–90.

Goldkamp, O. (1984). Treatment effectiveness in cerebral palsy. *Archives of Physical Medicine and Rehabilitation, 65*(5), 232–234.

Granger, C.V., Albrecht, G.L., & Hamilton, B.B. (1979). Outcome of comprehensive medical rehabilitation: Measurement by PULSES profile and the Barthel Index. *Archives of Physical Medicine and Rehabilitation, 60*(4), 145–154.

Granger, C.V., Greer, D.S., Liset, E., Coulombe, J., & O'Brien, E. (1975). Measurement of outcomes of care for stroke patients. *Stroke, 6*(1), 34–41.

Gresham, G.E., & Labi, M.L.C. (1984). Functional assessment instruments currently available for documenting outcomes in rehabilitation medicine. In C.V. Granger & G.E. Gresham (Eds.), *Functional assessment in rehabilitation medicine* (pp. 65–85). Baltimore: Williams & Wilkins.

Moskowitz, E., Fuhn, E.R., Peters, M.E., & Kearley, A.S. (1959). Aged infirm residents in a custodial institution. *Journal of the American Medical Association, 169*(17), 2009–2012.

Moskowitz, E., Goldman, J.J., Randall, E.H., Fox, R.I., & Brumfield, W.A. (1960). A controlled study of the rehabilitation potential of nursing home residents. *New York State Journal of Medicine, 60*(9), 1439–1444.

Moskowitz, E., Lightbody, F.E.H., & Freitag, N.S. (1972). Long-term follow-up of the post-stroke patient. *Archives of Physical Medicine and Rehabilitation, 53*(4), 167–172.

Moskowitz, E., & McCann, C.B. (1957). Classification of disability in the chronically ill and aging. *Journal of Chronic Diseases, 5*(3), 342–346.

O'Toole, D.M., Goldberg, R.T., & Ryan, B. (1985). Functional changes in vascular amputee patients: Evaluation by Barthel Index, PULSES Profile and ESCROW Scale. *Archives of Physical Medicine and Rehabilitation, 66*(8), 508–511.

Reynolds, F.W., Abramson, M., & Young, A. (1959). The rehabilitation potential of patients in chronic disease institutions. *Journal of Chronic Diseases, 10*(2), 152–159.

Exhibit A–4 PULSES Profile

P Physical condition including diseases of the viscera (cardiovascular, pulmonary, gastrointestinal, urologic, and endocrine) and cerebral disorders which are not enumerated in the lettered categories below.
   1. No gross abnormalities considering the age of the individual.
   2. Minor abnormalities not requiring frequent medical or nursing supervision.
   3. Moderately severe abnormalities requiring frequent medical or nursing supervision yet still permitting ambulation.
   4. Severe abnormalities requiring constant medical or nursing supervision confining individual to bed or wheelchair.
U Upper extremities including shoulder girdle, cervical, and upper dorsal spine.
   1. No gross abnormalities considering the age of the individual.
   2. Minor abnormalities with fairly good range of motion and function.
   3. Moderately severe abnormalities but permitting the performance of daily needs to a limited extent.
   4. Severe abnormalities requiring constant nursing care.
L Lower extremities including the pelvis, lower dorsal, and lumbosacral spine.
   1. No gross abnormalities considering the age of the individual.
   2. Minor abnormalities with fairly good range of motion and function.
   3. Moderately severe abnormalities permitting limited ambulation.
   4. Severe abnormalities confining the individual to bed or wheelchair.
S Sensory components relating to speech, vision, and hearing.
   1. No gross abnormalities considering the age of the individual.
   2. Minor deviations insufficient to cause any appreciable functional impairment.
   3. Moderate deviations sufficient to cause appreciable functional impairment.
   4. Severe deviations causing complete loss of hearing, vision, or speech.
E Excretory function, i.e. bowel and bladder control.
   1. Complete control.
   2. Occasional stress incontinence or nocturia.
   3. Periodic bowel and bladder incontinence or retention alternating with control.
   4. Total incontinence, either bowel or bladder.
S Social and mental status.
   1. No deviations considering the age of the individual.
   2. Minor deviations in mood, temperament, and personality not impairing environmental adjustment.
   3. Moderately severe variations requiring some supervision.
   4. Severe variations requiring complete supervision.

PROFILE

P	U	L	S	E	S

Source: Reprinted with permission from E. Moskowitz and C.B. McCann, Classification of Disability in the Chronically Ill and Aging, *Journal of Chronic Diseases*, Vol. 5, No. 3, p. 343, © 1957, Mosby-Yearbook, Inc.

Rankin Scale

The Rankin Scale (Rankin, 1957) was developed as a means of following the overall disability status of patients with stroke. It was part of the author's historic work that demonstrated that stroke is not a uniform disaster and that many survivors do remarkably well and go on to lead satisfying and productive lives. The scale is ordinal and contains five grades:

I. *No significant disability*: able to carry out all usual duties.
II. *Slight disability*: unable to carry out some of previous activities but able to look after own affairs without assistance.
III. *Moderate disability*: requiring some help but able to walk without assistance.
IV. *Moderately severe disability*: unable to walk without assistance and unable to attend to own bodily needs without assistance.
V. *Severe disability*: bedridden, incontinent, and requiring constant nursing care.

The Rankin Scale is clearly appropriate for stroke survivors, because it includes walking, basic activities of daily living, instrumental activities of daily living, cognitive function, and incontinence. Because it is an ordinal scale, the Rankin Scale should be treated in statistical manipulations with methods that are nonparametric. It can discern significant progress (or deterioration) in the overall function of individual patients, and by appropriate methods of aggregation and the use of nonparametric statistics, it can document the same in a group of patients. In spite of being one of the first global functional assessment instruments developed, the Rankin Scale is still popular. It enjoys continued use, particularly in the stroke literature (Censori et al., 1993; De Haan, Horn, Limburg, Van Der Meulin, & Bossuyt, 1993; The Dutch TIA Study Group, 1988; Granger & Gresham, 1993; Lodder, Bamford, Kappelle, & Boiten, 1994; Milandre, Brosset, Gouirand, & Khalil, 1992; Popa, Nistorescu, & Stanescu, 1992; Popa et al., 1989; van Swieten, Koudstaal, Visser, Schouten, & van Gijn, 1988; Wade, 1992; Wolfe, Taub, Woodrow, & Burney, 1991; Zorzon et al., 1993).

The Rankin Scale has also been used as a functional measure in cardiac disease (Visser et al., 1992). Wade (1992) pointed out three shortcomings of the Rankin Scale ("inherent insensitivity, mixing of objective and subjective items, and spanning impairment, disability, and handicap" [p. 91]). He did, however, concede that it has "the two great virtues of simplicity and reliability, making it ideal for large multi-centre trials" (p. 91). Wade (1992) included in his work the modifications to the original Rankin Scale that have evolved over the years. These include the addition of a sixth grade—0 for no symptoms at all—and some minor wording changes.

REFERENCES

Censori, B., Camerlingo, M., Casto, L., Ferraro, B., Gazzaniga, G.C., Cesana, B., & Mamoli, A. (1993). Prognostic factors in first-ever stroke in the carotid artery territory seen within 6 hours after onset. *Stroke, 24*(4), 532–535.

De Haan, R., Horn, J., Limburg, M., Van Der Meulen, J., & Bossuyt, P. (1993). A comparison of five stroke scales with measures of disability, handicap, and quality of life. *Stroke, 24*(8), 1178–1181.

The Dutch TIA Study Group (1988). The Dutch TIA trial: Protective effects of low-dose aspirin and atenolol in patients with transient ischemic attacks or non-disabling stroke. *Stroke, 19*(4), 512–517.

Granger, C.V., & Gresham, G.E. (1993). Functional assessment in rehabilitation medicine. Introduction and brief background. In C.V. Granger & G.E. Gresham (Eds.), *New developments in functional assessment* (pp. 417–423). Philadelphia: W.B. Saunders.

Lodder, J., Bamford, J., Kappelle, J., & Boiten, J. (1994). What causes false clinical prediction of small deep infarcts? *Stroke, 25*(1), 86–91.

Milandre, L., Brosset, C., Gouirand, R., & Khalil, R. (1992). Pure cerebellar infarction. Thirty cases (In French). *Presse Medicale-Paris, 21*(33), 1562–1565.

Popa, G., Nistorescu, A., & Stanescu, A. (1992). Outcome in ischaemic stroke: Carotid versus vertebro-basilar territory. *Romanian Journal of Neurology & Psychiatry, 30*(3), 181–188.

Popa, G., Popa, C., Stanescu, A., Ionescu, G., Logoji, G., Radula, D., & Popescu, A. (1989). Hemodilution therapy in acute ischaemic stroke. *Neurologie et Psychiatrie, 27*(2), 79–90.

Rankin, J. (1957). Cerebral vascular accidents in patients over the age of 60. II. Prognosis. *Scottish Medical Journal, 2*, 200–215.

van Swieten, J.C., Koudstaal, P.J., Visser, M.C., Schouten, H.J., & van Gijn, J. (1988). Inter-observer agreement for the assessment of handicap in stroke patients. *Stroke, 19*(5), 604–607.

Visser, M.C., Koudstaal, P.J., van Latum J.C., Frericks, H., Berenghollz-Zlochin, S.N., & van Gijn, J. (1992). Inter-observer variation in the application of 2 disability scales in heart patients (In Dutch). *Nederlands Tijdschrifft voor Geneeskunde, 136*(17), 831–834.

Wade D.T. (1992). *Measurement in neurological rehabilitation* (pp. 89–96, 231–258). Oxford, England: Oxford University Press.

Wolfe, C.D., Taub, N.A., Woodrow, E.J., & Burney, P.G. (1991). Assessment of scales of disability and handicap for stroke patients. *Stroke, 22*(10), 1242–1244.

Zorzon, M., Mase, G., Pozzi-Mucelli, F., Biasutti, E., Antonutti, L., Jona, L., & Cazzata, G. (1993). Increased density in the middle cerebral artery by non-enhanced computed tomograph: Prognostic value in acute cerebral infarction. *European Neurology, 33*(3), 256–259.

Activities of Daily Living (ADL) Instruments

Barthel Index

The Barthel Index (Mahoney & Barthel, 1965) was originally devised as a means of clearly differentiating patients who are dependent in ADL from those who are not. It is a 10-category, *weighted* index, which includes ambulation and stairs as well as self-care and has a perfect score of 100 (see Table A–2). As stated by the authors, a Barthel Index score of 100 means that a patient may not be able to live alone, for various reasons, but "he [or she] is able to get along without attendant care" (p. 2). The weights assigned to each of the 10 categories are arbitrary, but the authors' judgment in these has stood the test of time (Gresham & Labi, 1984). The Barthel Index has been used extensively throughout the world, and as late as 1992, it was described by Wade (1992) as "the best measure available" (p. 175).

The Barthel Index has been used in rehabilitation research and practice for more than 25 years. As pointed out by Mahoney and Barthel (1965), this instrument can be used to monitor the process of rehabilitation. It can "establish a functional baseline for a patient, follow his or her progress in a rehabilitation program, and identify a point of 'maximum benefit' after which improvement fails to occur. In addition . . . when functional dependence is due, in part, to environmental factors, the correction of these will immediately result in a higher . . . score" (Gresham & Labi, 1984, p. 71).

The original Barthel Index is shown in Table A–2. At least five versions (including the original) have been used. These include the Granger three-level modification (Granger, Albrecht, & Hamilton, 1979), Granger four-level modification (Fortinsky, Granger, & Seltzer, 1981), zero to 20-point scoring modification (Collin, Wade, Davies, & Horne, 1988), and Shah modification for greater sensitivity (Shah, Vanclay, & Cooper, 1989). These four particular modifications are shown in Tables A–3, A–4, A–5, and Exhibit A–5. Because these different formulations of the Barthel Index exist, it is important to specify precisely which one was used in any given study or project.

The biometric properties of the Barthel Index must be kept in mind. First, it is a weighted scale. Each subscale, as well as the entire Barthel Index, gives a numerical score. These scores, however, must be used with care when data are aggregated. The overall Barthel Index score can be compared only with other overall scores on one or more persons. Individual category subscores can be treated similarly, but the Barthel Index is neither a metric nor a true ordinal scale. Thus only nonparametric statistics can be used for any other type of statistical analysis and these statistics should be used with caution. In addition, it is important to remember that the perfect score of 100 is simply a numerical score and has nothing to do with percentage.

The validity of the Barthel Index has been addressed by a number of authors. Gresham and Labi (1984) summarized early work on the original version and Granger three- and four-level adaptations. Their review included a unique concurrent validity analysis, with the use of Framingham study data, that showed that the Barthel Index, Katz Index of ADL (Katz, Ford, Moskowitz, Jackson, & Jaffee, 1963), and Kenny Self-Care Evaluation (Schoening et al., 1965) all measure the same domain of ADL with similar overall results (Gresham, Phillips, & Labi, 1980). Wade and Collin (1988) reviewed predictive and construct validity as well, and Wade (1992) concluded that the validity of the Barthel Index "has been well established" (p. 75). Basmajian (1994) reviewed other positive evidence of Barthel Index validity, including its use as a comparison standard for other scales.

The reliability of the Barthel Index has been reviewed by Gresham and Labi (1984), Collin et al. (1988), Wade (1992), and Basmajian (1994). All concluded that the instrument had satisfactory reliability (regardless of which version was used). Wade (1992) did point out, however, that the Barthel Index has some limitations: it has "floor" and "ceiling" effects and lacks sensitivity (a problem addressed by Shah et al. in 1989). It remains, however, highly regarded for its usefulness and satisfactory biometric properties. For a functional assessment instrument, "floor" means some persons can score below the lowest category and "ceiling" (more common) means some persons can score above the highest category. With the Barthel Index, which measures basic ADL independence, persons can have a perfect score of 100 and still not be able to live independently (e.g., because of dementia). This disclaimer regarding the Barthel Index was made by the authors when the instrument was first published and appears in Appendix A as Table A–3.

Much functional assessment research has been carried out by using the Barthel Index. As discussed earlier in Appendix A, the Barthel Index was used with the PULSES Profile (Moskowitz & McCann, 1957) in the landmark 10-center study of medical rehabilitation by Granger, Albrecht, and Hamilton (1979). They clearly documented functional improvement in 307 medical rehabilitation patients between admission and discharge. This improvement was maintained for at least two years.

A review of the medical literature discloses many studies, in several languages (including French, German, Dutch, Japanese, and Chinese), in which the Barthel Index was used. In addition, the Barthel Index has been used as the measure of ADL in studies of several impairment groups.

Selected studies of stroke that used the Barthel Index include those of Becker et al. (1986); Davies, Bamford, and Warlow (1989); Dickstein, Hocherman, Pillar, and Shaham (1986); Granger, Dewis, Peters, Sherwood, and Barrett (1979); Matchar, Divine, Heyman, and Feussner (1992);

Novack, Haban, Graham, and Sutherfield (1987); Reding and Potes (1988); Sandin and Smith (1990); Shah, Vanclay, and Cooper (1990); and Wood-Dauphinee, Williams, and Shapiro (1990).

Studies of spinal cord injury with the Barthel Index include those of Anderson and Bohlman (1992); DeJong, Branch, and Corcoran (1984); Drewes, Olsson, Slot, and Andreasen (1989); Lazar et al. (1989); and Roth, Lawler, and Yarkony (1990). The Barthel Index has also been used in studies of hip fracture (Bentur & Eldar, 1993; Cameron, Lyle, & Quine, 1993); amputees (O'Toole, Goldberg, & Ryan, 1985), and traumatic brain injury (Tuel, Presty, Meythaler, Heinemann, & Katz, 1992), as well as in the rapidly growing field of geriatrics (Eagle et al., 1991; Harris, Mion, Patterson, & Frengley, 1988; Stone, Herbert, Chrisostomou, Vessey, & Horwood, 1993).

REFERENCES

Anderson, P.A., & Bohlman, H.H. (1992). Anterior decompression and arthrodesis of the cervical spine: Long-term motor improvement. Part II. Improvement in complete traumatic quadriplegia. *Journal of Bone and Joint Surgery—American Volume, 74*(5), 683–692.

Basmajian, J. (Ed.). (1994). *Physical rehabilitation outcome measures.* Toronto, Ontario, Canada: Canadian Physiotherapy Association in Co-operation with Health and Welfare Canada and the Canadian Communications Group-Publishing, Supply & Services Canada.

Becker, C., Howard, G., McLeroy, K.R., Yatsu, F.M., Toole, J.F., Coull, B., Feibel, J., & Walker, M.D. (1986). Community hospital-based stroke programs: North Carolina, Oregon and New York. II. Description of study populations. *Stroke 17*(2), 285–293.

Bentur, N., & Eldar, R. (1993). Quality of rehabilitation care in two inpatient geriatric settings. *Quality Assurance in Health Care, 5*(3), 237–242.

Cameron, I.D., Lyle, D.M., & Quine, S. (1993). Accelerated rehabilitation after proximal femoral fracture: A randomized controlled trial. *Disability and Rehabilitation, 15*(1), 29–34.

Collin, C., Wade, D.T., Davies, S., & Horne, V. (1988). The Barthel ADL Index: A reliability study. *International Disability Studies, 10*(2), 61–63.

Davies, P., Bamford, J., & Warlow, C. (1989). Remedial therapy and functional recovery in a total population of first-stroke patients. *International Disability Studies, 11*(1), 40–44.

DeJong, G., Branch, L.G., & Corcoran, P.J. (1984). Independent living outcome in spinal cord injury: Multivariate analysis. *Archives of Physical Medicine and Rehabilitation, 65*(2), 66–73.

Dickstein, R., Hocherman, S., Pillar, T., & Shaham, R. (1986). Stroke rehabilitation: Three exercise therapy approaches. *Physical Therapy, 66*(8), 1233–1238.

Drewes, A.M., Olsson, A.T., Slot, O., & Andreasen, A. (1989). Rehabilitation outcome for patients with spinal cord injury. *International Disability Studies, 11*(4), 178–180.

Eagle, D.J., Guyatt, G.H., Patterson, C., Turpie, J., Sackett, B., & Singer, J. (1991). Effectiveness of a geriatric day hospital. *Canadian Medical Association Journal, 144*(6), 699–704.

Fortinsky, R.H., Granger, C.V., & Seltzer, G.B. (1981). The use of functional assessment in understanding home care needs. *Medical Care, 19*(5), 489–497.

Granger, C.V., Albrecht, G.L., & Hamilton, B.B. (1979). Outcome of comprehensive medical rehabilitation: Measurement by PULSES Profile and the Barthel Index. *Archives of Physical Medicine and Rehabilitation, 60*(4), 145–154.

Granger, C.V., Dewis, L.S., Peters, N.C., Sherwood, C.C., & Barrett, J.E. (1979). Stroke rehabilitation: Analysis of repeated Barthel Index measures. *Archives of Physical Medicine and Rehabilitation, 60*(1), 14–17.

Gresham, G.E., & Labi, M.L.C. (1984). Functional assessment instruments currently available for documenting outcomes in rehabilitation medicine. In C.V. Granger & G.E. Gresham (Eds.), *Functional assessment in rehabilitation medicine* (pp. 71–73). Baltimore: Williams & Wilkins.

Gresham, G.E., Phillips, T.F., & Labi, M.L.C. (1980). ADL status in stroke: Relative merits of three standard indexes. *Archives of Physical Medicine and Rehabilitation, 61*(8), 355–358.

Harris, R.E., Mion, L.C., Patterson, M.B., & Frengley, J.D. (1988). Severe illness in older patients: The association between depression disorders and functional dependency during the recovery phase. *Journal of the American Geriatrics Society, 36*(10), 890–896.

Katz, S., Ford, A.B., Moskowtiz, R.W., Jackson, B.A., & Jaffee, M.W. (1963). Studies of illness in the aged. The index of ADL: A standardized measure of biological and psychosocial function. *Journal of the American Medical Association, 185*(12), 914–919.

Lazar, R.B., Yarkony, G.M., Ortolano, D., Heinemann, A.W., Perlow, E., Lovell, L., & Meyer, P.R. (1989). Prediction of functional outcome by motor capability after spinal cord injury. *Archives of Physical Medicine and Rehabilitation, 70*(12), 819–822.

Mahoney, F.I., & Barthel, D.W. (1965). Functional evaluation: The Barthel Index. *Maryland State Medical Journal, 14*, 61–65.

Matchar, D.B., Divine, G.W., Heyman, A., & Feussner, J.R. (1992). The influence of hyperglycemia and outcome of cerebral infarction. *Annals of Internal Medicine, 117*(6), 449–456.

Moskowitz, E., & McCann, C.B. (1957). Classification of disability in the chronically ill and aging. *Journal of Chronic Disability, 5*, 342–346.

Novack, T.A., Haban, G., Graham, K., & Sutherfield, W.T. (1987). Prediction of stroke rehabilitation outcome from psychological screening. *Archives of Physical Medicine and Rehabilitation, 68*(10), 729–734.

O'Toole, D.M., Goldberg, R.T., & Ryan B. (1985). Functional changes in vascular amputee patients: Evaluation by Barthel Index, PULSES Profile and ESCROW Scale. *Archives of Physical Medicine and Rehabilitation, 66*(8), 508–511.

Reding, M.J., & Potes, E. (1988). Rehabilitation outcome following initial unilateral hemispheric stroke. Life table analysis approach. *Stroke, 19*(11), 1354–1358.

Roth, E.J., Lawler, M.H., & Yarkony, G.M. (1990). Traumatic cord syndrome: Clinical features and functional outcomes. *Archives of Physical Medicine and Rehabilitation, 71*(1), 15–23.

Sandin, K.J., & Smith, B.S. (1990). The measure of balance in sitting in stroke rehabilitation prognosis. *Stroke, 21*(1), 82–86.

Schoening, H.A., Anderegg, L., Bergstrom, D., Fonda, M., Steinke, N., & Ulrich, P. (1965). Numerical scoring of self-care status of patients. *Archives of Physical Medicine and Rehabilitation, 46*(10), 689–697.

Shah, S., Vanclay, F., & Cooper, B. (1989). Improving the sensitivity of the Barthel Index for stroke rehabilitation. *Journal of Clinical Epidemiology, 42*(8), 703–709.

Shah, S., Vanclay, F., & Cooper, B. (1990). Efficiency, effectiveness and duration of stroke rehabilitation. *Stroke, 21*(2), 241–246.

Stone, S.P., Herbert, P., Chrisostomou, J., Vessey, C., & Horwood, C. (1993). The assessment of disability in patients on an acute medical ward for elderly. *Disability and Rehabilitation, 15*(1), 35–37.

Tuel, S.M., Presty, S.K., Meythaler, J.M., Heinemann, A.W., & Katz, R.T.

(1992). Functional improvement in severe head injury after readmission for rehabilitation. *Brain Injury, 6*(4), 363–372.

Wade, D.T. (1992). *Measurement in neurological rehabilitation.* Oxford, England: Oxford University Press.

Wade, D.T., & Collin, C. (1988). The Barthel Index: A standard measure of physical disability. *International Disability Studies, 10*(2), 64–67.

Wood-Dauphinee, S.L., Williams, J.J., & Shapiro, S.H. (1990). Examining outcome measures in a clinical study of stroke. *Stroke, 21*(5), 731–739.

Table A–2 Barthel Index

	With Help	Independent
1. Feeding (if food needs to be cut up—help)	5	10
2. Moving from wheelchair to bed and return (includes sitting up in bed)	5–10	15
3. Personal toilet (wash face, comb hair, shave, clean teeth)	0	5
4. Getting on and off toilet (handling clothes, wipe, flush)	5	10
5. Bathing self	0	5
6. Walking on level surface (or if unable to walk, propel wheelchair)	10	15
*Score only if unable to walk	0*	5*
7. Ascend and descend stairs	5	10
8. Dressing (includes tying shoes, fastening fasteners)	5	10
9. Controlling bowels	5	10
10. Controlling bladder	5	10

A patient scoring 100 on the BI is continent, feeds himself [or herself], dresses himself [or herself], gets up out of bed and chairs, bathes himself [or herself], walks at least a block, and can ascend and descend stairs. This does not mean that he [or she] is able to live alone: he [or she] may not be able to cook, keep house, and meet the public, but he [or she] is able to get along without attendant care.

Source: Reprinted with permission from F.J. Mahoney and D.W. Barthel, Functional Evaluation: The Barthel Index, *Maryland State Medical Journal,* Vol. 14, pp. 1–3, © 1965.

Table A–3 Three-Level Barthel Index

The following presents the items or tasks scored in the Barthel Index with the corresponding values for independent performance of the task:

	"Can do by myself"	*"Can do with help of someone else"*	*"Cannot do at all"*
Self-care Index			
1. Drinking from a cup	4	0	0
2. Eating	6	0	0
3. Dressing upper body	5	3	0
4. Dressing lower body	7	4	0
5. Putting on brace or artificial limb	0	−2	0 (not applicable)
6. Grooming	5	0	0
7. Washing or bathing	6	0	0
8. Controlling urination	10	5 (accidents)	0 (incontinent)
9. Controlling bowel movements	10	5 (accidents)	0 (incontinent)
Mobility Index			
10. Getting in and out of chair	15	7	0
11. Getting on and off toilet	6	3	0
12. Getting in and out of tub or shower	1	0	0
13. Walking 50 yards on the level	15	10	0
14. Walking up/down one flight of stairs	10	5	0
15. IF NOT WALKING: Propelling or pushing wheelchair	5	0	0 (not applicable)

BARTHEL TOTAL: BEST SCORE IS 100; WORST SCORE IS 0.

NOTE: Tasks 1–9, the self-care index (including control of bladder and bowel sphincters), have a total possible score of 53. Tasks 10–15, the mobility index, have a total possible score of 47. The 2 groups of tasks combined make up the total Barthel Index with a total possible score of 100. We customarily prefer to use the 4-level adaptation. The main difference between the 2 versions is that the 4-level describes independent function as either intact or with some limitation such as using an adaptive appliance. In the case of this study, review of the medical records did not consistently distinguish independent-intact from independent-limited. Therefore, the 3-level was used for this study. Both assessments of independent function receive the same Barthel scoring. Therefore, with either version, the Barthel index score sums are equivalent.

Source: Reprinted with permission from C.V. Granger, G.L. Albrecht, & B.B Hamilton. Outcome of Comprehensive Medical Rehabilitation: Measurement by PULSES Profile and the Barthel Index, *Archives of Physical Medicine and Rehabilitation*, Vol. 60, No. 4, pp. 145–154, © 1979, W.B. Saunders.

Table A–4 Granger "4-Level Modification"

Independent		Dependent		
I Intact	II Limited	III Helper	IV Null	
10	5	0	0	Drink from cup/feed from dish
5	5	3	0	Dress upper body
5	5	2	0	Dress low body
0	0	–2		Don brace or prosthesis
5	5	0	0	Grooming
4	4	0	0	Wash or bathe
10	10	5	0	Bladder continence
10	10	5	0	Bowel continence
4	4	2	0	Care of perineum/clothing at toilet
15	15	7	0	Transfer, chair
6	5	3	0	Transfer, toilet
1	1	0	0	Transfer, tub or shower
15	15	10	0	Walk on level 50 yards or more
10	10	5	0	Up and down stairs for one flight or more
15	5	0	0	Wheelchair/50 yards—only if not walking

Source: Reprinted with permission from R.H. Fortinsky, C.V. Granger, and G.B. Seltzer, The Use of Functional Assessment in Understanding Home Care Needs, *Medical Care*, Vol. 19, pp. 489–497, © 1981, Elsevier Science Inc.

Exhibit A–5 The Barthel ADL Index and Guidelines

The Barthel ADL Index

Bowels
  0 = incontinent (or needs to be given enemata)
  1 = occasional accident (once/week)
  2 = continent
Bladder
  0 = incontinent, or catheterized and unable to manage
  1 = occasional accident (max once per 24 hours)
  2 = continent (for over 7 days)
Grooming
  0 = needs help with personal care
  1 = independent face/hair/teeth/shaving (implements provided)
Toilet use
  0 = independent
  1 = needs some help, but can do something alone
  2 = independent (on and off, dressing, wiping)
Feeding
  0 = unable
  1 = needs help cutting, spreading butter, etc.
  2 = independent (food provided in reach)

Transfer
  0 = unable—no sitting balance
  1 = major help (one or two people, physical), can sit
  2 = minor help (verbal or physical)
  3 = independent
Mobility
  0 = immobile
  1 = wheel chair independent including corners, etc.
  2 = walks with help of one person (verbal or physical)
  3 = independent (but may use any aid, e.g., stick)
Dressing
  0 = dependent
  1 = needs help, but can do about half unaided
  2 = independent (including buttons, zips, laces, etc.)
Stairs
  0 = unable
  1 = needs help (verbal, physical, carrying aid)
  2 = independent up and down
Bathing
  0 = dependent
  1 = independent (or in shower)
  Total (0–20)

continues

Exhibit A–5 continues

The Barthel ADL Index Guidelines

General

The Index should be used as a record of *what a patient does*, NOT as a record of *what a patient could do*.

The main aim is to establish *degree of independence from any help*, physical or verbal, however minor and for whatever reason.

The need for *supervision* renders the patient, NOT *independent*.

A patient's performance should be established *using the best available evidence*. Asking the patient, friends/relatives and nurses will be the usual source, but direct observation and common sense are also important. However, *direct testing is not needed*.

Usually the performance over the preceding *24–48 hours** is important, but occasionally longer periods will be relevant.

Unconscious patients should score '0' throughout, even if not yet incontinent.

Middle categories imply that patient supplies *over 50% of the effort*.

Use of aids to be independent is *allowed*.

Bowels (preceding week)
If needs enema from nurse, then 'incontinent'*
Occasional* = once a week.

Bladder (preceding week)
Occasional = less than once a day
A catheterized patient who can completely manage the catheter alone is registered as 'continent'.

Grooming (preceding 24-48 hours)
Refers to personal hygiene: doing teeth, fitting false teeth, doing hair, shaving, washing face. Implements* can be provided by helper.

Toilet use
Should be able to reach toilet/commode, undress sufficiently, clean self, dress and leave.

With help = can wipe self, and do some other of above.*

Feeding
Able to eat any normal food (not only soft food*). Food cooked and served by others. But not cut up.
Help = food cut up, patient feeds self.*

Transfer
From bed to chair and back.
Dependent—NO sitting balance (unable to sit); two people to lift.
Major help = one strong/skilled, or two normal people. Can sit up.
Minor help = one person easily, OR needs any supervision for safety.

Mobility
Refers to mobility about house or ward, indoors. May use aid. If in wheelchair, must negotiate corners/doors unaided.
Help = by one, untrained person, including supervision/moral support.

Dressing
Should be able to select and put on all clothes, which may be adapted.
Half = help with buttons, zips etc., but can put on some garments alone.*

Stairs
Must carry any walking aid used to be independent.

Bathing
Usually the most difficult activity.
Must get in and out unsupervised, and wash self.
Independent in shower = 'independent' if unsupervised/ unaided.*

*Items added or modified after study; asterisk at end, whole item added; asterisk in middle, phrase added or clarified.

Source: Reprinted with permission from C. Collin, D.T. Wade, S. Davies, and V. Horne, The Barthel Index: A Reliability Study, *International Disability Studies*, Vol. 10, pp. 61–63, © 1988, Taylor and Francis Ltd.

Table A–5 Modified Scoring for the Barthel Index

	Code				
Items	1 Unable To Perform Task	2 Attempts Task But Unsafe	3 Moderate Help Required	4 Minimal Help Required	5 Fully Independent
Personal hygiene	0	1	3	4	5
Bathing self	0	1	3	4	5
Feeding	0	2	5	8	10
Toilet	0	2	5	8	10
Stair climbing	0	2	5	8	10
Dressing	0	2	5	8	10
Bowel control	0	2	5	8	10
Bladder control	0	2	5	8	10
Ambulation	0	3	8	12	15
Wheelchair*	0	1	3	4	5
Chair/bed transfer	0	3	8	12	15
Range	0				100

*Score only if Ambulation coded "1" and patient trained in wheelchair management.

Source: Reprinted by permission of the publisher from S. Shah, F. Vanclay, and B. Cooper, Improving the Sensitivity of the Barthel Index for Stroke Rehabilitation, *Journal of Clinical Epidemiology,* Vol. 42, No. 8, pp. 703–709, Copyright 1989 by Elsevier Science, Inc.

Katz Index of ADL

The Katz Index of ADL (see Exhibit A–6) resulted from a series of studies carried out at the Benjamin Rose Hospital in Cleveland, Ohio. It was used to summarize overall performance in activities of daily living (ADL) of 1,001 geriatric patients with hip fracture. Design of the instrument is based on the theory that when functional ability is lost, it is recovered in a specific developmental sequence on the basis of primary biological and psychosocial function (Kane & Kane, 1981).

The instrument includes six major functional categories scored from A to G or Other, with A being totally independent and G being totally dependent in ADL. Scoring is based on the patient's ability to perform a task without assistance of another person (Kane & Kane, 1981).

The six specific personal ADL variables measured with this instrument are bathing, dressing, going to toilet, transfer, continence, and feeding. The supplement to the Katz Index of ADL includes five instrumental activities of living: cooking, washing, transportation, cleaning, and shopping. The Katz Index of ADL requires the rater to use an ordinal scale, and the mode of scoring is dichotomous.

To study reliability, scalability, and validity of the expanded index, 85 mostly elderly persons who had consulted with an occupational therapist were assessed in their homes. Construct validity was established with a scalability coefficient well above the acceptance level. External validity was established when it was found that no person was dependent in personal ADL and totally independent in instrumental

ADL. Persons dependent in both basic and instrumental ADL were older and lived in sheltered accommodation more often than persons dependent only in instrumental ADL. Interobserver reliability was high (Asberg & Sonn, 1989).

The Katz Index of ADL can be used "to document the clinical course of disabling chronic conditions and to examine interrelationships of specific variables concurrently documented in a single group of subjects at a specific point in time" (Labi & Gresham, 1984, p. 88). It is used currently by caretakers in the home and hospital because of its common language of disability (Asberg, 1986) and this common language results in better communication between home and hospital care providers.

The Katz Index of ADL has been correlated with mobility and house confinement after discharge (Katz, Ford, Moskowitz, Jackson, & Jaffe, 1963). Predictive validity has been established in studies done in Sweden where the Katz Index of ADL is currently used as a valid tool for early prognosis of stroke outcome for better planning of care and rehabilitation (Asberg & Nydevik, 1991). The expanded scale has been used to describe a broader range of needs for elders living in the community, and it has been useful to clinicians, researchers, and health service planners (Spector, Katz, Murphy, & Fulton, 1987). Many investigators, however, have found the Katz Index of ADL is not very sensitive (Donaldson, Wagner, & Gresham, 1973; Gresham, Phillips, & Labi, 1980).

Advantages of the Katz Index of ADL are that it identifies broad functional categories, is short, and has been widely used. It can be used for teaching house officers and nursing students, as a basis for prognostic prediction, for comparing treatment and control groups in a clinical trial, for focusing attention on functional limitations, and to guide treatment (Gresham & Labi, 1984). Its popularity in geriatrics is attested to by its inclusion in *Assessing the Elderly* by Kane and Kane (1981).

Theoretical assumptions on which this instrument was developed are debatable. Its statistical manipulability is fairly limited because the overall score is not quantitative (Labi & Gresham, 1984).

REFERENCES

Asberg, K.H. (1986). Change in ADL and use of short-term hospital care. *Scandinavian Journal of Social Medicine, 14*(2), 105–111.

Asberg, K.H., & Nydevik, I. (1991). Early prognosis of stroke outcome by means of Katz Index of Activities of Daily Living. *Scandinavian Journal of Rehabilitation Medicine, 23*(4), 187–191.

Asberg, K.H., & Sonn, U. (1989). The cumulative structure of personal and instrumental ADL. A study of elderly people in a health service district. *Scandinavian Journal of Rehabilitation Medicine, 21*(4), 171–177.

Donaldson, S.W., Wagner, C.C., & Gresham, G.E. (1973). A unified ADL evaluation form. *Archives of Physical Medicine and Rehabilitation, 54*(4), 175–179.

Gresham, G.E., & Labi, M.L.C. (1984). Functional assessment instruments currently available for documenting outcomes in rehabilitation medicine. In C.V. Granger & G.E. Gresham (Eds.), *Functional assessment in rehabilitation medicine*. Baltimore: Williams & Wilkins.

Gresham, G.E., Phillips, T.F., & Labi, M.L. (1980). ADL status in stroke: Relative merits of three standard indexes. *Archives of Physical Medicine and Rehabilitation, 61*(8), 355–358.

Kane, R.A., & Kane, R.L. (1981). *Assessing the elderly*. Lexington, MA: Lexington Books.

Katz, S., Ford, A.B., Moskowitz, R.W., Jackson, B.A., & Jaffee, M.W. (1963). Studies of illness in the aged. The Index of ADL: A standardized measure of biological and psychosocial function. *Journal of the American Medical Association, 185*(12), 914–919.

Labi, M.L.C., & Gresham, G.E. (1984). Some research applications of functional assessment instruments used in rehabilitation medicine. In C.V. Granger & G.E. Gresham (Eds.), *Functional assessment in rehabilitation medicine* (pp. 86–98). Baltimore: Williams & Wilkins.

Spector, W.D., Katz, S., Murphy, J.B., & Fulton, J.P. (1987). The hierarchical relationship between activities of daily living and instrumental activities of daily living. *Journal of Chronic Diseases, 40*(6), 481–489.

Exhibit A–6 Katz Index of ADL

Index of Independence in Activities of Daily Living

The Index of Independence in Activities of Daily Living is based on an evaluation of the functional independence or dependence of patients in bathing, dressing, going to toilet, transferring, continence, and feeding. Specific definitions of functional independence and dependence appear below the index.

A — Independent in feeding, continence, transferring, going to toilet, dressing, and bathing.
B — Independent in all but one of these functions.
C — Independent in all but bathing and one additional function.
D — Independent in all but bathing, dressing, and one additional function.
E — Independent in all but bathing, dressing, going to toilet, and one additional function.
F — Independent in all but bathing, dressing, going to toilet, transferring, and one additional function.
G — Dependent in all six functions.
Other — Dependent in at least two functions, but not classifiable as C, D, E, or F.

Independence means without supervision, direction, or active personal assistance, except as specifically noted below. This is based on actual status and not on ability. A patient who refuses to perform a function is considered as not performing the function, even though he is deemed able.

Bathing (Sponge, Shower, or Tub)
Independent: assistance only in bathing a single part (as back or disabled extremity) or bathes self completely
Dependent: assistance in bathing more than one part of body; assistance in getting in or out of tub or does not bathe self

Dressing
Independent: gets clothes from closets and drawers; puts on clothes, outer garments, braces; manages fasteners; act of tying shoes is excluded
Dependent: does not dress self or remains partly undressed

continues

Exhibit A–6 continued

Going to Toilet

Independent: gets to toilet; gets on and off toilet; arranges clothes; cleans organs of excretion (may manage own bedpan used at night only and may or may not be using mechanical supports)

Dependent: uses bedpan or commode or receives assistance in getting to and using toilet

Transfer

Independent: moves in and out of bed independently and moves in and out of chair independently (may or may not be using mechanical supports)

Dependent: assistance in moving in or out of bed and/or chair; does not perform one or more transfers

Continence

Independent: urination and defecation entirely self-controlled

Dependent: partial or total incontinence in urination or defecation; partial or total control by enemas, catheters, or regulated use of urinals and/or bedpans

Feeding

Independent: gets food from plate or its equivalent into mouth (precutting of meat and preparation of food, as buttering bread, are excluded from evaluation

Dependent: assistance in act of feeding (see above); does not eat at all or parenteral feeding

---

Evaluation Form

Name _____   Date of evaluation _____

For each area of functioning listed below, check description that applies. (The word "Assistance" means supervision, direction or personal assistance.)

Bathing—either sponge bath, tub bath, or shower.

❑ Receives no assistance (gets in and out of tub by self if tub is usual means of bathing)

❑ Receives assistance in bathing only one part of the body (such as back or a leg)

❑ Receives assistance in bathing more than one part of the body (or not bathed)

Dressing—gets clothes from closets and drawers—including underclothes, outer garments and using fasteners (including braces if worn)

❑ Gets clothes and gets completely dressed without assistance

❑ Gets clothes and gets dressed without assistance except for assistance in tying shoes

❑ Receives assistance in getting clothes or in getting dressed, or stays partly or completed undressed

Toileting—going to the "toilet room" for bowel and urine elimination; cleaning self after elimination, and arranging clothes

❑ Goes to "toilet room," cleans self, and arranges clothes without assistance (may use object for support such as cane, walker, or wheelchair and may manage night bedpan or commode, emptying same in morning)

❑ Receives assistance in going to "toilet room" or in cleansing self or in arranging clothes after elimination or in use of night bedpan or commode

❑ Doesn't go to room termed "toilet" for the elimination process

Transfer—

❑ Moves in and out of bed as well as in and out of chair without assistance (may be using object for support such as cane or walker)

❑ Has occasional "accidents"

❑ Supervision helps keep urine or bowel control; catheter is used, or is incontinent

Feeding—

❑ Feeds self without assistance

❑ Feeds self except for getting assistance in cutting meat or buttering bread

❑ Receives assistance in feeding or is fed partly or completely by using tubes or intravenous fluids

Source: Reprinted with permission from S. Katz et al., Studies of Illness in the Aged, The Index of ADL: A Standardized Measure of Biological and Psychological Function. *Journal of the American Medical Association,* Vol. 185, pp. 914–919, Copyright 1963, American Medical Association.

Kenny Self-Care Evaluation

The Kenny Self-Care Evaluation (Schoening et al., 1965) (see Exhibit A–7) has merit from a historical viewpoint. In 1968 a need was recognized for more precise measurement of rehabilitation outcomes. Schoening and Iversen (1968) noted that "glib use of general phrases by the professionals in the field of rehabilitation implies to the uninitiated that 'rehabilitation' is a single, universally applicable process that can be purchased, prescribed, applied, or otherwise achieved with a minimum of thought and effort" (p. 221). Schoening and Iversen also noted that the many complex variables involved in the rehabilitation process make measurement of the rehabilitation process difficult. When cure could not be used as a univariate measure of success, rehabilitators often turned to other simple bases of measurement such as return to full-time work. Unfortunately, this criterion cannot be used with older individuals and many times cannot be applied to younger patients until years after their discharge from acute rehabilitation programs.

At the time of the development of the Kenny Self-Care Evaluation, the need for more global measures was identified to determine to what degree an individual functions independently within an open or closed environment. The Kenny Self-Care Evaluation, developed at the Kenny Rehabilitation Institute, is one such global measure (Schoening et al., 1965) and was constructed to measure a person's physical capacity to function in the home or other closed environments.

Nature of Items. The Kenny Self-Care Evaluation measures outcomes in six categories: bed activities, transfers, locomotion, dressing, personal hygiene, and feeding. Seventeen specific activities are included in these six categories. These items are rated on a five-point scale, ranging from zero to four with the high score indicating complete independence. Unique to this scale was an expanded central interval, "a catch all in which the patient's level cannot be specifically determined" (Schoening & Iversen, 1968, p. 226) and an interval in which the patient passes quickly on the way from zero to four.

The total self-care score is determined by adding the mean scores in each of the six categories. Therefore a patient with a score of 24 is completely independent in all categories. Although the categories are equally important, some categories have more activities listed. Thus the use of mean scores in each category seemed sound at the time (Schoening & Iversen, 1968).

Standardization. The Kenny Self-Care Evaluation was used routinely week after week for rating new patients and reevaluating old patients. Data were managed by a statistical services department (Schoening & Iversen, 1968). The physiatrist added data to help classify the patient, the physical therapist rated locomotion activities, the occupational thera-pist rated feeding activity, and the nurse was responsible for rating all other activities. The form is used for the rehabilitation conference when the patient's admission evaluation is complete. Data are sent to the statistical services department with printouts sent to each rater. The printouts are used during reevaluation so changes can be recorded on the form. The best observed performance for that week is recorded and presented at the weekly conference. The corrected form is sent to the statistical services department, which in turn distributes the updated printouts to the raters.

Validity. Much effort was devoted to appropriate definitions of levels of independence after initial difficulty in determining ratings. Criteria for definitions were that they must have good face validity and be simple and workable. Content and construct validity have not been reported (Basmajian, 1994). Correlations between the Kenny Self-Care Evaluation and the Barthel Index were moderate ($k = .42$; $r = .73$). More clients are rated as independent when the Barthel Index is used as compared with findings from the Kenny Self-Care Evaluation (Basmajian, 1994). Gresham, Phillips, and Labi (1980) documented concurrent validity by comparing the frequency of "perfect" ADL scores from concurrent testing of the same patients with the Katz Index of ADL, the Barthel Index, and the Kenny Self-Care Evaluation. They found no statistically significant differences among these scores and concluded that these instruments measured the same "universe of function."

Reliability. Internal consistency and test–retest reliability have not been reported (Basmajian, 1994). Inter-rater reliability was moderate (.67–.74) in two studies (Gordon, Drenth, Jarvis, Johnson, & Wright, 1978; Kerner & Alexander, 1981).

Sensitivity. Donaldson, Wagner, and Gresham (1973) compared the Kenny Self-Care Evaluation with the Katz Index of ADL and the Barthel Index and found the Kenny Self-Care Evaluation was the most sensitive of the three.

Strengths. Some of the strengths of the Kenny Self-Care Evaluation are simplicity in use for the rater and enough breadth to distinguish between patients and demonstrate progress in functional independence. No real problems have been cited in uniformity of rating among various rehabilitation personnel working with the patients tested. The test is short and concise, and it provides an easily accessible means of comparison on one form.

Examples of Use as Cited in Literature. The developers of the Kenny Self-Care Evaluation discovered that various disability groups learned self-care in apparently different manners. This finding suggests that when someone is physically able to begin learning and has an intact mind, he or she learns quickly. However, in a category such as personal hygiene—where adaptive equipment, physiological readiness, and psychological readiness are needed—learning is appreciably slowed. When learning curves of persons who were right hemiplegic, left hemiplegic, paraplegic, quadriplegic, or arthritic—or who had other disabilities—were examined, an abrupt type of learning curve predominated except in the case of the individual with left hemiplegia (Schoening & Iversen, 1968).

It was thought that the time-rating curve had some predictive value in determining how long it would take to achieve an expected outcome. The authors contend that the "problem of precise definition of points near the center of the abilities continuum can be effectively circumvented by not defining them at all (and by grouping them into a single rating level encompassing a relatively broad spectrum of the abilities continuum)" (Schoening & Iversen, 1968, p. 229).

This instrument has been used to measure outcomes in persons with a variety of disabilities. Labi, Phillips, & Gresham (1980) found that stroke survivors "do not return to a normal social life even after physical disability has ceased to be a serious obstacle" (p. 564). This instrument, along with the Katz Index of ADL and the Barthel Index, received the greatest use and study during the 1970s (Gresham & Labi, 1984). The original instruction book is available from Dr. Herbert A. Schoening, 4828 Pennsylvania Avenue South, Minneapolis, MN 55409.

REFERENCES

Basmajian, J. (Ed.). (1994). *Physical rehabilitation outcome measures.* Toronto, Ontario, Canada: Canadian Physiotherapy Association in co-operation with Health and Welfare Canada and the Canada Communications Group-Publishing, Supply & Services Canada.

Donaldson, S.W., Wagner, C.C., & Gresham, G.E. (1973). A unified ADL evaluation form. *Archives of Physical Medicine and Rehabilitation, 54*(4), 175–180.

Gordon, E.E., Drenth, V., Jarvis, L., Johnson, J., & Wright, V. (1978). Neurophysiologic syndromes in stroke as predictors of outcomes. *Archives of Physical Medicine and Rehabilitation, 59*(9), 399–409.

Gresham, G.E., & Labi, M.L.C. (1984). Functional assessment instruments currently available for documenting outcomes in rehabilitation. In C.V. Granger & G.E. Gresham (Eds.), *Functional assessment in rehabilitation medicine.* Baltimore: Williams & Wilkins.

Gresham, G.E., Phillips, T.F., & Labi, M.L. (1980). ADL status in stroke: Relative merits of three standard indexes. *Archives of Physical Medicine and Rehabilitation, 61*(8), 355–358.

Kerner, J.F., & Alexander, J. (1981). Activities of daily living: Reliability and validity of gross vs specific ratings. *Archives of Physical Medicine and Rehabilitation, 62*(4), 161–166.

Labi, M.L., Phillips, T.F., & Gresham, G.E. (1980). Psychosocial disability in physically restored long-term stroke survivors. *Archives of Physical Medicine and Rehabilitation, 61* (12), 561–565.

Schoening, H.A., Anderegg, L., Bergstrom, D., Fonda, M., Steinke, N., & Ulrich, P. (1965). Numerical scoring of self-care status of patients. *Archives of Physical Medicine and Rehabilitation, 46*(10), 689–697.

Schoening, H.A., & Iversen, I.A. (1968). Numerical scoring of self-care status: A study of the Kenny Self-Care Evaluation. *Archives of Physical Medicine and Rehabilitation, 49*(4), 221–229.

Exhibit A–7 Kenny Self-Care Evaluation

Kenny Self-Care
Admission/Evaluation
Data Transmittal Form

Hospital

Patient Name

Last, First, Middle Initial (Leave one space between each).
If married, female, use given rather than married name

Unit Number

Eight digit patient identification number

Admission Number
01 = First Admission
02 = Second Admission
Etc.

Serial Number

Six digit number uniquely identifying this admission
in the chronoligically ordered set of all admissions

Habitat immediately prior to
admission (Patient admitted from . . .)
1 = Home
2 = Nursing Home
3 = Hospital
4 = Other
5 = Undetermined

Sex
1 = Male
2 = Female

Race
0 = White
1 = Negro
2 = Latin
3 = Oriental
4 = Indian (American)
5 = Other

Type of Admission
0 = New
1 = Readmit (new problem)
2 = Readmit (same problem)
3 = Continuation (previous
    discharge provisional)
4 = Other

Age at Admission
(Calendar age)

Date of Onset of
Primary Impairment

Month   Day   Year

Reason for Admission
0 = Evaluation Only
1 = Treatment Only
2 = Evaluation & Treatment
3 = Other

Locomotion Status at Admission Evaluation
0 = Bedfast
1 = Locomotion limited to wheelchair
2 = Primarily wheelchair; ambulation short distances with aids or
    assistance
3 = Ambulation with aids (wheelchair, two crutches)
4 = Ambulation without aids (one cane or less)

Admission Date

Month   Day   Year

Length of Time—Onset to Admission—
Specify days, weeks, months, or years

Predicted Length of Stay (days)

SELF-CARE RATINGS

Diagnoses should be descriptive—Hemiplegia: please specify side involved, aphasia, or sensory loss if present. Arthritis: affected joint if monarticular; affected extremities if polyarticular. Paraplegia/Quadriplegia: neurologic level, incomplete or complete. Etc.

Predicted Discharge by Attending Physician		Admission Evaluation by R.T., O.T., & Nursing	Adm. Eval. Rater P.T., O.T. or Nurse		
			Initials	Code	
	BED ACTIVITIES				
	Move in Bed				
	Rise and Sit				
	TRANSFERS				
	Sitting				
	Standing		_____		
	Toilet				
	LOCOMOTION				
	Walking				
	Stairs		_____		
	Wheelchair				
	DRESSING				
	Upper Trunk, Arms				
	Lower Trunk, Legs		_____		
	Feet				
	PERSONAL HYGIENE				
	Face, Hair, Arms				
	Trunk, Perineum				
	Lower Extremities		_____		
	Bowel Program				
	Bladder Program				
	FEEDING				
	Feeding		_____		

Primary DX (Specific Impairment
Necessitating Current Admission)

Course of Pathology

Regressing

Static

Improving

Severity

Mild

Moderate

Severe

Etiology of Above Impairment

Other Diagnoses

Attending
Physician _____

K.R.I
Form 98-002
05-10-65

Klein–Bell Activities of Daily Living Scale

The Klein–Bell Activities of Daily Living Scale (Klein & Bell, 1982) (see Exhibits A–8 and A–9) was developed in an effort to provide a "reliable, quantitative and meaningful measure of independence in activities of daily living (ADL)" (Asher, 1989, p. 29) and to be universally applicable. It was designed to help determine a patient's current level of functioning, record progress, and enable health care professionals as well as family members to communicate in an understandable language. This scale allows for specific and comprehensive treatment planning, thus making it appropriate for clinical and research purposes (Asher, 1989).

The Klein–Bell Activities of Daily Living Scale is devised to identify observable behavior significant to all people, both with and without disabilities. An understandable generic language is used to express these behaviors. The scale is composed of 170 items in six areas of function: dressing, elimination, mobility, bathing/hygiene, eating, and emergency telephone communication (Klein & Bell, 1982). Each area is subdivided (e.g., dressing is subdivided into 10 areas such as shorts/pants), and each subdivision is again broken down into behavioral elements (e.g., for shorts/pants: get left leg into left leghole). The behavior element is monitored and scored as independent or dependent. Activities are scored as achieved (performs behavior without verbal or physical assistance) or failed (assistance is needed). When an individual uses adaptive equipment without verbal or physical assistance, he or she is assigned a full score. Raw scores of individual areas are summed, and percentages of total achievable score are calculated. Total points achieved within each ADL area are summed and then added with other areas to yield an overall ADL score for independence. Scores are plotted on a graph for ease of interpretation (Klein & Bell, 1982).

The instrument and items within it represent what Klein and Bell intended to measure. There was a consistent relationship (−.86, p <.01) when ADL scores at discharge and number of hours per week of assistance required were compared with scores and number of hours of assistance needed 5 to 10 months after discharge (Klein & Bell, 1982; Smith, Morrow, Heitman, Rardin, Powelson, & Von, 1986). Lower ADL scores indicated a need for more assistance. As ADL scores increased, the need for assistance decreased.

Inter-rater agreement was 92% when two occupational therapists and two rehabilitation nurses rated 20 patients independently (Asher, 1989; Klein & Bell, 1982).

The Klein–Bell Activities of Daily Living Scale is useful in determining the current level of ADL function and noting progress. It is also useful in communicating treatment plans and objective results to patients, families, and third-party payers (Klein & Bell, 1982). It has been used in research involving patients with stroke (Titus, Gall, Yerxa, Roberson, & Mack, 1991) and children with spina bifida (Unruh, Fairchild, & Versnel, 1993). The Klein–Bell Activities of Daily Living Scale can be used to teach a patient's family members, because it focuses on observable performance and thus enables family members to know exactly in what areas the patient requires assistance. The scale can also be used to reinforce staff because it helps identify gradual progress over time. Its sensitivity to small changes in function helps generate a sense of accomplishment for health care professionals. The scale has been used as a measure in cost benefit studies and hospital utilization analyses (Klein & Bell, 1982).

Scoring instructions, definitions, and further instructions are found in the manual that accompanies the Klein–Bell Activities of Daily Living Scale. The scale can be obtained from the University of Washington Medical School, Health Sciences Center for Educational Resources, Distribution Department, H.S. Building Box 357161, T281, Seattle, WA 98195–7161; Telephone (206) 685–1186.

REFERENCES

Asher, I.E. (1989). *An annotated index of occupational therapy evaluation tools.* Bethesda, MD: American Occupational Therapy Association.

Klein, R.M., & Bell, B. (1982). Self-care skills: Behavior measurements with the Klein–Bell ADL Scale. *Archives of Physical Medicine and Rehabilitation, 63*(7), 335–338.

Smith, R.O., Morrow, M.E., Heitman, J.K., Rardin, W.J., Powelson, J.L., & Von, T. (1986). The effects of introducing the Klein–Bell ADL Scale in a rehabilitation service. *American Journal of Occupational Therapy, 40*(6), 420–424.

Titus, M.N.D., Gall, N.G., Yerxa, E.J., Roberson, T.A., & Mack W. (1991). Correlation of perceptual performance and activities of daily living in stroke patients. *American Journal of Occupational Therapy, 45*(5), 410–418.

Unruh, A.M., Fairchild, S., & Versnel, J. (1993). Parents' and therapists' ratings of self-care skills in children with spina bifida (journal, research, tables/charts). *Canadian Journal of Occupational Therapy–Revue Canadienne D Ergotherapie, 60*(3), 145–158.

Exhibit A–8 Klein–Bell Activities of Daily Living Scale

DRESSING:

A. Obtain clothing from bureau

1. Grasp drawer	(1)					
2. Pull drawer open	(2)					
3. Reach into drawer	(2)					
4. Grasp clothes	(1)					
5. Shut drawer	(1)					

B. Obtain clothing from closet

6. Grasp clothing hung in closet	(1)					
7. Place clothes within reach for dressing	(1)					

C. Socks

8. Grasp sock	(1)					
9. Reach sock to R foot	(2)					
10. Reach sock to L foot	(2)					
11. Pull sock over R toes	(2)					
12. Pull sock over L toes	(2)					
13. Pull sock over R foot with heel to heel	(2)					
14. Pull sock over L foot with heel to heel	(2)					
15. Pull sock up to full extension on R leg	(2)					
16. Pull sock up to full extension on L leg	(2)					

D. Shoes

17. Place R toe into R shoe	(2)					
18. Place R heel into R shoe	(2)					
19. Place L toe into L shoe	(2)					
20. Place L heel into L shoe	(2)					
21. Fasten R shoe	(2)					
22. Fasten L shoe	(2)					

continues

Exhibit A–8 continued

E. Shorts/pants

23. Reach shorts to foot	(2)					
24. Get R leg into R leghole	(2)					
25. Get L leg into L leghole	(2)					
26. Pull pants up to waist	(2)					
27. Zip zipper	(2)					
28. Fix fastener	(2)					

F. Pullover shirt

29. Reach shirt to top of head	(2)					
30. Pull head through neck hole	(2)					
31. Put R hand through R armhole	(2)					
32. Put R elbow into sleeve	(2)					
33. Put L hand through L armhole	(2)					
34. Put L elbow into sleeve	(2)					
35. Pull shirt down over trunk	(2)					

G. Button shirt/sweater/coat/jacket

36. Put R hand through R armhole	(2)					
37. Put R elbow into sleeve	(2)					
38. Put L hand through L armhole	(2)					
39. Put L elbow into sleeve	(2)					
40. Bring collar to neck	(2)					
41. Button front	(2)					
42. Fasten R cuff	(2)					
43. Fasten L cuff	(2)					
44. Tuck shirt into pants	(2)					
45. Fasten zipper	(2)					
46. Zip zipper	(2)					
47. Apply sufficient pressure to close snaps	(2)					

continues

Exhibit A–8 continued

H. Bra

48. Approximate two ends (ends touching each other while around body) (2)					
49. Fasten bra (2)					
50. Rotate to proper orientation (2)					
51. Put R strap on R shoulder (2)					
52. Put L strap on L shoulder (2)					

I. Hat

53. Grasp hat (1)					
54. Place hat on top of head (1)					

J. Extra devices (3 points total for all necessary devices)

55. Glasses					
56. Belt					
57. Hearing aid					
58. Sling					
59. Eye patch					
60. Orthoses					
61. Splints					
62. Body jacket					
63. Stump wrapping					
64. Prosthesis					
65. Other					

ELIMINATION:

A. Voiding control

66. Produce when appropriate (3)					
67. Withhold when appropriate (3)					

Exhibit A–8 continued

B. Urination

68. Undo clothing	(2)					
69. Achieve urinating position	(2)					

C. Wiping

70. Grasp toilet paper	(1)					
71. Rip off toilet paper	(1)					
72. Reach genital area	(2)					

D. Manage menstrual needs

73. Grasp device	(1)					
74. Insert or apply device	(2)					
75. Remove device	(2)					

E. Redo clothing

76. Pull pants/panties up to waist from knees	(2)					
77. Fasten pants	(2)					
78. Resume ambulation position	(2)					

F. Bowel control

79. Produce when appropriate	(3)					
80. Withhold when appropriate	(3)					

G. Defecation

81. Achieve defecating position	(2)					
82. Undo clothing	(2)					

H. Wiping

83. Reach anal area for wiping	(2)					
84. Apply sufficient pressure to clean anal area	(2)					

continues

Exhibit A–8 continued

I. Redo clothing

85. Pull pants/panties up to waist from knees	(2)					
86. Fasten pants	(2)					
87. Resume ambulation position	(2)					

J. Flushing

88. Depress lever sufficiently to initiate flush	(1)					

MOBILITY:

A. Bed mobility

89. Turn from supine to one side for 30 seconds	(3)					
90. Turn from side to prone	(3)					
91. Turn from prone to side	(3)					
92. Go from supine to at least 70 degrees sitting for one minute	(3)					

B. Ambulation

93. Transfer from sitting to ambulation position	(2)					
94. Maintain ambulation position for 10 seconds	(2)					
95. Mobility on straight flat surface for 20 feet without falling or hitting an obstacle	(2)					
96. Mobility on 20 degree incline without falling or hitting an obstacle	(3)					
97. Mobility 12 stairs up without falling or hitting an obstacle	(3)					
98. Mobility 12 stairs down without falling or hitting an obstacle	(3)					
99. Mobility on uneven surface for 20 feet without falling	(3)					
100. Achieve resting position	(2)					
101. Transfer from floor to ambulation position	(3)					
102. Transfer from sitting position in chair to lying in bed	(2)					

continues

Exhibit A–8 continued

C. Get into car

103. Open door	(2)					
104. Get seat into car	(2)					
105. Get feet into car	(2)					
106. Load necessary equipment	(3)					
107. Close door	(2)					

D. Get out of car

108. Open door	(2)					
109. Get feet out of car	(2)					
110. Get seat out of car	(2)					
111. Assume ambulation position	(2)					
112. Unload necessary equipment	(3)					
113. Close door	(1)					

E. Mobility through doors

114. Operate doorknob	(1)					
115. Open door toward self	(2)					
116. Open door away from self	(2)					
117. Close door toward self	(2)					
118. Close door away from self	(1)					

BATHING/HYGIENE:

A. Achieve bathing position

119. Achieve bathing position	(3)					

B. Accomplish set up

120. Obtain soap, towels, washcloth, shampoo; bring to bathing area	(2)					

C. Adjust water

121. Turn on water	(2)					
122. Regulate temperature	(2)					

continues

Exhibit A–8 continued

D. Apply water to body

123. Apply water to body	(2)					

E. Lather body

124. Grasp soap and/or washcloth	(1)					
125. Lather front of body from head to knees	(3)					
126. Lather back of body from head to knees	(3)					
127. Lather from knees to feet, front and back	(2)					

F. Dry body

128. Dry front of body from head to knees	(2)					
129. Dry back of body from head to knees	(2)					
130. Dry from knees to feet	(2)					

G. Brushing teeth

131. Grasp toothbrush	(1)					
132. Put toothpaste on brush	(2)					
133. Brush teeth	(2)					
134. Release toothbrush	(1)					
135. Rinse/mouthwash	(2)					

H. Comb hair

136. Grasp comb/brush	(1)					
137. Comb top hair	(2)					
138. Comb back hair	(2)					
139. Release comb/brush	(1)					

I. Shaving

140. Grasp shaving device	(1)					
141. Bring shaver to face	(1)					
142. Apply appropriate pressure to shave	(2)					
143. Release shaver	(1)					
144. Apply shaving aids	(2)					

continues

Exhibit A–8 continued

J. Nose blowing

145. Grasp handkerchief	(1)					
146. Bring handkerchief to nose	(1)					
147. Wipe nose	(2)					

K. Clip nails

148. Clip nails	(2)					

L. Take medication

149. Take medication	(3)					

EATING:

A. Eat solid food

150. Grasp knife	(1)					
151. Grasp fork/spoon	(1)					
152. Cut food (sufficient force)	(2)					
153. Spear food portion with fork	(2)					
154. Place portion inside mouth	(2)					
155. Chewing	(3)					
156. Swallowing	(3)					

B. Eat semi-solid food

157. Scoop food portion onto utensil	(2)					
158. Place food inside mouth	(2)					

C. Eat liquid food

159. Scoop food portion from bowl	(2)					
160. Place portion inside mouth	(2)					

continues

Exhibit A–8 continued

D. Drink

161. Grasp container	(1)					
162. Bring container to mouth	(2)					
163. Intake liquid without spilling	(2)					
164. Swallow liquid without choking	(3)					

EMERGENCY TELEPHONE COMMUNICATION:

A. Telephone

165. Grasp receiver	(1)					
166. Bring receiver to ear	(2)					
167. Dial (standard) number	(2)					
168. Hold receiver in place for 60 seconds	(2)					
169. Verbalize (standard) message into telephone	(2)					
170. Replace receiver on telephone	(1)					

Source: Courtesy of Ronald M. Klein, PhD.

Exhibit A–9 Klein–Bell Activities of Daily Living Scale Score Sheet

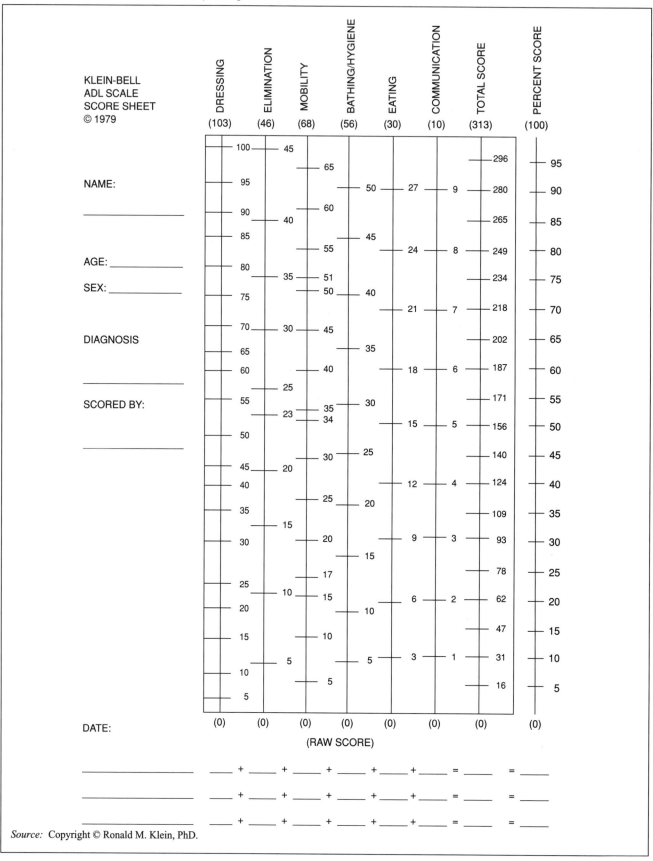

Source: Copyright © Ronald M. Klein, PhD.

Time Care Profile

An unusual approach to the functional assessment of activities of daily living is seen in the Time Care Profile (Halstead & Hartley, 1975). It "utilizes a diary method to record the amount of time the patient receives assistance during the course of a normal day as an index of dependency" (p. 110). This design is in contrast to most instruments used to measure activities of daily living, which assess only the patient's ability to perform specific tasks and completely ignore the time element.

Results of initial validity studies showed that frequency of assistance provided was a more dependable measure, when the diary method versus length-of-time measurements were compared. The authors noted that the amount of service a patient requires is related to fatigue, motivation, and other factors and is not necessarily fully reflected by instruments that determine only whether the patient can perform an activity (perhaps at an ideal time and under the most favorable circumstances).

Initial evaluation of the instrument was conducted on five patients with stroke by using six areas of ADL for two days. The individual patient diaries were completed by caregivers for 24-hour periods. Concurrent observer assessments of time and type of caregiving were also performed. Findings were as described above. Although not widely used, this approach is of great theoretical and practical interest.

REFERENCE

Halstead, L., & Hartley, R.B. (1975). Time Care Profile: An evaluation of a new method of assessing ADL dependence. *Archives of Physical Medicine and Rehabilitation, 56*(3), 110–115.

Instrumental Activities of Daily Living

The Instrumental Activities of Daily Living (IADL Scale) (Lawton & Brody, 1969) (see Exhibit A–10) was designed to provide a simple, reliable, comprehensive assessment of elderly people in skills necessary for independent living in the community. The scale can be used to suggest interventions or serve in the evaluation of progress.

There are eight areas of assessment on the IADL Scale: ability to use a telephone, shopping, food preparation, housekeeping, laundry, mode of transportation, responsibility for own medications, and ability to handle finances. Scores are based on observation of behavior and need for assistance. The eight categories are rated according to three to five levels of independence. Higher scores indicate increased need for assistance (Lawton & Brody, 1969).

Validity of the IADL Scale was established by correlating it with the Physical Self-Maintenance Scale, developed at the Langley-Porter Neuropsychiatric Institute (Lowenthal, 1964), by using the following three measures:

1. Physical Classification, a six-point rating scale of functional health rated by the physician with the use of medical history, physical examination, and laboratory study findings (Waldman & Fryman, 1964)
2. Mental Status Questionnaire, a 10-item test of orientation and memory (Kahn, Goldfarb, Pollock, & Gerber, 1960)
3. Behavior and Adjustment Rating Scales, four six-point scales measuring intellectual, personal, behavioral, and social adjustment (Waldman & Fryman, 1964, revised by Brody & Lawton in Lawton & Brody, 1969)

The IADL Scale, Physical Self-Maintenance Scale, and above-listed three instruments each measure different levels of functioning in an individual. The IADL Scale is more suitable for women. When administered to men, food prepara-tion, housekeeping, and laundry categories are eliminated, and the instrument is consequently much shorter (Lawton & Brody, 1969). According to Lawton and Brody (1969), "competence at one level is likely to be roughly related to competence at another, with the amount of shared variance differing as a direct function of the proximity of the pair of levels to each other in the hierarchy of complexity" (p. 183). Lawton (1983) developed a hierarchy of behavioral competence, which included health, functional health, cognition, time use, and social behavior. Within these groups were possible behaviors ranging from simple to more complex. In the functional health category, the example of the simplest behavior was physical activities of daily living (ADL), followed by instrumental ADL, financial management, and, at the more complex level, paid employment.

A rough regularity of relationships was demonstrated between the Physical Self-Maintenance Scale and IADL Scale and three other functional measures, giving support to the validity of the measures (Lawton & Brody, 1969). Extensive reliability studies have not been done.

The IADL Scale has been used and adapted for inclusion in the Older Adult Resources and Services (OARS) instrument (Duke University, 1978). Some of the items have also been used in the Supplement on Aging in the National Health Interview Survey administered by the National Center for Health Statistics (Dawson et al., 1987; Kovar & LaCroix, 1987). The items in the IADL Scale have also been included in an adapted format and scoring in the Philadelphia Geriatric Center Multilevel Assessment Instrument (MAI) (Lawton, Moss, Fulcomer, & Kleban, 1982) and the Self-Evaluation of Life Function (SELF) Scale (Linn & Linn, 1984). According to Lawton (1988), "the Lawton and Brody ADL adds a greater range of scores and therefore may have greater sensitivity, although this has not been demonstrated. The three-point scale versions of ADL that are used in the OARS and the MAI have the advantage of having more psychometric information available" (p. 613).

REFERENCES

Dawson, D., Hendershot, G., & Fulton, J. (1987, June 10). *Aging in the eighties, functional limitations of individuals age 65 years and over, data from the Supplement on Aging to the National Health Interview Survey: United States, 1984.* Hyattsville, MD: U.S. Department of Health and Human Services, Public Health Service.

Duke University Center for the Study of Aging and Human Development (1978). *Functional assessment: The OARS methodology.* Durham, NC: Duke University.

Kahn, R.I., Goldfarb, A.I., Pollock, M., & Gerber, I.E. (1960, August). The relationship of mental and physical status in institutionalized aged persons. *American Journal of Psychiatry, 117,* 120–124.

Kovar, M.G., & LaCroix, A.Z. (1987, May 8). *Aging in the eighties, ability to perform work-related activities, data from the Supplement on Aging to the National Health Interview Survey: United States, 1984.* Hyattsville, MD: U.S. Department of Health and Human Services, Public Health Service.

Lawton, M.P. (1983). Environment and other determinants of well-being in older people. *Gerontologist, 23*(4), 349–357.

Lawton, M.P. (1988). Scales to measure competence in everyday activities. *Psychopharmacology Bulletin, 24*(4), 609–614.

Lawton, M.P., & Brody, E.M. (1969). Assessment of older people: Self-maintaining and instrumental activities of daily living. *Gerontologist, 9,* 179–186.

Lawton M.P., Moss, M., Fulcomer, M., & Kleban, M.H. (1982). A research and service-oriented multilevel assessment instrument. *Journal of Gerontology, 37*(1), 91–99.

Exhibit A–10 Scale for Instrumental Activities of Daily Living

MALE SCORE		FEMALE SCORE
	A. Ability to use telephone	
1	1. Operates telephone on own initiative—looks up and dials numbers, etc.	1
1	2. Dials a few well-known numbers.	1
1	3. Answers telephone but does not dial.	1
0	4. Does not use telephone at all.	0
	B. Shopping	
1	1. Takes care of all shopping needs independently.	1
0	2. Shops independently for small purchases.	0
0	3. Needs to be accompanied on any shopping trip.	0
0	4. Completely unable to shop.	0
	C. Food preparation	
	1. Plans, prepares, and serves adequate meals independently.	1
	2. Prepares adequate meals if supplied with ingredients.	0
	3. Heats and serves prepared meals, or prepares meals but does not maintain adequate diet.	0
	4. Needs to have meals prepared and served.	0
	D. Housekeeping	
	1. Maintains house alone or with occasional assistance (e.g., "heavy work-domestic help").	1
	2. Performs light daily tasks such as dishwashing, bedmaking.	1
	3. Performs light daily tasks but cannot maintain acceptable level of cleanliness.	1
	4. Needs help with all home maintenance tasks.	1
	5. Does not participate in any housekeeping tasks.	0
	E. Laundry	
	1. Does personal laundry completely.	1
	2. Launders small items—rinses socks, stockings, etc.	1
	3. All laundry must be done by others.	0
	F. Mode of transportation	
1	1. Travels independently on public transportation or drives own car.	1
1	2. Arranges own travel via taxi, but does not otherwise use public transportation.	1
0	3. Travels on public transportation when assisted or accompanied by another.	1
0	4. Travel limited to taxi or automobile with assistance of another.	0
0	5. Does not travel at all.	0
	G. Responsibility for own medications	
1	1. Is responsible for taking medication in correct dosages at correct time.	1
0	2. Takes responsibility if medication is prepared in advance in separate dosages.	0
0	3. Is not capable of dispensing own medication.	0
	H. Ability to handle finances	
1	1. Manages financial matters independently (budgets, writes checks, pays rent, bills, goes to bank), collects and keeps track of income.	1
1	2. Manages day-to-day purchases, but needs help with banking, major purchases, etc.	1
1	3. Incapable of handling money.	0

Source: Copyright © M. Powell Lawton, PhD.

Linn, M.W., & Linn, B.S. (1984). Self-Evaluation of Life (SELF) Scale: A short comprehensive self-report of health for the elderly. *Journal of Gerontology, 39*(5), 603–612.

Lowenthal, M.F. (1964). *Lives in distress.* New York: Basic Books.

Waldman, A., & Fryman, E. (1964). Classification in homes for the aged. In H. Shore & M. Leeds (Eds.), *Geriatric institutional management.* New York: Putnam's.

Outpatient Functional Status Monitoring Instrument

Medical Rehabilitation Follow Along (MRFA™ Instrument)

The Medical Rehabilitation Follow Along (MRFA™ instrument) was designed for medical rehabilitation outpatient settings to assess and monitor the functional status of patients with identified disability problems (Baker, Granger, & Fiedler, in press). The formats cover physical functioning, pain experience, affective well-being, and cognitive functioning. Rasch analysis was used to construct nonredundant, unidimensional, linear, equal interval measures. These assessments reflect the quality of daily living of persons with disability. They can also assist in screening and early identification of problems in functioning to prevent secondary complications.

There are three formats of the MRFA™ instrument: musculoskeletal, neurologic, and multiple sclerosis forms, covering the relevant domains of overall quality of daily living.

The musculoskeletal form consists of 31 patient report items and includes the three domains of physical functioning, experience of pain, and affective well-being. Component scales include body movement and control, perceived effort, painfree, a visual analog rating scale, placid, and satisfaction with life in general. Elements are derived from the Functional Assessment Screening Questionnaire (Granger & Wright, 1993), the Oswestry Scale (Fairbank, Couper, Davies, & O'Brien, 1980), and the Short Form McGill Pain Questionnaire (Melzack, 1987). This form is rated by the patient.

The neurologic form of the MRFA™ instrument uses 39 elements selected from the Functional Independence Measure (FIM℠ instrument) and Mini-Mental State Examination (MMSE), as well as items to evaluate instrumental activities of daily living (see FIM℠ and MMSE descriptions). It includes a limitations component to provide an overview of the degree to which function is limited by various types of impairment. Domains include physical functioning, experience of pain, cognition, and affective well-being. This form is rated by the clinician with input from the patient (and caregiver when appropriate). The multiple sclerosis form is derived from elements in the neurologic form.

Administration. The patient report components of the MRFA™ instrument may be self-administered or conducted with an interview format. The neurologic form is administered through the clinician by interview with the patient and caregiver. The multiple sclerosis form is administered by the clinician or the patient.

Psychometric Properties. The initial reliability study of the musculoskeletal form of the MRFA™ instrument demonstrated overall high test-retest reliability. Intraclass correlation coefficient, a reliability coefficient assessing the stability of responses, showed values ranging from $r = .74$ to $r = .97$ for the physical functioning domain. The intraclass correlation coefficient values for the items assessing pain and psychological well-being ranged from .36 to .93. The item with the lowest value (fearful pain) has been dropped from the measure.

Validity studies for the musculoskeletal form have been completed by using both raw scoring and Rasch measures. Content, construct, and criterion validity have been addressed in these studies. The results provide support for the validity of inferences made from the raw scores and Rasch measures of the MRFA™ instrument for persons with musculoskeletal problems. Additional studies are being conducted with other types of problems in outpatient medical rehabilitation settings (Baker, Granger, & Ottenbacher, 1996; Granger, Ottenbacher, Baker, & Sehgal, 1995). Reliability and validity studies are being conducted on the neurologic form of the MRFA™ instrument.

Assessments of quality of daily living in the MRFA™ instrument series are the first disability instruments designed through Rasch analysis to assess the specific types of problems encountered with medical rehabilitation outpatients. By assessing patients early, it may be possible to prevent later secondary complications.

REFERENCES

Baker, J.G., Granger, C.V., & Fiedler, R.C. (in press). A brief outpatient functional assessment measure: Validity using Rasch measures. *American Journal of Physical Medicine and Rehabilitation.*

Baker, J.G., Granger, C.V., & Ottenbacher K.J. (1996). Validity of a brief outpatient functional assessment measure. *American Journal of Physical Medicine and Rehabilitation.*

Fairbank, J.C., Couper, J., Davies, J.B., & O'Brien, J.P. (1980). The Oswestry Low Back Pain Disability Questionnaire. *Physiotherapy, 66,* 271–273.

Granger, C.V., Ottenbacher, K.J., Baker, J.G., & Sehgal, A. (1995). Reliability of a brief outpatient functional outcome assessment measure.

American Journal of Physical Medicine and Rehabilitation, 74(6), 469–475.

Granger, C.V., & Wright, B.D. (1993). Looking ahead to the use of functional assessment in ambulatory physiatric and primary care: The Functional Assessment Screening Questionnaire. *Physical Medicine and Rehabilitation Clinics of North America, 4,* 1–11.

Melzack, R. (1987). The Short Form McGill Pain Questionnaire. *Pain, 30,* 191–197.

Cognitive Function and Affect Measures

Agitated Behavior Scale

The Agitated Behavior Scale (ABS) (Corrigan, 1989) (see Exhibit A–11) was developed at Ohio State University. This 14-item scale was designed to assess agitation in individuals with traumatic brain injury during the acute stage of recovery. It has been tested on an independent sample of 35 subjects with head injuries.

To ensure that the full domain of agitation was included in scale items, descriptors in the literature were identified. In addition, items were elicited from representatives of rehabilitation disciplines of the traumatic brain injury unit in a selected facility. The rehabilitation professionals were asked to list behaviors seen in agitated patients. These lists were collected, and one week later the professionals participated in a structured elicitation technique described by Kelly (1955). The structured and unstructured techniques elicited 39 initial descriptors in an initial item pool, which was then used by registered nurses on the traumatic head injury unit. Their 67 observations were analyzed to select items for the ABS. Corrigan (1989) was guided by the recommendations of Nunnally (1978) and Carmines and Zeller (1979), which included the intent to sample the "full domain of agitation while eliminating items that could not be reliably rated, were not related to the construct, or contributed minimal variance to its observation" (Corrigan, 1989, pp. 263–264). The original pool was reduced to 14 items, and a new sample was used to validate the instrument.

Each item of the ABS is scored on a scale of one to four as follows: 1 = absent, 2 = present to a slight degree, 3 = present to a moderate degree, and 4 = present to an extreme degree. A person was considered agitated if the total score for an eight-hour shift was above 21, the mean score for all patients with head injury (Corrigan, 1989).

Reliability was determined by measures of internal consistency and qualitative findings from principal components factor analysis. Cronbach's alpha was above .80 for ratings by two registered nurses, one occupational therapist, and one physical therapist (Corrigan, 1989). Results of the principal factor analysis indicated that the ABS had adequate internal consistency.

Four measures were used to evaluate concurrent validity: the Braintree Agitation Scale (Weinberg, Auerbach, & Moore, 1983) as well as three linear combinations of ratings made by four independent observers. Correlations were consistently high ($p < .0001$) and of practical and statistical significance. According to Corrigan, "the lowest correlation identified was between the ABS score for PTs [physical therapists] and the Braintree Agitation Scales completed by medical residents" (Corrigan, 1989, p. 273).

Corrigan and Bogner (1994) investigated the underlying factor structure of the ABS and determined the systematic effects of time-of-day on occurrence of agitation. Two-hundred twelve patients who exhibited agitation while receiving treatment on a brain injury unit for traumatic or recently acquired brain injury were studied. The factor analysis indicated that three factors represented the general construct of agitation: aggression, disinhibition, and lability. Overall level of agitation was lowest during the night shift when rated by registered nurses.

Objective measures of agitation in clinical settings are necessary to determine and monitor interventions. The ABS is simple to administer yet yields a wealth of data. It can be used to answer specific questions about agitation after acquired brain injury. This instrument seems to be a valid and reliable measure of agitation.

The ABS can be obtained from Dr. J.D. Corrigan, Department of Physical Medicine and Rehabilitation, The Ohio State University, 480 West 9th Avenue, Columbus, OH 43210.

REFERENCES

Carmines, E.G., & Zeller, R.A. (1979). *Reliability and validity assessment.* Beverly Hills, CA: Sage.

Corrigan, J.D. (1989). Development of a scale for assessment of agitation following traumatic brain injury. *Journal of Clinical and Experimental Neuropsychology, 11*(2), 261–277.

Corrigan, J.D., & Bogner, J.A. (1994). Factor structure of the Agitated Behavior Scale. *Journal of Clinical and Experimental Neuropsychology, 16*(3), 386–392.

Kelly, G.A. (1955). *The psychology of personal constructs,* Vol. I. New York: Norton.

Nunnally, J.C. (1978). *Psychometric theory.* New York: McGraw-Hill.

Weinberg, R.M., et al. (1983, October). Management of the agitated patient. Paper presented at the Fourth Annual Traumatic Brain Injury Conference, Braintree, MA.

Exhibit A–11 Agitated Behavior Scale

Patient _____   Period of Observation:

                                                                                      a.m.

Observ. Environ. _____   From: _____   p.m.___/___/___

                                                                                      a.m.

Rater/Disc. _____   To: _____   p.m.___/___/___

At the end of the observation period indicate whether each behavior was present and, if so, to what degree: slight, moderate or extreme. The degree can be based on either the frequency of the behavior or the severity of a given incident. Use the following numerical values for every behavior listed. DO NOT LEAVE BLANKS.

      1 = absent
      2 = present to a slight degree
      3 = present to a moderate degree
      4 = present to an extreme degree

____   1. Short attention span, easy distractibility, inability to concentrate.

____   2. Impulsive, impatient, low tolerance for pain or frustration.

____   3. Uncooperative, resistant to care, demanding.

____   4. Violent and/or threatening violence toward people or property.

____   5. Explosive and/or unpredictable anger.

____   6. Rocking, rubbing, moaning or other self-stimulating behavior.

____   7. Pulling at tubes, restraints, etc.

____   8. Wandering from treatment areas.

____   9. Restlessness, pacing, excessive movement.

____ 10. Repetitive behaviors, motor and/or verbal.

____ 11. Rapid, loud or excessive talking.

____ 12. Sudden changes of mood.

____ 13. Easily initiated or excessive crying and/or laughter.

____ 14. Self-abusiveness, physical and/or verbal.

____ Total Score

Source: Reprinted with permission from J.D. Corrigan, Development of a Scale for Assessment of Agitation Following Traumatic Brain Injury. *Journal of Clinical and Experimental Psychology,* Vol. 11, No. 2, pp. 261–277, © 1989, Swets and Zeitlinger.

Mini-Mental State Examination (MMSE)

The Mini-Mental State Examination (MMSE) (Folstein, Folstein, & McHugh, 1975) (see Exhibit A–12) was developed to assess the cognitive state of psychogeriatric patients (older persons with psychiatric problems) with delirium or dementia syndromes. The test focuses on cognitive aspects of mental function only and excludes questions concerning mood, abnormal mental experiences, and form of thinking. It is, however, thorough in examination of the cognitive realm. The MMSE is not a substitute for a full mental status examination, nor a neuropsychological examination, because of the aforementioned excluded areas (Cockrell & Folstein, 1988).

The MMSE consists of two parts, with a maximum score of 21 on the first and a maximum score of 9 on the second (total possible score = 30). The first part requires vocal response and tests orientation, memory, and attention. Ability to name, follow verbal and written commands, write a sentence spontaneously, and copy two overlapping pentagons are tested in the second part. Patients are required to read and write when taking the second part, so individuals with impaired vision may have difficulties taking the MMSE. These difficulties can be overcome with the use of large print (Folstein et al., 1975). The test is not timed, and instructions accompany the MMSE. The scale used in this test is a ratio scale in which a score for each component is obtained by summing the correct item responses within the components of each section. The MMSE takes from 5 to 10 minutes to administer.

The MMSE separates patients with cognitive disturbance from those without and has been deemed a valid test to determine cognitive function (Folstein et al., 1975). Scores rise when and if cognitive state improves. Concurrent validity was determined by correlating the MMSE scores with scores on the Wechsler Adult Intelligence Scale. There is a significant correlation between the two tests. It should be emphasized that data from the MMSE, cognitive ability indicated in the psychiatric history, results of a full mental status examination, physical examination findings, and relevant laboratory data all contribute to accurate diagnosis (Folstein et al., 1975). Findings from the MMSE also correlate with those from computed tomography of the brain (Tsai & Tsuang, 1979) and electroencephalography (Tune & Folstein, 1986).

According to Folstein et al. (1975), "the test is reliable on 24 hour or 28 day retest by single or multiple examiners. When the MMSE was given twice 24 hours apart by the same tester on both occasions, the correlation by Pearson coefficient was 0.887. Scores were not significantly different using a Wilcoxon T" (p. 194). To determine examiner effect on 24-hour test–retest reliability, the MMSE was given twice but by two different examiners. The Pearson product-moment correlation (r) demonstrated a continued high correlation at .83. When elderly depressed and demented patients—who were chosen for their clinical stability—were given the MMSE twice, an average of 28 days apart, the Pearson product-moment correlation of test 1 vs. test 2 was .98 (Folstein et al., 1975).

Although the MMSE cannot carry the diagnostic responsibility alone, the objective data support or negate vague and subjective impressions of cognitive disability formed during the course of the history and physical examination. The few minutes required for completion of the MMSE are a definite advantage, given the information provided in return. In addi-

tion, the MMSE can be given a second time during an illness with little demonstrated practice effect, which is improved performance due solely to increased familiarity with instrument and absence of any real change in cognitive function. It is also useful in teaching psychiatry residents to become skilled in evaluating the cognitive aspects of mental status (Folstein et al., 1975).

The MMSE has been used in evaluating the cognitive status of individuals with Alzheimer's disease in which orientation and recall sections demonstrated the most importance (Allen, Namazi, Patterson, Crozier, & Groth, 1992; Ashford, Kolm, Colliver, Bekian, & Hsu, 1989; Ashford et al., 1992; Galasko et al., 1990), in patients with multiple sclerosis (Franklin, Heaton, Nelson, Filley, & Seibert, 1988; Grigsby, Kravcisin, Ayarbe, & Busenbark, 1993), and for the preliminary screening diagnosis and serial assessment of psychogeriatric patients (Cockrell & Folstein, 1988). The MMSE can be very useful when performance on each item, rather than the total score, is noted (Wade, 1992).

The MMSE also has some limitations. Although designed for elderly patients who are often unable to tolerate lengthy examinations, the MMSE overestimates cognitive impairments in this group and in persons with less than nine years of education. It has also been reported that it lacks sensitivity in persons with right hemisphere dysfunction, as well as with milder forms of cognitive dysfunction regardless of cortical origin (Naugle & Kawczak, 1989). Wade (1992) points out that "it attempts to compress assessment of too many functions into one test, making interpretation of an isolated score difficult" (p. 62). Thus researchers and clinicians must be aware of the situations in which this test may produce misleading data.

REFERENCES

Allen, P.A., Namazi, K.H., Patterson, M.B., Crozier, L.C., & Groth, K.E. (1992). Impact of adult age and Alzheimer's disease on levels of neural noise for letter matching. *Journal of Gerontology 47*(5), 344–349.

Ashford, J.W., Kolm, P., Colliver, J.A., Bekian, C., & Hsu, L.N. (1989). Alzheimer patient evaluation and the Mini-Mental State: Item characteristic curve analysis. *Journal of Gerontology, 44*(5), 239–246.

Ashford, J.W., Kumar, V., Barringer, M., Becker, M., Bice, J., Ryan, N., & Vicari, S. (1992, Summer). Assessing Alzheimer severity with a global clinical scale. *International Psychogeriatrics 4*(1), 55–74.

Cockrell, J.R., & Folstein, M.F. (1988). Mini-Mental State Examination (MMSE). *Psychopharmacology Bulletin, 24*(4), 689–692.

Folstein, M.F., Folstein, S.E., & McHugh, P.R. (1975). "Mini-Mental State": A practical method for grading the cognitive state of patients for the clinician. *Journal of Psychiatric Research, 12*(3), 189–198.

Franklin, G.M., Heaton, R.K., Nelson, L.M., Filley, C.M., & Seibert, C. (1988). Correlation of neuropsychological and MRI findings in chronic/progressive multiple sclerosis. *Neurology, 38*(12), 1826–1829.

Galasko, D., Klauber, M.R., Hofstetter, R., Salmon, D.P., Lasker, B., & Thal, L.J. (1990). The Mini-Mental State Examination in the early diagnosis of Alzheimer's disease. *Archives of Neurology, 47*(1), 49–52.

Grigsby, J., Kravcisin, N., Ayarbe, S.D., & Busenbark, D. (1993). Prediction of deficits in behavioral self-regulation among persons with multiple sclerosis. *Archives of Physical Medicine and Rehabilitation, 74*(12), 1350–1353.

Naugle, R.I., & Kawczak, K. (1989). Limitations of the Mini-Mental State Examination. *Cleveland Clinic Journal of Medicine, 56*(3), 277–281.

Tsai, L., & Tsuang, M.T. (1979). The Mini-Mental State Test and computerized tomography. *American Journal of Psychiatry, 136*(4A), 436–438.

Tune, L., & Folstein, M.F. (1986). Post-operative delirium. *Advances in Psychosomatic Medicine, 15*, 51–68.

Wade, D.T. (1992). *Measurement in neurological rehabilitation.* New York: Oxford University Press.

Exhibit A–12 Mini-Mental State Examination (MMSE)

INSTRUCTIONS FOR ADMINISTRATION OF THE
MINI-MENTAL STATE EXAMINATION

ORIENTATION

1) Ask for the date. Then ask specifically for parts omitted, e.g., "Can you also tell me what season it is?" One point for each correct.
2) Ask in turn "Can you tell me the name of this hospital?" (town, county, etc.) One point for each correct.

REGISTRATION

Ask the patient if you can test his (sic) memory. Then say the names of 3 unrelated objects, clearly and slowly, about one second for each. After you have said all 3, ask him (sic) to repeat them. This first repetition determines his (sic) score (0–3) but keep saying them until he (sic) can repeat all 3, up to 7 trials. If he (sic) does not eventually learn all 3, recall cannot be meaningfully tested.

ATTENTION AND CALCULATION

Ask the patient to begin with 100 and count backwards by 7. Stop after 5 subtractions (93, 86, 79, 72, 65). Score the total number of correct answers.

If the patient cannot or will not perform this task, ask him (sic) to spell the word "world" backwards. The score is the number of letters in correct order, e.g. dlrow = 5, dlorw = 3.

RECALL

Ask the patient if he (sic) can recall the 3 words you previously asked him to remember, score 0–3.

LANGUAGE

Naming: Show the patient a wrist watch and ask him (sic) what it is. Repeat for pencil. Score 0–2.

Repetition: Ask the patient to repeat the sentence after you. Allow only one trial. Score 0 or 1.

3-Stage command: Give the patient a piece of plain blank paper and repeat the command. Score 1 point for each part correctly executed.

Reading: On a blank piece of paper print the sentence "close your eyes," in letters large enough for the patient to see clearly. Ask him (sic) to read it and do what it says. Score 1 point only if he (sic) actually closes his (sic) eyes.

Writing: Give the patient a blank piece of paper and ask him (sic) to write a sentence for you. Do not dictate a sentence; it is to be written spontaneously. It must contain a subject and verb and be sensible. Correct grammar and punctuation are not necessary.

Copying: On a clean piece of paper, draw intersecting pentagons, each side about 1 in., and ask him (sic) to copy it exactly as it is. All 10 angles must be present and 2 must intersect to score 1 point. Tremor and rotation are ignored.

Estimate the patient's level of sensorium along a continuum, from alert on the left to coma on the right.

MINI-MENTAL STATE EXAMINATION (MMSE)

		Score	*Points*
Orientation			
1. What is the	Year?	_____	1
	Season?	_____	1
	Date?	_____	1
	Day?	_____	1
	Month?	_____	1
2. Where are we?	State?	_____	1
	County?	_____	1
	Town or city?	_____	1
	Hospital?	_____	1
	Floor?	_____	1

continues

Exhibit A–12 continued

	Score	Points

Registration

3. Name three objects, taking one second to say each. Then ask the patient all three after you have said them. Give one point for each correct answer. Repeat the answers until the patient learns all three.   _____   3

Attention and calculation

4. Serial sevens. Give one point for each correct answer. Stop after five answers. *Alternate*: Spell WORLD backwards.   _____   5

Recall

5. Ask for names of three objects learned in question 3. Give one point for each correct answer.   _____   3

Language

6. Point to a pencil and a watch. Have the patient name them as you point.   _____   2
7. Have the patient repeat "No ifs, ands, or buts."   _____   1
8. Have the patient follow a three-stage command. "Take the paper in your right hand. Fold the paper in half. Put the paper on the floor."   _____   3
9. Have the patient read and obey the following: "CLOSE YOUR EYES." (Write it in large letters.)   _____   1
10. Have the patient write a sentence of his or her own choice. (The sentence should contain a subject and a verb and should make sense.) Ignore spelling errors when scoring.   _____   1
11. Have the patient copy the figure below. (Give two overlapping pentagons and one point if all sides and angles are preserved and if the intersecting sides form a quadrangle).   _____   1

    _____   Total = 30

Source: Copyright © Marshall Folstein, M.D.

Hamilton Rating Scale for Depression

The Hamilton Rating Scale for Depression was developed to assess severity of illness in patients already diagnosed with depressive illness. Multiple versions of the instrument exist. The initial 17-item scale relates to symptoms associated with depression, such as depressed mood, insomnia, general somatic symptoms, insight, and loss of weight (Hamilton, 1960). It was later revised to include 21 items (Hamilton, 1967). The interviewer elicits information about commonly occurring symptoms. Scoring is done by an observer after completing an interview. Symptoms are rated on a three-point scale (0–2) ranging from absent to clearly present, or a five-point scale (0–4) ranging from absent to severe (Hamilton, 1967). The three-point scale is used when quantification of a variable is difficult or impossible. Most of the items are graded on the five-point scale (Hamilton,

1974). Hamilton (1960) states that "no distinction is made between intensity and frequency of symptom, the rater having to give due weight to both of them in making his [or her] judgement (sic)" (p. 57).

Preliminary studies in which two physicians scored the same patient's responses were used in attempts to establish inter-rater reliability. Correlations for the successive addition of 10 patients at a time ranged from .84 to .90, with the last correlation as the total for 70 patients (Hamilton, 1960). Hamilton (1969) reports inter-rater reliability of different raters for the same interview as ranging between .80 and .90.

The Hamilton Rating Scale for Depression has been used extensively in drug trials, to examine differences in depressive illness in men and women (Hamilton, 1967), and in studying depression in individuals challenged by a stroke (U.S. Department of Health and Human Services, 1995). It has been translated into several languages as well as used as a basis for several other scales.

According to Wade (1992), "the scale was designed to help psychiatrically trained observers standardize clinical judgements (sic) but not to diagnose severity of depression. It requires a psychiatrically trained observer, and simply standardizes clinical judgements (sic)" (p. 270). Advantages of this scale are that it is easy to use, is observer rated, and requires minimal additional training to produce reliable results. In addition, it can be completed as a result of a routine clinical interview. A disadvantage is the time it takes for an interview, but this time is necessary to get to know the patient and establish rapport (Hamilton, 1969). Another disadvantage is that multiple differing versions compromise interobserver reliability (U.S. Department of Health and Human Services, 1995).

REFERENCES

Hamilton, M. (1960, February). A rating scale for depression. *Journal of Neurology and Neurosurgical Psychiatry, 23*, 56–62.

Hamilton, M. (1967). Development of a rating scale for primary depressive illness. *British Journal of Social and Clinical Psychology, 6*(4), 278–296.

Hamilton, M. (1969). Standardized assessment and recording of depressive symptoms. *Psychiatria, Neurologia, Neurochirurgia, 72*(2), 201–205.

Hamilton, M. (1974). General problems of psychiatric rating scales (especially for depression). *Modern Problems of Pharmacopsychiatry, 7*, 125–138.

U.S. Department of Health and Human Services. (1995, May). *Post-stroke rehabilitation: Assessment, referral, and patient management* (AHCPR Publication No. 95-0663). Rockville, MD: Author.

Wade, D.T. (1992). *Measurement in neurological rehabilitation*. Oxford, England: Oxford University Press.

Self-rating Depression Scale

The Self-rating Depression Scale (SDS) (see Exhibit A–13) developed by Zung (1965), is a short and simple instrument designed to assess depression in persons with a primary diagnosis of depressive disorder. It includes all symptoms of the illness, is self-administered, and indicates the patient's own response at the time the scale is administered (Zung, 1965). Verbatim records of patient interviews and statements that were most representative of particular symptoms were used to develop items for inclusion (Zung, 1965). The commonly found characteristics of depression accounted for in this instrument are divided into "pervasive affect, physiological equivalents or concomitants, and psychological concomitants" (p. 63).

The SDS contains 20 items, 10 worded positively and 10 worded negatively. The patient responds to each item by marking in one of four columns indicating "a little of the time," "some of the time," "good part of the time," or "most of the time." This ordinal scale is scored by assigning numerical values from one to four, respectively, for positively worded items and from four to one, respectively, for negatively worded items. The scores for the 20 items are summed to arrive at a raw score. The raw score is divided by 80, the maximum raw score for the 20 responses. The less depression experienced by the patient, the higher will be his or her score. Zung (1967) later found that multiplying the SDS score by 100 to give a whole number made analysis less cumbersome. Indexes for use with the SDS then were mild to moderate depression = 50 and above, moderate to severe depression = 60 and above, and severe depression = 70 and above (Zung, 1967).

Reliability intercorrelations on SDS items were .73 ($p < .01$) (Zung, 1972). Zung (1967) found that outcome of the SDS was not affected by the patient's age, sex, marital status, educational level, financial status, or intelligence level. Zung (1973) reported further that the SDS had shown significant correlations when compared with other depression scales, thereby establishing concurrent validity. No significant differences in accuracy were found when the SDS was compared with the Hamilton Rating Scale for Depression ($r = .79$, $p < .01$) (Brown & Zung, 1972). Measures of central tendency, particularly mean scores, are used to analyze data.

The Depression Status Inventory was introduced in 1972 as an adjunct to the SDS (see Exhibit A–14) (Zung, 1972). This 20-item scale allows an interviewer to record clinical observations to use with patient-reported data on the SDS items.

The SDS performs well clinically, as opposed to diagnostically, when change in symptoms is observed over time (Magruder-Habib et al., 1989). The SDS should not be used exclusively to select treatment modalities (Zung & Wonnacott, 1970), nor for setting up therapy (Colucci, Luciano, & Citarella, 1974).

In addition to its use in English-speaking cultures, the SDS has been used in Italian and French (Colucci et al., 1974), Korean (Kim & Park, 1989), Serbo-Croatian (Smiljkovic & Ocic, 1989), and German (Zerfass, Kretzschmar, & Forstl, 1992) cultures. A guidebook is not available.

REFERENCES

Brown, G.L., & Zung, W.W.K. (1972). Depression scales: Self or physician rating? A validation of certain clinically observable phenomena. *Comprehensive Psychiatry, 13*(4), 361–367.

Colucci, D.C.C., Luciano, L.R., & Citarella, S. (1974). Studies in critical evaluations of Zung's "Self-rating Depression Scale" in a group of patients with depression. (Italian and French). *Acta Neurologica, 29*(5), 574–581.

Kim, K.S., & Park, K.O. (1989). A study on factors related to daily activities of post myocardial infarction patients. *Kanho Hakho Chi, 19*(1), 108–117.

Magruder-Habib, K., Zung, W.W.K., Fuessner, J., Alling, W., Saunders, W., & Stevens, H. (1989). Management of general medical patients with symptoms of depression. *General Hospital Psychiatry, 11*(3), 201–221.

Smiljkovic, P., & Ocic, G. (1989). Thinking disorders in patients with Parkinson's disease. *Srpski Archiv Za Celokupno Lekarstvo, 117*(5–6), 291–300.

Zerfass, R., Kretzschmar, K., & Forstl, H. (1992). Depressive disorders after cerebral infarct. Relations to infarct site, brain atrophy and cognitive deficits. *Nervenrzt, 63*(3), 163–168.

Zung, W.W.K. (1965). A self-rating depression scale. *Archives of General Psychiatry, 12*(1), 63–70.

Zung, W.W.K. (1967). Factors influencing the Self-rating Depression Scale. *Archives of General Psychiatry, 16*(5), 543–547.

Zung, W.W.K. (1972). The Depression Status Inventory: An adjunct to the Self-rating Depression Scale. *Journal of Clinical Psychology, 28*(4), 539–543.

Zung, W.W.K. (1973). From art to science: The diagnosis and treatment of depression. *Archives of General Psychiatry, 29*(3), 328–337.

Zung, W.W.K., & Wonnacott, T.H. (1970). Treatment prediction in depression using a self-rating scale. *Biological Psychiatry, 2*(4), 321–329.

Exhibit A–13 Self-rating Depression Scale

	A Little of the Time	Some of the Time	Good Part of the Time	Most of the Time
1. I feel down-hearted and blue				
2. Morning is when I feel the best				
3. I have crying spells or feel like it				
4. I have trouble sleeping at night				
5. I eat as much as I used to				
6. I still enjoy sex				
7. I notice that I am losing weight				
8. I have trouble with constipation				
9. My heart beats faster than usual				
10. I get tired for no reason				
11. My mind is as clear as it used to be				
12. I find it easy to do the things I used to				
13. I am restless and can't keep still				
14. I feel hopeful about the future				
15. I am more irritable than usual				
16. I find it easy to make decisions				
17. I feel that I am useful and needed				
18. My life is pretty full				
19. I feel that others would be better off if I were dead				
20. I still enjoy the things I used to do				

Source: Copyright © Elizabeth Zung.

The CES–D Scale. The CES–D (Center for Epidemiologic Studies Depression) Scale (see Exhibit A–15) was developed to measure depressive symptoms in the general population (Radloff, 1977). Whereas other scales such as the Hamilton Rating Scale for Depression (Hamilton, 1960) were designed to measure severity of symptoms, the CES–D Scale was designed to measure current depressive symptoms. Items for this instrument were chosen from previously validated scales designed to measure depression (Beck, Ward, Mendelson, Mock, & Erbaugh, 1961; Raskin, Schulterbrandt, Reatig, & McKeon, 1969; Zung, 1965). Review of the psychiatric literature validated the major components of depressive symptoms, including depressed mood, feelings of guilt and worthlessness, feelings of helplessness and hopelessness, psychomotor retardation, loss of appetite, and sleep distur-

bance (Radloff, 1977). Four of 20 items included in this instrument were worded in a positive direction to break response set tendencies. Items were scored on a four-point scale from zero to three, with zero indicating occurrence of a depressive symptom "rarely or none of the time (less than 1 day)" to three indicating "most or all of the time (5–7 days)." Total scores ranged from zero to 60.

Three field surveys were conducted to develop this instrument. The first survey included a structured interview with more than 300 items selected from other scales and standard sociodemographic items. The interviews were conducted in randomly selected households in Kansas City, Missouri (response rate, 75%) and Washington County, Maryland (response rate, 80%). The second survey used a slightly revised and shortened version of the questionnaire in Washington

Exhibit A–14 Depression Status Inventory

Signs & Symptoms of Depression	Interview Guide for Depression Status Inventory (DSI)	Severity of Observed or Reported Responses			
		None	*Mild*	*Mod*	*Sev*
1. Depressed mood	Do you ever feel sad or depressed?	1	2	3	4
2. Crying spells	Do you have crying spells or feel like it?	1	2	3	4
3. Diurnal variation: symptoms worse in a.m.	Is there any part of the day when you feel worst? best?	1	2	3	4
4. Sleep disturbance	How have you been sleeping?	1	2	3	4
5. Decreased appetite	How is your appetite?	1	2	3	4
6. Weight loss	Have you lost any weight?	1	2	3	4
7. Decreased libido	How about your interest in the opposite sex?	1	2	3	4
8. Constipation	Do you have trouble with constipation?	1	2	3	4
9. Tachycardia	Have you had times when your heart was beating faster?	1	2	3	4
10. Fatigue	How easily do you get tired?	1	2	3	4
11. Psychomotor agitation	Do you find yourself restless and can't sit still?	1	2	3	4
12. Psychomotor retardation	Do you feel slowed down in doing the things you usually do?	1	2	3	4
13. Confusion	Do you ever feel confused and have trouble thinking?	1	2	3	4
14. Emptiness	Do you feel life is empty for you?	1	2	3	4
15. Hopelessness	How hopeful do you feel about the future?	1	2	3	4
16. Indecisiveness	How are you at making decisions?	1	2	3	4
17. Irritability	How easily do you get irritated?	1	2	3	4
18. Dissatisfaction	Do you still enjoy the things you used to do?	1	2	3	4
19. Personal devaluation	Do you ever feel useless and not wanted?	1	2	3	4
20. Suicidal ruminations	Have you had thoughts about doing away with yourself?	1	2	3	4

Source: Copyright © Elizabeth Zung.

County only. Major differences in these two surveys were length of interview (60 versus 30 minutes); time (weekly versus four weeks), and site (two sites versus one site). In the third field survey, subjects in surveys one and two were reinterviewed. On reinterview, subjects had significantly lower scores (correlation coefficient .40 or greater), and it was suggested that this finding warranted further analysis. In addition, two clinical validation studies were done: one in Washington County (Craig & Van Natta, 1976) and one in New Haven, Connecticut. Distribution of scores was skewed in the control group and symmetrical in the patient group. In all subgroups used in the field and clinical trials described, coefficient alphas were .80 or greater. Subgroups did not differ from each other or the total population in the factor structure.

Interobserver reliability was determined by using a research nurse and a psychiatric research assistant to administer the test to 27 nonaphasic individuals. The reliability coefficient was .76. Spearman rho correlations between each item and the total test score were calculated for the data obtained by the nurse. All but one were significant ($p > .05$) and ranged from .39 to .75 (Shinar et al., 1986). The CES–D Scale was acceptable to general and clinical populations.

The CES–D Scale correlated highly and significantly with the Present State Examination (Wing, Cooper, & Sartorius, 1974) modified to assess affective mood and anxiety, the Hamilton Rating Scale for Depression (Hamilton, 1960), and the Zung Self-Rating Depression Scale (DeForge & Sobal, 1988; Zung, 1965). The Johns Hopkins Functioning Inventory (Robinson & Benson, 1981; Robinson & Szetela, 1981) was used to assess degree of functional physical impairment, and the Mini-Mental State Examination (MMSE) (Folstein, Folstein, & McHugh, 1975) was used to assess degree of cognitive impairment. Social function was assessed by using the Social Ties Checklist and the Social Functioning Examination (Robinson, Bolduc, Kubos, Starr, & Price, 1985; Starr, Robinson, & Price, 1983). Scores did not correlate with measures of cognitive, physical, or social functioning (Shinar et al., 1986).

In another study (Parikh, Eden, Price, & Robinson, 1988), the sensitivity and specificity of The CES–D Scale was evaluated over a two-year period in a sample of 80 poststroke patients. Significant correlations with diagnoses of depression in the *Diagnostic and Statistical Manual of Mental Disorders* (third edition) were found at three months, six months, and one year but not at two-year follow-up, "reflecting the natural course of these depressions, as well as the predictive validity of the CES-D" (p. 169). The CES–D Scale had a specificity of 90%, a sensitivity of 86%, and positive predictive value of 80% when used with this sample.

Radloff (1977) cautions that the instrument should not be used for clinical diagnoses nor should interpretations of individual scores be made. The scale has a "high internal consistency, acceptable test–retest stability, excellent concurrent validity by clinical and self-report criteria, and substantial evidence of construct validity.... It is suitable for use in Black and White English-speaking American populations of both sexes with a wide range of age and socioeconomic status for the epidemiologic study of depression" (p. 400).

REFERENCES

Beck, A.T., Ward, C.H., Mendelson, M., Mock, J., & Erbaugh, J. (1961). An inventory for measuring depression. *Archives of General Psychiatry, 4*(6), 561–571.

Craig, T.J., & Van Natta, P.A. (1976). Recognition of depressed affect in hospitalized psychiatric patients: Staff and patient perceptions. *Diseases of the Nervous System, 37*(10), 561–566.

DeForge, B.R., & Sobal, J. (1988). Self-report depression scales in the elderly: The relationship between the CES-D and the Zung. *International Journal of Psychiatry in Medicine, 18*(4), 325–338.

Folstein, M.F., Folstein, S.E., & McHugh, P.R. (1975). "Mini-Mental State": A practical method for grading the cognitive state of patients for the clinician. *Journal of Psychiatric Research, 12*(3), 189–198.

Hamilton, M. (1960, February). A rating scale for depression. *Journal of Neurology and Neurosurgical Psychiatry, 23*, 56–62.

Parikh, R.M., Eden, D.T., Price, T.R., & Robinson, R.G. (1988). The sensitivity and specificity of the Center for Epidemiologic Studies Depression Scale in screening for post-stroke depression. *International Journal of Psychiatry in Medicine, 18*(2), 169–181.

Radloff, L.S. (1977). The CES–D Scale: A self-report depression scale for research in the general population. *Applied Psychological Measurement, 1*(3), 365–411.

Raskin, A., Schulterbrandt, J.G., Reatig, N., & McKeon, J.J. (1969). Replication of factors of psychopathology in interview, ward behavior and self-report ratings of hospitalized depressives. *Journal of Nervous and Mental Disease, 148*(1), 87–98.

Robinson, R.G., & Benson, D.F. (1981). Depression in aphasic patients: Frequency, severity and clinical-pathological correlations. *Brain & Language, 14*(2), 282–291.

Robinson, R.G., Bolduc, P.L., Kubos, K.L., Starr, L.B., & Price, T.R. (1985). Social functioning assessment in stroke patients: Responses of patient and other informant and relationship of initial evaluation to six months follow-up. *Archives of Physical Medicine and Rehabilitation, 66*(8), 496–500.

Robinson, R.G., & Szetela, B. (1981) Mood change following left hemispheric brain injury. *Annals of Neurology, 9*(5), 447–453.

Shinar, D., Gross, C.R., Price, T.R., Banko, M., Bolduc, P.L., & Robinson, R.G. (1986). Screening for depression in stroke patients: The reliability and validity of the Center for Epidemiologic Studies Depression Scale. *Stroke, 17*(2), 241–245.

Starr, L.B., Robinson, R.G., & Price, T.R. (1983). Reliability, validity, and clinical utility of the Social Functioning Exam in the assessment of stroke patients. *Experimental Aging Research, 9*(2), 101–106.

Wing, J.K., Cooper, J.E., & Sartorius, N. (1974). *Measurement and classification of psychiatric symptoms*. London, England: Cambridge University Press.

Zung, W.W.K. (1965). A self-rating depression scale. *Archives of General Psychiatry, 12*(1), 63–70.

Exhibit A–15 The CES–D Scale

INSTRUCTIONS FOR QUESTIONS: Below is a list of the ways you might have felt or behaved. Please tell me how often you have felt this way during the past week.

    Rarely or None of the Time (Less than 1 Day)
    Some or a Little of the Time (1–2 Days)
    Occasionally or a Moderate Amount of Time (3–4 Days)
    Most or All of the Time (5–7 Days)

During the past week:	Less than 1 day	1–2 days	3–4 days	5–7 days
1. I was bothered by things that usually don't bother me.	0	1	2	3
2. I did not feel like eating; my appetite was poor.	0	1	2	3
3. I felt that I could not shake off the blues even with help from my family or friends.	0	1	2	3
4. I felt that I was just as good as other people.	0	1	2	3
5. I had trouble keeping my mind on what I was doing.	0	1	2	3
6. I felt depressed.	0	1	2	3
7. I felt that everything I did was an effort.	0	1	2	3
8. I felt hopeful about the future.	0	1	2	3
9. I thought my life had been a failure.	0	1	2	3
10. I felt fearful.	0	1	2	3
11. My sleep was restless.	0	1	2	3
12. I was happy.	0	1	2	3
13. I talked less than usual.	0	1	2	3
14. I felt lonely.	0	1	2	3
15. People were unfriendly.	0	1	2	3
16. I enjoyed life.	0	1	2	3
17. I had crying spells.	0	1	2	3
18. I felt sad.	0	1	2	3
19. I felt that people dislike me.	0	1	2	3
20. I could not get "going."	0	1	2	3

Source: Reprinted from Center for Epidemiological Studies at DHHS.

Functional Communication Instruments

American Speech-Language-Hearing Association Functional Assessment of Communication Skills for Adults (ASHA FACS)

The American Speech-Language-Hearing Association Functional Assessment of Communication Skills for Adults (ASHA FACS) was developed by the American Speech-Language-Hearing Association and further refined, pilot tested, and field tested at 10 rehabilitation facilities representative of each mainland United States region. In addition, two Veterans Administration Medical Centers were used in the trials. The reliability and validity studies were supported by a three-year grant from the U.S. Department of Education's National Institute on Disability and Rehabilitation Research. The project director was Dr. Carol Frattali, former Director of Health Services Division.

The initial goal of this project was to offer a more sensitive analysis of functional communication to complement the use of other widely used measures such as the Functional Independence Measure (FIM℠ instrument). Other instruments to assess communication (see Table A–6) were developed for measurement of specific populations, namely persons with aphasia, even though some instruments such as the Communicative Abilities in Daily Living were applicable to other populations as well (Frattali, Thompson, Holland, Wohl, & Ferketic, 1995). The ASHA FACS measures functional communication across four domains: social communication; communication of basic needs; reading, writing, and number concepts; and daily planning, as well as four qualitative dimensions: adequacy, appropriateness, promptness, and communication sharing. The 43 items included in this instrument are measured on a seven-point scale of communication independence. According to a summary of ASHA FACS Field Test Results, "a more global rating of functional performance in each assessment domain is conducted on the basis of a five-point Scale of Qualitative Dimensions of Communication" (C.M. Frattali, C.K. Thompson, A.L. Holland, C.B. Wohl, & M.M. Ferketic, personal communication, July 1995). Both mean and overall domain and dimension scores are summarized to yield a profile of communication performance.

Subjects for the field test included 131 adults with aphasia as a result of left hemisphere stroke and 54 adults with cognitive communication impairments as a result of traumatic brain injury. All were fluent in English and had adequate hearing and vision. In addition, all had adequate basic reading and writing ability before onset of impairment. A summary of the field test results written by Frattali and others (C. M. Frattali et al., personal communication, July 1995) and transmitted to the editors of this book by ASHA follows and is used with permission.

Summary of Field Test Results

Reliability. Inter-rater reliability for the four communication independence mean scores ranged from .88 to .92. The inter-rater reliability of overall communication independence scores was .95. Percent score agreement across items ranged from 67% to 100% with a mean overall agreement of 91%. Inter-rater reliability for the four qualitative dimension scores ranged from .72 to .84. Inter-rater agreement of overall qualitative dimension scores was .88.

Intra-rater reliability for communication independence scores ranged from .95 to .99; intra-rater agreement of overall communication independence scores was .99. Intra-rater reliability on qualitative dimension scores also was high; correlations ranged from .94 to .99 across qualitative dimensions with overall qualitative dimension scores correlating at .99.

External Validity. For the aphasia group, a correlation of .73 was found between Western Aphasia Battery (WAB) Aphasia Quotients (AQs) and ASHA FACS overall scores. Correlations ranging from .62 to .80 were found between AQs and communication independence scores. Correlations between the ASHA FACS overall communication independence scores and select scales of the Functional Independence Measure (FIM^{SM} Instrument) ranged from .61 to .83. Correlations between ASHA FACS communication independence scores and FIM^{SM} scores ranged from .54 to .87. ASHA FACS overall qualitative dimension scores correlated with WAB AQs at .78.

For the TBI [traumatic brain injury] group, a correlation of .78 was found between ASHA FACS overall communication independence scores and Scale of Cognitive Abilities for Traumatic Brain Injury (SCATBI) severity scores. Correlations between overall communication independence scores

and FIM^{SM} instrument scores ranged from .72 to .86; correlations between communication independence scores and FIM^{SM} instrument scores ranged from .61 to .87. ASHA FACS overall qualitative dimension scores correlated with SCATBI severity scores at .79.

External validity data suggest that the ASHA FACS, which provides more in-depth and detailed information concerning functional communication ability than the FIM^{SM} instrument, can augment FIM^{SM} instrument measurements.

Internal Consistency. All communication independence mean scores correlated with overall independence scores between .89 and .99; all qualitative dimension mean scores correlated with overall dimension scores between .91 and .96.

Factor analysis through principal components resulted in one predominant factor (considered to be functional communication) shared by all ASHA FACS items, accounting for 59% of the underlying variability. All 43 items, treated as independent variables, shared high, positive correlations with this principal factor, implying that the ASHA FACS items measure the same latent construct. More than 73% of the total variance of item scores was accounted for by four "factors" or unifying concepts underlying the ASHA FACS items (i.e., Social Communication; Communication of Basic Needs; Reading, Writing, Number Concepts; Daily Planning).

Measure Sensitivity. A series of analysis of variance determined measure sensitivity. Communication independence and qualitative dimension scores and overall scores all showed significantly different means (at the .001 level of significance) for each of the severity groups (i.e., mild, moderate, severe) in both the aphasia and TBI populations. Thus, the ASHA FACS was found to be sufficiently sensitive to degrees of impairment severity for both populations. TBI subjects showed consistently higher communication independence scores and overall scores than the aphasia subjects. However, the spread of item scores (ranging from 3 to 7), spread of overall communication independence scores (ranging from 5.6 to 7), and spread of overall qualitative dimension scores (ranging from 3.2 to 5) for the mild TBI population suggested the absence of a ceiling effect.

Social Validity. Moderate correlations, ranging from .58 to .73, were found between overall functional communication ratings by clinicians and overall ratings by family members/friends/caregivers. However, family members/friends/caregivers neither consistently overrated nor underrated performance when compared to clinician ratings. This finding supports the need for clinicians to work closely with significant others during the clinical intervention process and to regard them as integral members of the interdisciplinary treatment team.

A consumer survey, in which family members/friends/caregivers rated the importance of ASHA FACS items to functional communication, was completed by 179 respondents. All items were considered either important or some-what important for functional communication by a majority (69% to 99%) of consumers.

Usability. A usability questionnaire was completed by 32 examiners following field testing. Examiners believed administration, rating, and score calculation instructions were clear and easy to follow; few items were problematic and should be deleted; and most items were considered to be sensitive to age, gender, ethnicity, socioeconomic status, and cultural differences. Most examiners believe that the ASHA FACS yields more, better, or different information than other available functional communication measures. On average,

examiners reported that the ASHA FACS takes approximately 20 minutes to administer (C.M. Frattali et al., personal communication, 1995).

A 100-page manual accompanies the instrument. Background information on the measure and administration procedures are included in the manual. Both paper and pencil version and computerized version of the instrument are included with instructions for use. Also included is a rating key on a 5" x 7" card for easy reference. This product is available for $95.00 (1996) plus shipping and handling for ASHA members. Shipping and pricing information can be obtained by calling (301) 897–5700, ext. 218.

REFERENCES

Blomert, L., Kean, M. L., Koster, C., & Schokker, D. (1994). Amsterdam-Nijmagen Everyday Language Test: Construction, reliability, and validity. *Aphasiology, 8*(4), 381–407.

Frattali, C., Thompson C., Holland, A., Wohl, C., & Ferketic, M. (1995). American Speech-Language-Hearing Association Functional Assessment of Communication Skills for Adults (ASHA FACS). Rockville, MD: ASHA.

Goodglass, H., & Kaplan, E. (1984). *Assessment of aphasia and related disorders* (2nd ed.). Baltimore: Williams & Wilkins.

Holland, A.L. (1980). *Communicative Abilities in Daily Living: Manual.* Baltimore: University Park Press.

Jacobson, B., Johnson, A., Silbergleit, A., & Benniger, M. (in press). *Voice Handicap Index,* Detroit: Henry Ford Hospital.

Lomas, J., Pickard, L., Bester, S., Elbard, H., Finlayson, A., & Zoghaib, D. (1989). The Communicative Effectiveness Index: Development and psychometric evaluation of a functional communication for adult aphasia. *Journal of Speech and Hearing Disorders, 54*(1), 113–124.

Payne, J. (1994). *Communication Profile: A Functional Skills Survey.* Tucson, AZ: Communication Skill Builders.

Porch, B.E. (1971). *The Porch Index of Communicative Ability.* Palo Alto, CA: Consulting Psychologists Press.

Sarno, M.T. (1969). *The Functional Communication Profile: Manual of directions.* New York: Institute of Rehabilitation Medicine.

Schow, R., & Nerbonne, M. (1982). Communication screening profile uses with elderly clients. *Ear and Hearing, 3,* 133–147.

Ventry, I.W., & Weinstein, B.E. (1982). The Hearing Handicap Inventory for the Elderly: A new tool. *Ear and Hearing, 3,* 128–134.

Wirz, S.L., Skinner, C., & Dean, E. (1990). *Revised Edinburgh Functional Communication Profile.* Tucson, AZ: Communication Skill Builders.

Table A-6 Characteristics of Selected Functional Communication Instruments

Instrument (Reference)	Communication Components	Assessment Method	Applicable Populations	Reliability/Validity
Functional Communication Profile (FCP; Sarno, 1969)	45 communication behaviors in these areas: movement (e.g., gestures), speaking, understanding, reading, miscellaneous (e.g., writing, calculation)	9-point scale	Adults with aphasia	Concurrent and predictive validity (correlates with measures of auditory memory span and CADL); high interexaminer reliability; test–retest reliability described as significant
Communicative Abilities in Daily Living (CADL; Holland, 1980)	68 items incorporating everyday language activities in these areas: content/form (production, comprehension), cognition, use (role-playing, speech acts)	3-point scoring system. (0 = wrong, 1 = adequate, 2 = correct)	Adults with aphasia, mental retardation or Alzheimer's disease; experienced hearing aid users	Concurrent validity (correlates with Boston Diagnostic Aphasia Examination [Goodglass & Kaplan, 1984], Porch Index of Communicative Ability [Porch, 1971], FCP, and direct observations of communication behavior); high interexaminer and test–retest reliability
Hearing Handicap Inventory for the Elderly (HHIE; Ventry & Weinstein, 1982)	25-item self-assessment questionnaire to identify perceived problems caused by hearing loss (i.e., emotional consequences and social and situational effects)	3-point scale (4 = yes; 2 = sometimes; 0 = no)	Adults with hearing loss	Reported reliability (by assessing internal consistency) as well as construct and content validity
Self-Assessment of Communication (SAC; Schow & Nerbonne, 1982)	10 self-assessment items addressing perceived difficulties in various communication situations, feelings about communication, and the reactions of others to one's hearing	5-point scale (1 = almost never/never; 5 = practically always/always)	Adults with hearing loss	High test–retest reliability and internal consistency, and is predictive of the extent of hearing impairment
Communicative Effectiveness Index (CETI; Lomas et al., 1989)	16 communication items categorized by social need, life skill, basic need, health threat	10-cm visual analogue scale from "not at all able" to "as able as before the stroke"	Adults with aphasia secondary to stroke	Based on evaluation of 22 aphasic patients (11 recovering, 11 stable); has good test–retest and inter-rater reliability; face and construct validity (correlates with global ratings of language and communication by spouses)
Revised Edinburgh Functional Communication Profile (EFCP; Wirz, Skinner, & Dean, 1990)	Communication functions and modalities used: greetings, acknowledging, responding, requesting, initiating	5-point effectiveness scale, and modality used is noted	Adults with aphasia, developmental disorders, mental retardation, cerebral palsy who use AAC systems	No concurrent validity; content validity evaluated by scoring 16-minute language samples and comparing with 10 exchanges; inter-rater reliability on 14 patients

Test	Description	Population	Psychometric Characteristics
Amsterdam-Nijmegen Everyday Language Test (ANELT; Blomert, Kean, Koster, & Schokker, 1994)	Two parallel versions, each consisting of 10 items constructed as scenarios of familiar daily life activities	Adults with aphasia	Psychometric analysis showed perfect parallelism for both test versions. Based on 60 adult subjects with no history of neurological impairment and 60 subjects with aphasia, inter-rater reliability ranged from .70 to .92. Concurrent validity (correlates with Aachen Aphasia Test–Communicative Behavior Scale) is reported. Two 5-point scales: A-scale (understandability of the message) and B-scale (intelligibility of the utterance). Points on rating scale: not at all, a little, medium, reasonable, and good
Communication Profile: A Functional Skills Survey (Payne, 1994)	26 daily communication skills involving speaking, reading comprehension, verbal comprehension, writing, and math comprehension	Adults with language impairments from diffuse neurological disorders, hearing impairments, mental retardation, stroke, and traumatic brain injury	On the basis of administration with 257 elderly people (143 African Americans, 144 Caucasians), internal consistency of items was .82. Group differences were found for living arrangement, type of job, and personal income. 5-point scale (face-to-face interview) that rates communication skills from "very important" to "not important at all"
Voice Handicap Index (Jacobson, Johnson, Sibergleit, & Benninger, in press)	30 items evenly distributed across 3 subscales: physical symptomatology, functional, and emotional	Adults with voice disorders	Based on 65 subjects, internal consistency of items was .95. Internal consistency reliability of subscales was high. Test–retest reliability was .92. Validity between total score and patient self-assessment of severity was .63. 5-point interval-level scale from always to never

Source: Reprinted with permission from C. Frattali et al., *Characteristics of Selected Functional Assessment Measures.* © 1995, American-Speech-Language-Hearing Association.

Tests of Sensorimotor Function

Fugl-Meyer Assessment

The Fugl-Meyer Assessment (or Fugl-Meyer Numerical Scoring System) was developed to provide a "system for evaluation of motor function, balance, some sensation qualities and joint function in hemiplegic patients" (Fugl-Meyer, Jääskö, Leyman, Olsson, & Steglind, 1975, p. 13). After reviewing the work of Twitchell (1951), Bard and Hirschberg (1965), Reynolds, Archibald, Brunnström, and Thompson (1958), Brunnström (1966), Vallbo (1971), and Bobath (1965), as well as the earlier work of Fugl-Meyer and Steglind (1972), the authors produced a comprehensive assessment instrument that is proving to be a valuable resource for clinical investigators.

The assessment "comprises three different but interdependent areas: (1) motor function and balance, (2) some sensation qualities, and (3) passive range of motion and occurrence of joint pain" (Fugl-Meyer et al., 1975, p. 14) (see Exhibits A–16 through A–18). The scoring method for each of the sections is an ordinal three-point graded scale, with zero as minimum and two as maximum. The assessment is extensive but very clear and the components are shown in the exhibits with these categories (upper extremity, lower extremity, sensation, and passive joint motion/joint pain). The maximum motor score is 66 for upper extremity and 34 for lower extremity (total, 100). Other totals are balance, 14; sensation, 24; position sense, 24; range of motion, 44; and joint pain, 44 (total possible Fugl-Meyer Assessment score, 250). The precise methods for the testing maneuvers and scoring are extensive and require the user to refer to the original text (Fugl-Meyer et al., 1975).

Fugl-Meyer and colleagues (1975) performed their initial feasibility study on 28 carefully selected patients with hemiplegia due to stroke. The group was reassessed monthly for six months and then at one year. Progressive motor recovery was documented in most patients, and the stages of recovery were sequential as hypothesized. The interrelationships of all variables and sequences were analyzed in great detail. They concluded that the Fugl-Meyer Assessment displayed both validity and reliability. Subsequent research to test biometric properties of the Fugl-Meyer Assessment has been extensive (Berglund & Fugl-Meyer, 1986; Duncan, Propst, & Nelson, 1983; Fugl-Meyer et al., 1975).

Dettmann, Linder, and Sepic (1987) found the complementary aspects of the Fugl-Meyer Assessment and the Barthel Index useful as quantitative measures of function in patients with hemiplegia. Arsenault and colleagues (1988) used the Fugl-Meyer Assessment in evaluating the Bobath approach to treatment of 62 patients with hemiplegia. Crisostomo, Duncan, Propst, and Dawson (1988) used the instrument in a double-blind study of the effect of amphet-amine on motor recovery in patients with cerebral infarction. A modified form of the Fugl-Meyer Assessment was introduced in 1988 and found to perform well in several studies of various aspects of stroke recovery (Lindmark & Hamrin, 1988). Poole and Whitney (1988) used the Motor Assessment Measure (MAS) as a comparison measure for establishing concurrent validity and inter-rater reliability of the motor function assessment aspect of the Fugl-Meyer Assessment in patients with stroke.

The 1990s brought continued productive use of the Fugl-Meyer Assessment. Di Fabio and Badke (1990) used the Fugl-Meyer Assessment to determine concurrent validity of a sensory organization balance test and found significant correlations. Wood-Dauphinee, Williams, and Shapiro (1990), studying 167 patients with stroke, found significant correlations with the Barthel Index and the activities of daily living and cognition subscales of the Level of Rehabilitation Scale (LORS). Filiatrault, Arsenault, Dutil, and Bourbonnais (1991) compared the Fugl-Meyer Assessment, the Barthel Index, and The Functional Test for the Hemiplegic Paretic Upper Extremity in 18 subjects. Disparities were deemed consistent with the use of compensatory techniques. Horner, Matchar, Divine, and Feussner (1991) used the Fugl-Meyer Assessment and the Barthel Index to study racial differences in stroke outcome. In 145 patients with ischemic stroke, Blacks seemed to have greater residual deficits than Whites.

Duncan, Goldstein, Matchar, Divine, and Feussner (1992) performed an innovative study, using the Fugl-Meyer Assessment in 104 patients with stroke, from which they concluded that "most of the variability in motor recovery can be explained by 30 days after stroke" (p. 1084). The Fugl-Meyer Assessment was also used in studies of spastic hypertonia (Katz, Rovai, Brait, & Rymer, 1992), electrical stimulation treatments for arm and hand function (Kraft, Fitts, & Hammond, 1992), and the association between level of glycemia and outcome of acute stroke (Matchar, Divine, Heyman, & Feussner, 1992).

The Fugl-Meyer Assessment has remained a popular and useful research instrument. Ferrucci and colleagues (1993) used it to study the pattern of functional status recovery in 50 patients with stroke. Gowland and associates (1993) used it to test concurrent validity of the Chedoke–McMaster Stroke Assessment, and Sanford, Moreland, Swanson, Stratford, and Gowland (1993) conducted further study of the biometric and clinical merits of the instrument. Further studies in 1994 used the Fugl-Meyer Assessment in a clinical trial of ganglioside GM1 in acute ischemic stroke (Anonymous, 1994), as well as in a study of motor recovery after stroke in upper and lower extremities conducted with 95 patients (Duncan et al., 1994). Thus the Fugl-Meyer Assessment has become a widely used and highly productive research tool.

REFERENCES

Anonymous. (1994). Ganglioside GM1 in acute ischemic stroke: The SASS trial. *Stroke, 25*(6), 1141–1148.

Arsenault, A.B., Dutil, E., Lambert, J., Corriveau, H., Guarna, F., & Drouin, G. (1988). An evaluation of the hemiplegic subject based on the Bobath approach. Part III. A validation study. *Scandinavian Journal of Rehabilitation Medicine, 20*(1), 13–16.

Bard, G., & Hirschberg, G.G. (1965). Recovery of voluntary motion in upper extremity following hemiplegia. *Archives of Physical Medicine and Rehabilitation, 46*(8), 567–572.

Berglund, K., & Fugl-Meyer, A.R. (1986). Upper extremity function in hemiplegia: A cross-validation study of two assessment methods. *Scandinavian Journal of Rehabilitation Medicine, 18*(4), 155–157.

Bobath, B. (1965). *Abnormal postural reflex activity caused by brain lesions.* London, England: William Heinemann Medical Books.

Brunnström, S. (1966). Motor testing procedures in hemiplegia. *Journal of the American Physical Therapy Association, 46*(4), 357–375.

Crisostomo, E.A., Duncan, P.W., Propst, M., Dawson, D.V., & Davis, J.N. (1988). Evidence that amphetamine with physical therapy promotes recovery of motor function in stroke patients. *Annals of Neurology, 23*(1), 94–97.

Dettmann, M.A., Linder, M.T., & Sepic, S.B. (1987). Relationships among walking performance, postural stability, and functional assessments of the hemiplegic patient. *American Journal of Physical Medicine, 66*(2), 77–90.

Di Fabio, R.P., & Badke, M.B. (1990). Relationship of sensory organization to balance function in patients with hemiplegia. *Physical Therapy, 70*(9), 542–548.

Duncan, P.W., Goldstein, L.B., Horner, R.D., Landsman, P.B., Samsa, G.P., & Matchar, D.B. (1994). Similar motor recovery of upper and lower extremities after stroke. *Stroke, 25*(6), 1181–1188.

Duncan, P.W., Goldstein, L.B., Matchar, D., Divine, G.W., & Feussner, J. (1992). Measurement of motor recovery after stroke: Outcome assessment and sample size requirements. *Stroke, 23*(8), 1084–1089.

Duncan, P.W., Propst, M., & Nelson, S.G. (1983). Reliability of the Fugl-Meyer Assessment of sensorimotor recovery following cerebrovascular accident. *Physical Therapy, 63*(10), 1606–1610.

Ferrucci, L., Bandinelli, S., Guralnik, J.M., Lamponi, M., Bertini, C., Falchini, M., & Baroni, A. (1993). Recovery of functional status after stroke: A post-rehabilitation follow-up study. *Stroke 24*(2), 200–205.

Filiatrault, J., Arsenault, A.B., Dutil, E., & Bourbonnais, D. (1991). Motor function and activities of daily living assessments: A study of three tests for persons with hemiplegia. *American Journal of Occupational Therapy, 45*(9), 806–810.

Fugl-Meyer, A.R., Jääskö, L., Leyman, I., Olsson, S., & Steglind, S. (1975). The poststroke hemiplegic patient. I. A method for evaluation of physical performance. *Scandinavian Journal of Rehabilitation Medicine, 7*(1), 13–31.

Fugl-Meyer, A.R., & Steglind, S. (1972). *Postural effects on the activity of spastic muscles in hemiplegic patients.* Paper presented at the Sixth International Conference of Physical Medicine, Barcelona, Spain.

Gowland, C., Stratford, P., Ward, M., Moreland, J., Torresin, W., Van Hullenaar, S., Sanford, J., Barreca, S., Vanspall, B., & Plews, N. (1993). Measuring physical impairment and disability with the Chedoke–McMaster Stroke Assessment. *Stroke, 24*(1), 58–63.

Horner, R.D., Matchar, D.B., Divine, G.W., & Feussner, J.R. (1991). Racial variations in ischemic stroke-related physical and functional impairments. *Stroke, 22*(12), 1497–1501.

Katz, R.T., Rovai, G.P., Brait, C., & Rymer, W.Z. (1992). Objective quantification of spastic hypertonia: Correlation with clinical findings. *Archives of Physical Medicine and Rehabilitation, 73*(4), 339–347.

Kraft, G.H., Fitts, S.S., & Hammond, M.C. (1992). Techniques to improve function of the arm and hand in chronic hemiplegia. *Archives of Physical Medicine and Rehabilitation, 73*(3), 220–227.

Lindmark, B., & Hamrin, E. (1988). Evaluation of functional capacity after stroke as a basis for active intervention. Validation of a modified chart for motor capacity assessment. *Scandinavian Journal of Rehabilitation Medicine, 20*(3), 111–115.

Matchar, D.B., Divine, G.W., Heyman, A., & Feussner, J.R. (1992). The influence of hyperglycemia on outcome of cerebral infarction. *Annals of Internal Medicine, 117*(6), 449–456.

Poole, J.L., & Whitney, S.L. (1988). Motor assessment scale for stroke patients: Concurrent validity and interrater reliability. *Archives of Physical Medicine and Rehabilitation, 69*(3 Pt. 1), 195–197.

Reynolds, G., Archibald, K.C., Brunnström, S., & Thompson, N. (1958). Preliminary report on neuromuscular function testing of the upper extremity in adult hemiplegia patients. *Archives of Physical Medicine and Rehabilitation, 39*(5), 303.

Sanford, J., Moreland, J., Swanson, L.R., Stratford, P.W., & Gowland, C. (1993). Reliability of the Fugl-Meyer Assessment for testing motor performance in patients following stroke. *Physical Therapy, 73*(7), 447–454.

Twitchell, T.E. (1951). The restoration of motor function following hemiplegia in man. *Brain, 74*, 443.

Vallbo, A.B. (1971). Muscle spindle response at the onset of isometric voluntary contractions in man: Time difference between fusimotor and skeletomotor effects. *Journal of Physiology, 218*(2), 405–431.

Wood-Dauphinee, S.L., Williams, J.I., & Shapiro, S.H. (1990). Examining outcome measures in a clinical study of stroke. *Stroke, 21*(5), 731–739.

Exhibit A–16 Fugl-Meyer Assessment

Test Form for Assessment of Motor Function of Upper Extremity in Hemiplegia

UPPER EXTREMITY

A SHOULDER/ELBOW/FOREARM

I	Reflex-activity	Flexors
		Extensors
II a	Shoulder	Retraction
		Elevation
		Abduction
		Outwards rotation
	Elbow	Flexion
	Forearm	Supination
b	Shoulder	Adduction/Inward rotation
	Elbow	Extension
	Forearm	Pronation

III Hand to lumbar spine

Shoulder	Flexion 0°–90°
Elbow 90°	Pronation/Supination

IV Shoulder

	Abduction 0°–90°
	Flexion 90°–180°
Elbow 0°	Pronation/Supination

V Normal reflex-activity

B WRIST

Elbow 90°	Wrist-stability
Elbow 90°	Wrist-flexion/extension
Elbow 0°	Wrist-stability
Elbow 0°	Wrist-flexion/extension
Circumduction	

C HAND

Fingers Massflexion
Fingers Massextension
Grasp a
Grasp b
Grasp c
Grasp d
Grasp e

D COORDINATION/SPEED

Tremor
Dysmetria
Time

Source: Courtesy of Dr. Axel R. Fugl-Meyer, Institute of Rehabilitation Medicine, University of Göteborg, Göteborg, Sweden.

Exhibit A–17 Fugl-Meyer Assessment

Test Form for Recording Lower Extremity Motor Function and Balance in Hemiplegia

LOWER EXTREMITY

E HIP/KNEE/ANKLE

I	Reflex-activity	Flexors
		Extensors
II a	Hip	Flexion
	Knee	Flexion
	Ankle	Dorsiflexion
b	Hip	Extension
		Adduction
	Ankle	Dorsiflexion
	Knee	Extension
	Ankle	Plantarflexion
III	Knee	Flexion
	Ankle	Dorsiflexion
IV	Knee	Flexion
	Ankle	Dorsiflexion
V	Normal reflex-activity	

F COORDINATION/SPEED

Tremor
Dysmetria
Time

G Balance

Sit without support
Protective reaction non-affected side
Protective reaction affected side
Stand with support
Stand without support
Stand on non-affected leg
Stand on affected leg

Source: Courtesy of Dr. Axel R. Fugl-Meyer, Institute of Rehabilitation Medicine, University of Göteborg, Göteborg, Sweden.

Exhibit A–18 Fugl-Meyer Assessment

Test Form for Assessment of Some Sensation Qualities, Passive Range of Motion, and Occurrence of Joint Pain in Hemiplegia

H SENSATION

a Light touch	Arm	Elbow	Flexion
	Vola		Extension
	Leg	Forearm	Pronation
	Plantar		Supination
b Position	Shoulder	Wrist	Flexion
	Elbow		Extension
	Wrist	Fingers	Flexion
	Thumb		Extension
	Hip	Hip	Flexion
	Knee		Abduction
	Ankle		Outward rotation
	Toes		Inward rotation
		Knee	Flexion
J PASSIVE JOINT MOTION/JOINT PAIN			Extension
Shoulder	Flexion	Ankle	Dorsiflexion
	Abduction ———→ 90°		Plantarflexion
	Outward rotation	Foot	Pronation
	Inward rotation		Supination

Source: Courtesy of Dr. Axel R. Fugl-Meyer, Institute of Rehabilitation Medicine, University of Göteborg, Göteborg, Sweden.

Standardized Test of Patient Mobility

The Standardized Test of Patient Mobility (Jebsen et al., 1970) is a well-designed and standardized functional assessment instrument that addresses not only a person's ability to perform specific tasks but also the time required for, and ease of, performance. These dimensions are also considered in the Time Care Profile (Halstead & Hartley, 1975), and Jebsen Test of Hand Function (Jebsen, Taylor, Trieschmann, Trotter, & Howard, 1969), as well as, along with pain, in arthritis-specific scales.

In the Standardized Test of Patient Mobility, Jebsen and coworkers (1970) incorporated the mobility variables of bed mobility, wheelchair activities, transfer activities, and ambulation. Specific activity subtests were designed to assess performance in each of these areas. Each of these subtests is thoroughly detailed, and performance directions are highly specific. The scoring mechanism is the time required by the patient to complete each of the standardized tests (which suggests careful selection of subjects who can actually perform the specified maneuvers).

In the standardization process, norms were established for 100 subjects without mobility deficits from age 20 to 69 years, 10 for each decade. Then reliability studies were conducted on 18 individuals with "stable disabilities affecting mobility" (Jebsen et al., 1970, p. 172). Ambulation aids were allowed. Normative data showed age, but not gender, differences. Age became a factor only in subjects age 50 years and older. Further standardization documented reliability over time, no significant practice effect (better performance as a result of repetition), and ability to discriminate between persons with and without impaired mobility. Administration time ranged from 30 to 60 minutes. As the authors point out, the Standardized Test of Patient Mobility provides an additional dimension (time) in assessing the degree of a patient's dependence in mobility activities.

Although this well-designed test has not been used extensively in published studies in clinical research, Mikulic, Griffith, and Jebsen (1976) published four case reports that illustrate the value of its use in documenting progress of individual patients over time.

REFERENCES

Halstead, L., & Hartley, R.B. (1975). Time Care Profile: An evaluation of a new method of assessing ADL dependence. *Archives of Physical Medicine and Rehabilitation, 56*(3), 110–115.

Jebsen, R.H., Taylor, N., Trieschmann, R.B., Trotter, M.J., & Howard, L.A. (1969). An objective and standardized test of hand function. *Archives of Physical Medicine and Rehabilitation, 50*(6), 311–319.

Jebsen, R.H., Trieschmann, R.B., Mikulic, M.A., Hartley, R.B., McMillan,

J.A., & Snook, M.E. (1970). Measurement of time in a standardized test of patient mobility. *Archives of Physical Medicine and Rehabilitation, 51*(3), 170–175.

Mikulic, M.A., Griffith, E.R., & Jebsen, R.H. (1976). Clinical applications of a standardized mobility test. *Archives of Physical Medicine and Rehabilitation, 57*(3), 143–146.

Test of Hand Function

Jebsen Test of Hand Function

The Jebsen Test of Hand Function (Jebsen, Taylor, Trieschmann, Trotter, & Howard, 1969) was developed to fulfill the need for a short, objective test of hand function and created by professionals interested in restoration of hand function. The test was designed to assess the broad aspects of hand function commonly used in activities of daily living. It provides objective measurements of standardized tasks with norms for comparison. It also allows documentation along a continuum of ability and can be administered in a short time by using readily available equipment and materials (Jebsen et al., 1969). Lynch and Bridle (1989) report that the Jebsen Test of Hand Function "is easy to administer and can be completed quickly" (p. 317).

Labi and Gresham (1984) noted that Jebsen and colleagues did not use traditional descriptors such as those found in scales for activities of daily living. Instead, they developed a set of specific tasks that "simulate various common activities involving hand use, e.g. writing, simulated feeding, holding objects, turning cards or pages as in reading, etc" (p. 97). The dimension used to measure each function is the length of time taken to complete each of the tasks. In contrast to most instruments used to measure activities of daily living, only time to accomplish tasks, not the amount of assistance required, is considered.

The Jebsen Test of Hand Function (Jebsen et al., 1969) contains seven subtests meant to be administered in a set sequence by using both the dominant and nondominant hand. The broad sampling of hand functions includes writing, turning cards, picking up small common objects, simulated feeding, stacking checkers, and picking up large light and heavy objects. Information on how these subtests were chosen was not published, but specific materials, equipment, and administration instructions were provided. Each of the seven subtests is timed by using a standard stopwatch, which allows for documentation of a continuum of ability score. The

time scale is considered a ratio scale, which means all mathematical and statistical operations are permissible (Portney & Watkins, 1993).

The test–retest reliability of the Jebsen Test of Hand Function ranged from .60 to .99 ($p < .01$), suggesting that the test is fairly reliable over time (Jebsen et al., 1969). Hackel, Wolfe, Bang, and Canfield (1992) also report that the Jebsen Test of Hand Function is "reliable and easily performed" (p. 377), with a test–retest reliability of .84 to .85 and an intertester reliability of .82 to 1.00. Both sets of results confirm absence of a practice effect (better performance due to repetition) resulting from multiple administrations of this test. However, Stern (1992) found less stable test–retest results in two of the subtests: writing and simulated feeding. Improvements in these two areas should be interpreted cautiously because they are the weaker subtests.

Few validity studies have been done with the Jebsen Test of Hand Function. However, in a recent validity study the relationship between the Jebsen Test of Hand Function and Klein–Bell Activities of Daily Living Scale was significant ($r = -.635, p < .01$). This was especially evident in three of six areas of function in the Klein–Bell Scale that required functional use of hands; that is, dressing, bathing/hygiene, and eating (Lynch & Bridle, 1989).

The Jebsen Test of Hand Function has been particularly useful in monitoring the ability of boys with Duchenne muscular dystrophy in performing tasks involving arm, wrist, and hand function (Hiller & Wade, 1992; Wagner, Vignos, Carlozzi, & Hull, 1993). The body of research available with use of the Jebsen Test of Hand Function has grown (Stern, 1992). Future research concerning reliability and validity of the instrument remains a priority.

Jebsen and associates (1969) tested 300 persons with no clinical evidence of abnormality of upper extremity structure, mobility, strength, sensation, or coordination and 26 persons with stable hand disabilities. Scores for men and women were not combined because there were significant differences between the scores for men and women on several subtests. Data were divided into two distinct age groups: persons 20 to 59 years of age and persons 60 to 94 years of age. Data were presented by hand (dominant or nondominant), sex, and subtest for the two different age groups (Jebsen et al., 1969).

Hackel and coworkers (1992) determined that significant differences existed for persons older than 60 years as a result of the aging process. Mean subtest scores were established by 10-year increments for 121 persons aged 60 to 89 years. These normative values differ from those published by Jebsen et al. (1969).

The Jebsen Test of Hand Function has also been useful in documenting more convincingly that "while the impact of hand osteoarthritis (OA) on some parameters of hand function may be statistically significant, the resulting function limitation overall is relatively insignificant" (Labi, Gresham, & Rathey, 1982, p. 440). The test has been used to measure the effects on function of the uninvolved hand in patients with stroke, and results demonstrated that patients with hemiparesis show decreased function in the unaffected as well as involved hand (Jebsen, Griffith, Long, & Fowler, 1971). It has been reported that subsets of the Jebsen Test of Hand Function successfully identify persons who are functionally disabled, as well as discriminate various degrees of disability (Hackel et al., 1992; Jebsen et al., 1969).

The Jebsen Test of Hand Function is available as it was originally published in 1969 in the *Archives of Physical Medicine and Rehabilitation*, volume 50, issue six, pages 311 to 319. As of 1994, it has not been published in another journal, nor in a language other than English.

REFERENCES

Hackel, M.E., Wolfe, G.A., Bang, S.M., & Canfield, J.S. (1992). Changes in hand function in the aging adult as determined by the Jebsen Test of Hand Function. *Physical Therapy, 72*(5), 373–377.

Hiller, L.B., & Wade, C.K. (1992). Upper extremity functional assessment scales in children with Duchennne muscular dystrophy: A comparison. *Archives of Physical Medicine and Rehabilitation, 73*(6), 527–534.

Jebsen, R.H., Griffith, E.R., Long, E.W., & Fowler, R., (1971). Function of "normal" hand in stroke patients. *Archives of Physical Medicine and Rehabilitation, 52*(4), 170–174.

Jebsen, R.H., Taylor, N., Trieschmann, R.B., Trotter, M.J., & Howard, L.A. (1969). An objective and standardized test of hand function. *Archives of Physical Medicine and Rehabilitation, 50*(6), 311–319.

Labi, M.L.C., & Gresham, G.E. (1984). Some research applications of functional assessment instruments used in rehabilitation medicine. In C.V. Granger & G.E. Gresham (Eds.), *Functional assessment in rehabilitation medicine* (pp. 86–98). Baltimore: Williams & Wilkins.

Labi, M.L., Gresham, G.E., & Rathey, U.K. (1982). Hand function in osteoarthritis. *Archives of Physical Medicine and Rehabilitation, 63*(9), 438–440.

Lynch, K.B., & Bridle, M.J. (1989). Validity of the Jebsen–Taylor Hand Function Test in predicting activities of daily living. *The Occupational Journal of Research, 9*(5), 316–318.

Portney, L.G., & Watkins, M.P. (1993). *Foundations of clinical research: Applications to practice.* Norwalk, CT: Appleton & Lange.

Stern, E.B. (1992). Stability of the Jebsen–Taylor Hand Function Test across three test sessions. *American Journal of Occupational Therapy, 64*(7), 647–649.

Wagner, M.B., Vignos, P.J., Jr., Carlozzi, C., & Hull, A.L. (1993). Assessment of hand function in Duchenne muscular dystrophy. *Archives of Physical Medicine and Rehabilitation, 74*(8), 801–804.

Medical Diagnosis–Specific Functional Assessment Instruments

Arthritis Impact Measurement Scales and Functional Status Index

Prime examples of medical diagnosis–specific functional assessment instruments are those designed for use in assessing persons with arthritis (any form). Two well-known ones are described here: Arthritis Impact Measurement Scales (AIMS) (Meenan, Gertman, & Mason, 1980) (see Exhibit A–19) and Functional Status Index (FSI) (Jette, 1980). Both contain the variable of pain, which is of primary importance in patients with arthritis (affecting their function as well), in contrast to most other impairment categories in which pain, per se, is not a major factor limiting functional abilities and quality of life (Himmel, 1984).

AIMS. The AIMS (Meenan et al., 1980) resulted from a systematic and historic analysis of the variables needed for adequate assessment of the patient with arthritis in reflecting disease activity and psychological status as well as physical function. The authors wished to devise an instrument that would be a "comprehensive, practical, and clinically relevant arthritis status index" (p. 147). Components of the Index of Well-Being (Kaplan, Bush, & Berry, 1976; Patrick, Bush, & Chen, 1973) and Rand's Health Insurance Study batteries (Brook et al., 1979; Ware, 1976) were incorporated into the initial construction of the instrument. The component variables of the AIMS are mobility, physical activity, dexterity, social role, social activity, activities of daily living, pain, depression, and anxiety. Each component is rated on an ordinal scale specific for that variable. Initial standardization was performed on a target sample of 100 eligible subjects from two "large rheumatology practice sites" (Meenan et al., 1980, p. 147). Final scaling and format were completed and construct validity, reliability, and feasibility were established. As finally formulated, the AIMS is self-administered (in any setting) and takes about 20 minutes to complete.

Meenan and colleagues used the AIMS to study patients with recent-onset rheumatoid arthritis (Meenan, Kazis, Anthony, & Wallin, 1991) and the impact of rheumatoid arthritis on household work performance of women (Allaire, Meenan, & Anderson, 1991). They also developed a revised and expanded version of the instrument, the AIMS2 (see Exhibit A–20), and documented reliability and validity by using a population of 408 subjects: 299 with rheumatoid arthritis and 109 with osteoarthritis (Meenan, Mason, Anderson, Guccione, & Kazis, 1992).

The AIMS2 contained revisions of some scale items:

Some items with low reliability and/or sensitivity were eliminated so that all scales now have four or five items. Three items were removed from the household physical activities scale because they dealt with cognitive functions rather than physical functions. The number of response options per item was also standardized, eliminating all yes/no responses. (R.F. Meenan, personal communication, January 1995)

Three new scales were added: arm function, work, and social support.

The authors used the AIMS2 in a study comparing self-report symptoms and health status information with data on these variables collected concurrently. They found that the information obtained was complementary, rather than duplicative (Mason, Meenan, & Anderson, 1992). Meenan and colleagues concluded that the AIMS2 had "excellent measurement properties that should be useful in arthritis clinical trials and in outcome research" (Meenan et al., 1992, p. 1). Because measurement properties of the AIMS2 have proved to be similar to those in the original instrument, the investigators believed that the AIMS2 did not need "to be retested for reliability or validity in all those groups or settings in which the original AIMS had already been tested" (R.F. Meenan, personal communication, January 1995). An example was demonstrated by Kovar et al. (1992) in a randomized trial of fitness walking in patients with osteoarthritis of the knee. Results of the trial showed that functional status in these patients could be improved without increasing pain or other symptoms.

A user's guide for the AIMS2 is available from Robert F. Meenan, M.D., Professor of Medicine, Dean of School of Public Health, Boston University, 80 East Concord Street, Boston, MA 02118–2394.

The *Functional Status Index* (FSI) (Jette, 1980) was developed to assess chronic disabling diseases such as arthritis. Previous work in this area was reviewed, including that of Taylor (1937) and Steinbrocker, Traiger, and Batterman (1949), the latter having led to the American Rheumatism Association Functional Classifications.

The FSI was originally designed as a program evaluation instrument for older persons with osteoarthritis (Jette, 1980). Jette and Deniston (1978) continued to refine the instrument and standardized the final format in 1980 (Jette, 1980).

The FSI addresses three dimensions: degree of dependence, degree of difficulty, and amount of pain experienced in performing specific activities of daily living. These three dimensions are assessed in five functional status categories:

1. *Gross Mobility* (walking inside, stair climbing, chair transfers)
2. *Personal Care* (washing all parts of the body, putting on pants, putting on a shirt, buttoning a shirt)
3. *Hand Activities* (opening containers, writing, dialing a phone)

4. *Home Chores* (doing laundry, reaching into low cupboards, doing yard work, vacuuming a rug)
5. *Interpersonal Activities* (driving a car, visiting family or friends, attending meetings, performing your job)

The standardized FSI thus examines three functional dimensions in each of 18 specific daily activities. This version was standardized with a group of 149 adults with rheumatoid arthritis and found to have internal consistency reliability levels from .66 to .91 and average test–retest and inter-observer reliability levels from .65 to .81 (Jette, 1980). It has subsequently been used in evaluation of total joint arthroplasty (Liang, Fossel, & Larson, 1990) and effects of a specific quantitative exercise program for persons with osteoarthritis of the knee (Fisher, Gresham, & Pendergast, 1993), as well as in 47 patients with hip fracture (Jette, 1987) and 10 women with vertical compression fractures in a case and matched control study (Lyles et al., 1993).

REFERENCES

AIMS and AIMS2

Allaire, S.H., Meenan, R.F., & Anderson, J.J. (1991). The impact of rheumatoid arthritis on the household work performance of women. *Arthritis and Rheumatism, 34*(6), 669–678.

Brook, R.H., Ware, J.E., Davis-Avery, A., Stewart, A.L., Donald, C.A., Rodgers, W.H., Williams, K.N., & Johnston, S.A. (1979). Overview of adult health status measures fielded in Rand's Health Insurance Study. *Medical Care, 17*(Suppl. 7), 1–131.

Himmel, P.B. (1984). Functional assessment strategies in clinical medicine: The case of the arthritic patient. In C.V. Granger & E. Gresham (Eds.), *Functional assessment in rehabilitation medicine* (pp. 343–363). Baltimore: Williams & Wilkins.

Kaplan, R.M., Bush, J.W., & Berry, C.C. (1976). Health status: Types of validity and the Index of Well-Being. *Health Service Research, 11*(4) 478–507.

Kovar, P.A., Allegrante, J.P., MacKenzie, C.R., Peterson, M.G.E., Gutlin, B., & Charlson, M.E. (1992). Supervised fitness walking in patients with osteoarthritis of the knee. *Annals of Internal Medicine, 116*(7), 529–534.

Mason, J.H., Meenan, R.F., & Anderson, J.J. (1992). Do self-reported arthritis symptoms (RADAR) and health status (AIMS2) data provide duplicative or complementary information? *Arthritis Care and Research, 5*(3), 163–172.

Meenan, R.F., Gertman, P.M., & Mason, J.H. (1980). Measuring health status in arthritis: The Arthritis Impact Measurement Scales. *Arthritis and Rheumatism, 23*(2), 146–152.

Meenan, R.F., Kazis, L.E., Anthony, J.M., & Wallin, B.A. (1991). The clinical and health status of patients with recent-onset rheumatoid arthritis. *Arthritis and Rheumatism, 34*(6), 761–765.

Meenan, R.F., Mason, J.H., Anderson, J.J., Guccione, A.A., & Kazis, L.E. (1992). AIMS2: The content and properties of a revised and expanded Arthritis Impact Measurement Scales Health Questionnaire. *Arthritis and Rheumatism, 35*(1), 1–10.

Patrick, D.L., Bush, J.W., & Chen, M.M. (1973). Methods for measuring levels of well-being for a health status index. *Health Service Research, 8*(3), 228–245.

Ware, J.E. (1976). *The conceptualization and measurement of health for policy relevant research and medical care delivery.* Santa Monica: Rand Corporation.

FSI

Fisher, N.M., Gresham, G.E., & Pendergast, D.R. (1993). Effects of a quantitative progressive rehabilitation program applied unilaterally to the osteoarthritic knee. *Archives of Physical Medicine and Rehabilitation, 74*(12), 1319–1326.

Jette, A.M. (1980). Functional Status Index: Reliability of a chronic disease evaluation instrument. *Archives of Physical Medicine and Rehabilitation, 61*(9), 395–401.

Jette, A.M. (1987). The Functional Status Index: Reliability and validity of a self-report functional disability measure. *Journal of Rheumatology, 14*(Suppl. 15), 15–21.

Jette, A.M., & Deniston, O.L. (1978). Inter-observer reliability of a functional status assessment instrument. *Journal of Chronic Diseases, 31*(9–10), 573–580.

Liang, M.H., Fossel, A.H., & Larson, M.G. (1990). Comparisons of five health status instruments for orthopedic evaluation. *Medical Care, 28*(7), 632–642.

Lyles, K.W., Bold, D.T., Shipp, K.M., Pieper, C.F., Martinez, S., & Mulhausen, P.L. (1993). Association of osteoporotic vertebral compression fractures with impaired functional status. *American Journal of Medicine, 94*(6), 595–601.

Steinbrocker, O., Traiger, C.H., & Batterman, R.C. (1949). Therapeutic criteria in rheumatoid arthritis. *Journal of the American Medical Association, 140*(8), 659–662.

Taylor, D. (1937). Table for degree of involvement in chronic arthritis. *Canadian Medical Association Journal, 36*(6), 608–610.

Exhibit A–19 Arthritis Impact Measurement Scale

Mobility

4 Are you in bed or chair for most or all of the day because of your health?

3 Are you able to use public transportation?

2 When you travel around your community, does someone have to assist you because of your health?

1 Do you have to stay indoors most or all of the day because of your health?

Physical Activity

5 Are you unable to walk unless you are assisted by another person or by a cane, crutches, artificial limbs, or braces?

4 Do you have any trouble either walking one block or climbing one flight of stairs because of your health?

3 Do you have any trouble either walking several blocks or climbing a few flights of stairs because of your health?

2 Do you have trouble bending, lifting, or stooping because of your health?

1 Does your health limit the kind of vigorous activities you can do such as running, lifting heavy objects, or participating in strenuous sports?

Dexterity

5 Can you easily write with a pen or pencil?

4 Can you easily turn a key in a lock?

3 Can you easily button articles of clothing?

2 Can you easily tie a pair of shoes?

1 Can you easily open a jar of food?

Social Role

7 If you had to take medicine, could you take all your own medicine?

6 If you had a telephone, would you be able to use it?

5 Do you handle your own money?

4 If you had a kitchen, could you prepare your own meals?

3 If you had laundry facilities (washer, dryer, etc.) could you do your own laundry?

2 If you had the necessary transportation, could you go shopping for groceries or clothes?

1 If you had household tools and appliances (vacuum, mops, etc.) could you do your own housework?

Social Activity

5 About how often were you on the telephone with close friends or relatives during the past month?

4 Has there been a change in the frequency or quality of your sexual relationships during the past month?

3 During the past month, about how often have you had friends or relatives to your home?

2 During the past month, about how often did you get together socially with friends or relatives?

1 During the past month, how often have you visited with friends or relatives at their homes?

Activities of Daily Living

4 How much help do you need to use the toilet?

3 How well are you able to move around?

2 How much help do you need in getting dressed?

1 When you bathe, either a sponge bath, tub or shower, how much help do you need?

Pain

4 During the past month, how often have you had severe pain from your arthritis?

3 During the past month, how would you describe the arthritis pain you usually have?

2 During the past month, how long has your morning stiffness usually lasted from the time you wake up?

1 During the past month, how often have you had pain in two or more joints at the same time?

Depression

6 During the past month, how often did you feel that others would be better off if you were dead?

5 How often during the past month have you felt so down in the dumps that nothing could cheer you up?

4 How much of the time during the past month have you felt downhearted and blue?

3 How often during the past month did you feel that nothing turned out for you the way you wanted it to?

2 During the past month, how much of the time have you been in low or very low spirits?

1 During the past month, how much of the time have you enjoyed the things you do?

Anxiety

6 During the past month, how much of the time have you felt tense or "high strung"?

5 How much have you been bothered by nervousness, or your "nerves" during the past month?

4 How often during the past month did you find yourself having difficulty trying to calm down?

3 How much of the time during the past month were you able to relax without difficulty?

2 How much of the time during the past month have you felt calm and peaceful?

1 How much of the time during the past month did you feel relaxed and free of tension?

Source: Reprinted with permission from R.F. Meenan, P.M. Gertman, and J.H. Mason, Measuring Health Status in Arthritis: The Arthritis Impact Measurement Scale, *Arthritis and Rheumatism*, Vol. 23, pp. 146–152, © 1980, American College of Rheumatology.

Exhibit A–20   Arthritis Impact Measurement Scales 2

Instructions: Please answer the following questions about your health. Most questions ask about your health during the past month. There are no right or wrong answers to the questions and most can be answered with a simple check (X). Please answer every question.

Please begin by providing the following information about yourself.

NAME: _____

ADDRESS: _____
             Number   Street   Apt#

PHONE: (   ) _____ TODAY'S DATE: _____
      Area code   Number   Month   Day   Year

Please check (X) the most appropriate answer for each question.

These questions refer to **MOBILITY LEVEL.**

DURING THE PAST MONTH . . .	All Days (1)	Most Days (2)	Some Days (3)	Few Days (4)	No Days (5)
1. How often were you physically able to drive a car or use public transportation?	___	___	___	___	___
2. How often were you out of the house for at least part of the day?	___	___	___	___	___
3. How often were you able to do errands in the neighborhood?	___	___	___	___	___
4. How often did someone have to assist you to get around outside your home?	___	___	___	___	___
5. How often were you in a bed or chair for most or all of the day?	___	___	___	___	___

These questions refer to **WALKING AND BENDING.**

DURING THE PAST MONTH . . .	All Days (1)	Most Days (2)	Some Days (3)	Few Days (4)	No Days (5)
6. Did you have trouble doing vigorous activities such as running, lifting heavy objects, or participating in strenuous sports?	___	___	___	___	___
7. Did you have trouble either walking several blocks or climbing a few flights of stairs?	___	___	___	___	___
8. Did you have trouble bending, lifting or stooping?	___	___	___	___	___
9. Did you have trouble either walking one block or climbing one flight of stairs?	___	___	___	___	___
10. Were you unable to walk unless assisted by another person or by a cane, crutches, or walker?	___	___	___	___	___

continues

Exhibit A–20 continued

Please check (X) the most appropriate answer for each question.

These questions refer to **HAND AND FINGER FUNCTION.**

DURING THE PAST MONTH . . .	All Days (1)	Most Days (2)	Some Days (3)	Few Days (4)	No Days (5)
11. Could you easily write with a pen or pencil?	___	___	___	___	___
12. Could you easily button a shirt or blouse?	___	___	___	___	___
13. Could you easily turn a key in a lock?	___	___	___	___	___
14. Could you easily tie a knot or bow?	___	___	___	___	___
15. Could you easily open a new jar of food?	___	___	___	___	___

These questions refer to **ARM FUNCTION.**

DURING THE PAST MONTH . . .	All Days (1)	Most Days (2)	Some Days (3)	Few Days (4)	No Days (5)
16. Could you easily wipe your mouth with a napkin?	___	___	___	___	___
17. Could you easily put on a pullover sweater?	___	___	___	___	___
18. Could you easily comb or brush your hair?	___	___	___	___	___
19. Could you easily scratch your low back with your hand?	___	___	___	___	___
20. Could you easily reach shelves that were above your head?	___	___	___	___	___

These questions refer to **SELF-CARE TASKS.**

DURING THE PAST MONTH . . .	Always (1)	Very Often (2)	Sometimes (3)	Almost Never (4)	Never (5)
21. Did you need help to take a bath or shower?	___	___	___	___	___
22. Did you need help to get dressed?	___	___	___	___	___
23. Did you need help to use the toilet?	___	___	___	___	___
24. Did you need help to get in or out of bed?	___	___	___	___	___

These questions refer to **HOUSEHOLD TASKS.**

DURING THE PAST MONTH . . .	Always (1)	Very Often (2)	Sometimes (3)	Almost Never (4)	Never (5)
25. If you had the necessary transportation, could you go shopping for groceries without help?	___	___	___	___	___
26. If you had kitchen facilities, could you prepare your own meals without help?	___	___	___	___	___
27. If you had household tools and appliances, could you do your own housework without help?	___	___	___	___	___
28. If you had laundry facilities, could you do your own laundry without help?	___	___	___	___	___

These questions refer to **SOCIAL ACTIVITY.**

DURING THE PAST MONTH . . .	All Days (1)	Most Days (2)	Some Days (3)	Few Days (4)	No Days (5)
29. How often did you get together with friends or relatives?	___	___	___	___	___
30. How often did you have friends or relatives over to your home?	___	___	___	___	___
31. How often did you visit friends or relatives at their homes?	___	___	___	___	___
32. How often were you on the telephone with close friends or relatives?	___	___	___	___	___
33. How often did you go to a meeting of a church, club, team, or other group?	___	___	___	___	___

continues

Exhibit A–20 continued

Please check (X) the most appropriate answer for each question.

These questions refer to **SUPPORT FROM FAMILY AND FRIENDS.**

DURING THE PAST MONTH . . .	Always (1)	Very Often (2)	Sometimes (3)	Almost Always (4)	Never (5)
34. Did you feel that your family or friends would be around if you needed assistance?	——	——	——	——	——
35. Did you feel that your family or friends were sensitive to your personal needs?	——	——	——	——	——
36. Did you feel that your family or friends were interested in helping you solve problems?	——	——	——	——	——
37. Did you feel that your family or friends understood the effects of your arthritis?	——	——	——	——	——

These questions refer to **ARTHRITIS PAIN.**

DURING THE PAST MONTH . . .	Severe (1)	Moderate (2)	Mild (3)	Very Mild (4)	None (5)
38. How would you describe the arthritis pain you usually had?	——	——	——	——	——

DURING THE PAST MONTH . . .	All Days (1)	Most Days (2)	Some Days (3)	Few Days (4)	No Days (5)
39. How often did you have severe pain from your arthritis?	——	——	——	——	——
40. How often did you have pain in two or more joints at the same time?	——	——	——	——	——
41. How often did your morning stiffness last more than one hour from the time you woke up?	——	——	——	——	——
42. How often did your pain make it difficult for you to sleep?	——	——	——	——	——

These questions refer to **WORK.**

DURING THE PAST MONTH . . .	Paid Work (1)	House Work (2)	School Work (3)	Unemployed (4)	Disabled (5)	Retired (6)
43. What has been your main form of work?	——	——	——	——	——	——

If you answered unemployed, disabled or retired, please skip the next four questions and go to the next page.

DURING THE PAST MONTH . . .	All Days (1)	Most Days (2)	Some Days (3)	Few Days (4)	No Days (5)
44. How often were you unable to do any paid work, house work or school work?	——	——	——	——	——
45. On the days that you did work, how often did you have to work a shorter day?	——	——	——	——	——
46. On the days that you did work, how often were you unable to do your work as carefully and accurately as you would like?	——	——	——	——	——
47. On the days that you did work, how often did you have to change the way your paid work, house work or school work is usually done?	——	——	——	——	——

continues

Exhibit A–20 continued

Please check (X) the most appropriate answer for each question.

These questions refer to **LEVEL OF TENSION.**

DURING THE PAST MONTH . . .	Always (1)	Very Often (2)	Sometimes (3)	Almost Never (4)	Never (5)
48. How often have you felt tense or high strung?	___	___	___	___	___
49. How often have you been bothered by nervousness or your nerves?	___	___	___	___	___
50. How often were you able to relax without difficulty?	___	___	___	___	___
51. How often have you felt relaxed and free of tension?	___	___	___	___	___
52. How often have you felt calm and peaceful?	___	___	___	___	___

These questions refer to **MOOD.**

DURING THE PAST MONTH . . .	Always (1)	Very Often (2)	Sometimes (3)	Almost Never (4)	Never (5)
53. How often have you enjoyed the things you do?	___	___	___	___	___
54. How often have you been in low or very low spirits?	___	___	___	___	___
55. How often did you feel that nothing turned out the way you wanted it to?	___	___	___	___	___
56. How often did you feel that others would be better off if you were dead?	___	___	___	___	___
57. How often did you feel so down in the dumps that nothing would cheer you up?	___	___	___	___	___

These questions refer to satisfaction with each health area.

DURING THE PAST MONTH . . .	Very Satisfied (1)	Somewhat Satisfied (2)	Neither Satisfied Nor Dissatisfied (3)	Somewhat Dissatisfied (4)	Very Dissatisfied (5)
58. How satisfied have you been with each of these areas of your health?					
MOBILITY LEVEL (example: do errands)	___	___	___	___	___
WALKING AND BENDING (example: climb stairs)	___	___	___	___	___
HAND AND FINGER FUNCTION (example: tie a bow)	___	___	___	___	___
ARM FUNCTION (example: comb hair)	___	___	___	___	___
SELF-CARE (example: take bath)	___	___	___	___	___
HOUSEHOLD TASKS (example: housework)	___	___	___	___	___
SOCIAL ACTIVITY (example: visit friends)	___	___	___	___	___
SUPPORT FROM FAMILY (example: help with problems)	___	___	___	___	___
ARTHRITIS PAIN (example: joint pain)	___	___	___	___	___
WORK (example: reduce hours)	___	___	___	___	___
LEVEL OF TENSION (example: felt tense)	___	___	___	___	___
MOOD (example: down in dumps)	___	___	___	___	___

continues

Exhibit A–20 continued

Please check (X) the most appropriate answer for each question.

These questions refer to arthritis impact on each area of health.

DURING THE PAST MONTH . . .	Not a Problem for Me (0)	Due Entirely to Other Causes (1)	Due Largely to Other Causes (2)	Due Partly to Arthritis and Partly to Other Causes (3)	Due Largely to My Arthritis (4)	Due Entirely to My Arthritis (5)
59. How much of your problem in each area of health was due to your own arthritis?						
MOBILITY LEVEL (example: do errands)	___	___	___	___	___	___
WALKING AND BENDING (example: climb stairs)	___	___	___	___	___	___
HAND AND FINGER FUNCTION (example: tie a bow)	___	___	___	___	___	___
ARM FUNCTION (example: comb hair)	___	___	___	___	___	___
SELF-CARE (example: take bath)	___	___	___	___	___	___
HOUSEHOLD TASKS (example: housework)	___	___	___	___	___	___
SOCIAL ACTIVITY (example: visit friends)	___	___	___	___	___	___
SUPPORT FROM FAMILY (example: help with problems)	___	___	___	___	___	___
ARTHRITIS PAIN (example: joint pain)	___	___	___	___	___	___
WORK (example: reduce hours)	___	___	___	___	___	___
LEVEL OF TENSION (example: felt tense)	___	___	___	___	___	___
MOOD (example: down in dumps)	___	___	___	___	___	___

You have now answered questions about different AREAS OF YOUR HEALTH. These areas are listed below. Please check (X) up to THREE AREAS in which you would MOST LIKE TO SEE IMPROVEMENT. Please read all 12 areas of health choices before making your decision:

60. AREAS OF HEALTH	THREE AREAS FOR IMPROVEMENT
MOBILITY LEVEL (example: do errands)	_____
WALKING AND BENDING (example: climb stairs)	_____
HAND AND FINGER FUNCTION (example: tie a bow)	_____
ARM FUNCTION (example: comb hair)	_____
SELF-CARE (example: take bath)	_____
HOUSEHOLD TASKS (example: housework)	_____
SOCIAL ACTIVITY (example: visit friends)	_____
SUPPORT FROM FAMILY (example: help with problems)	_____
ARTHRITIS PAIN (example: joint pain)	_____
WORK (example: reduce hours)	_____
LEVEL OF TENSION (example: felt tense)	_____
MOOD (example: down in dumps)	_____

Please make sure that you have checked no more than THREE AREAS for improvement.

continues

Exhibit A–20 continued

Please check (X) the most appropriate answer for each question.

These questions refer to your **CURRENT AND FUTURE HEALTH.**

	Excellent (1)	Good (2)	Fair (3)	Poor (4)
61. In general would you say that your **HEALTH NOW** is excellent, good, fair or poor?	___	___	___	___

	Very Satisfied (1)	Somewhat Satisfied (2)	Neither Satisfied Nor Dissatisfied (3)	Somewhat Dissatisfied (4)	Very Dissatisfied (5)
62. How satisfied are you with your **HEALTH NOW**?	___	___	___	___	___

	Not a Problem for Me (0)	Due Entirely to Other Causes (1)	Due Largely to Other Causes (2)	Due Partly to Arthritis and Partly to Other Causes (3)	Due Largely to My Arthritis (4)	Due Entirely to My Arthritis (5)
63. How much of your problem with your **HEALTH NOW** is due to your arthritis?	___	___	___	___	___	___

	Excellent (1)	Good (2)	Fair (3)	Poor (4)
64. In general do you expect that your **HEALTH 10 YEARS FROM NOW** will be excellent, good, fair or poor?	___	___	___	___

	No Problem At All (1)	Minor Problem (2)	Moderate Problem (3)	Major Problem (4)
65. How big a problem do you expect your arthritis to be **10 YEARS FROM NOW**?	___	___	___	___

These questions refer to your **OVERALL ARTHRITIS IMPACT.**

	Very Well (1)	Well (2)	Fair (3)	Poor (4)	Very Poorly (5)
66. **CONSIDERING ALL THE WAYS THAT YOUR ARTHRITIS AFFECTS YOU**, how well are you doing compared to other people your age?	___	___	___	___	___

67. What is the main kind of arthritis that you have?

Rheumatoid Arthritis	___
Osteoarthritis/Degenerative Arthritis	___
Systemic Lupus Erythematosus	___
Fibromyalgia	___
Scleroderma	___
Psoriatic Arthritis	___
Reiter's Syndrome	___
Gout	___
Low Back Pain	___
Tendonitis/Bursitis	___
Osteoporosis	___
Other	___

68. How many years have you had arthritis?   ___

continues

Exhibit A–20 continued

Please check (X) the most appropriate answer for each question.

DURING THE PAST MONTH . . .	All Days (1)	Most Days (2)	Some Days (3)	Few Days (4)	No Days (5)
69. How often have you had to take MEDICATION for your arthritis?	____	____	____	____	____

70. Is your health currently affected by any of the following medical problems?

	Yes (1)	No (2)
High blood pressure _____	____	____
Heart disease _____	____	____
Mental illness _____	____	____
Diabetes _____	____	____
Cancer _____	____	____
Alcohol or drug use _____	____	____
Lung disease _____	____	____
Kidney disease _____	____	____
Liver disease _____	____	____
Ulcer or other stomach disease _____	____	____
Anemia or other blood disease _____	____	____

	Yes (1)	No (2)
71. Do you take medicine every day for any problem other than your arthritis?	____	____

	Yes (1)	No (2)
72. Did you see a doctor more than three times last year for any problem other than arthritis?	____	____

Please provide the following information about yourself.

73. What is your age at this time? ____

74. What is your sex?
  Male (1) ____
  Female (2) ____

75. What is your racial background?
  White (1) ____
  Black (2) ____
  Hispanic (3) ____
  Asian or Pacific Islander (4) ____
  American Indian or Alaskan Native (5) ____
  Other (6) ____

76. What is your current marital status?
  Married (1) ____
  Separated (2) ____
  Divorced (3) ____
  Widowed (4) ____
  Never married (5) ____

continues

Exhibit A–20 continued

77. What is the highest level of education you received?
Less than seven years of school (1)   _____
Grades seven through nine (2)   _____
Grades ten through eleven (3)   _____
High school graduate (4)   _____
One to four years of college (5)   _____
College graduate (6)   _____
Professional or graduate school (7)   _____

78. What is your approximate family income including wages, disability payment, retirement income, and welfare?
Less than $10,000 (1)   _____
$10,000 - $19,999 (2)   _____
$20,000 - $29,999 (3)   _____
$30,000 - $39,999 (4)   _____
$40,000 - $49,999 (5)   _____
$50,000 - $59,999 (6)   _____
$60,000 - $69,999 (7)   _____
More than $70,000 (8)   _____

Thank you for completing this questionnaire.

Source: Reprinted with permission from R.F. Meenan, J.H. Manson, J.J. Anderson, et al., The Content and Properties of a Revised and Expanded Arthritis Impact Measurement Scales Health Questionnaire, *Arthritis and Rheumatism*, Vol. 35, pp. 1–10, © 1992, American College of Rheumatology.

Frenchay Activities Index

The Frenchay Activities Index (FAI) (Holbrook & Skilbeck, 1983) (see Exhibit A–21) is a brief scale designed to measure activities of daily life in individuals who have suffered a stroke. This scale was developed by Holbrook and Skilbeck (1983) to measure quality of life beyond the necessary skills for basic activities of daily living. The developers found the literature lacking a scale that would accurately represent lifestyle as opposed to self-care and activities of daily living. Thus the FAI quantifies aspects of lifestyle that represent levels of higher independence and social survival (Schuling, de Haan, Limburg, & Groenier, 1993). Specifically, the FAI was developed to "a) provide accurate information on premorbid lifestyle of stroke patients, and b) record changes in activities following stroke, at specific intervals" (Holbrook & Skilbeck, 1983, p. 167) Factor analysis of the 15 items yielded three factor structures in the scale: domestic chores, leisure/work, and outdoor activities.

The FAI is an ordinal scale. It consists of 15 items, and scores can range from 15 (inactive) to 60 (highly active) (Bond, Harris, Smith, & Clark, 1992). Patients are scored on a scale of one to four. The scores are based on frequency of performance. Although scores on ordinal measurement scales can be rank ordered, equal distances between categories do not necessarily exist. As mentioned in Chapter 3, values from ordinal scales do not have arithmetic properties and cannot be added, subtracted, multiplied, or divided. Thus controversy has developed regarding what methods are best used in analysis of data collected by using functional assessment instruments with ordinal scales.

Schuling and colleagues (1993) indicated that by using principal-components analysis, the FAI measures both disability and handicap (societal limitations). The neurological impairments resulting from a stroke have an impact on a patient's functional performance with daily activities, indicating disability.

Correlations among the FAI, Barthel Index, and Sickness Impact Profile (SIP) support construct validity (range of Cronbach's alpha coefficients, .78 to .87). The reliability of two subscales (i.e., reading books and gainful work) was weak. Schuling and coworkers (1993) suggested that the reliability of the instrument could be improved by deleting these two items. Most patients are already retired at the time of the stroke, so these items give little useful information.

Bond and colleagues (1992) suggested that the FAI should distinguish between indoor/outdoor and work/leisure activities. They administered the scale to a group of older persons who had not suffered a stroke to evaluate the underlying factor structure of the FAI. Data were collected during two separate time intervals and analyzed, yielding three factors termed indoor domestic chores, outdoor domestic chores, and outdoor social activities—a difference from the defined factors of domestic chores, leisure/work, and outdoor activities of Holbrook and Skilbeck (1983). Bond and colleagues (1992) argued that a useful distinction must exist between work and leisure and between indoor and outdoor activities.

de Haan, Aaronson, Limburg, Hewer, and van Crevel (1993) reviewed instruments used to measure quality of life and found the FAI was easy to administer (can be completed by direct interview within a few minutes and also as a mailed questionnaire by the patient or significant other) and measured lifestyle in terms of more complex activities after a stroke. They recommended additional studies of reliability and validity. Responsiveness of the test over time and ability of the scale to differentiate patient groups were studied with inconsistent results. Factor analysis supported the domains and demonstrated construct validity. The scale was sensitive to levels of function and health deterioration both before and after stroke. de Haan and colleagues (1993) suggested that data should be collected from a control sample of persons who had not suffered a stroke and research conducted to distinguish between loss of function associated with a stroke and loss of abilities due to the aging process.

Schuling and others (1993) examined a group who had experienced a stroke and a control group with use of the FAI and reported functional losses in both groups. Losses of function, however, were more substantial in the group with stroke.

The FAI has also been used in studies with community-based geriatric populations and found to be an effective measure of functional abilities (Cockburn, Smith, & Wade, 1990). Findings from the Cockburn et al. study indicated that the levels of activity in community-dwelling older people were related to cognitive abilities. They noted that the FAI may lack sensitivity in patients who are not community dwelling. In another study of the outcomes of prosthetic management of persons with bilateral lower-limb amputations, no significant difference was found in above-knee prosthesis users versus nonusers when the FAI was administered (Datta, Nair, & Payne, 1992).

The FAI has guidelines that address specific items, including domestic chores, shopping, social activities, walking, leisure activities, driving a car, travel, gardening, and household maintenance. The guidelines stress the importance of some initiative from the patient (Wade, 1992).

REFERENCES

Bond, M.L., Harris, R.D., Smith, D.S., & Clark, M.S. (1992). An examination of the factor structure of the Frenchay Activities Index. *Disability and Rehabilitation, 14*(1), 27–29.

Cockburn, J., Smith, P.T., & Wade, D.T. (1990). Influence of cognitive function on social, domestic, and leisure activities of community-dwelling older people. *International Disability Studies, 12*(4), 169–172.

Datta, D., Nair, P.M., & Payne, J. (1992). Outcome of prosthetic management of bilateral lower-limb amputees. *Disability and Rehabilitation, 14*(2), 98–102.

de Haan R., Aaronson, N., Limburg, M., Hewer, R.L., & van Crevel, H. (1993). Measuring quality of life in stroke. *Stroke, 24*(2), 320–327.

Holbrook, M., & Skilbeck, C.E. (1983). An activities index for use with stroke patients. *Age and Ageing, 12*(2), 166–170.

Schuling, J., de Haan, R., Limburg, M., & Groenier, K.H. (1993). The Frenchay Activities Index: Assessment of functional status in stroke patients. *Stroke, 24*(8), 1173–1177.

Wade, D.T. (1992). *Measurement in neurological rehabilitation.* New York: Oxford University Press.

Exhibit A–21 Frenchay Activities Index

Score	Activity	Code (score)
	In the last three months	
		1 = Never
_____	Preparing main meals	2 = Under once weekly
_____	Washing up	3 = 1–2 times/week
		4 = Most days
_____	Washing clothes	
_____	Light housework	
_____	Heavy housework	1 = Never
_____	Local shopping	2 = 1–2 times in three months
_____	Social occasions	3 = 3–12 times in three months
_____	Walking outside >15 mins	4 = At least weekly
_____	Actively pursuing hobby	
_____	Driving car/going on bus	
	In the last six months	
		1 = Never
_____	Travel outings/car rides	2 = 1–2 times in 6 months
		3 = 3–12 times in 6 months
		4 = At least twice weekly
		1 = Never
_____	Gardening	2 = Light
_____	Household/car maintenance	3 = Moderate
		4 = All necessary
		1 = None
		2 = One in 6 months
_____	Reading books	3 = Less than one in a fortnight
		4 = Over one each fortnight
		1 = None
		2 = Up to 10 hours/week
_____	Gainful work	3 = 10–30 hours/week
		4 = Over 30 hours/week

Source: Reproduced with permission from J. Shuling et al., The Frenchay Activities Index, Assessment of Functional Status in Stroke Patients, *Stroke*, Vol. 24, No. 8, pp. 1173–1177, © American Heart Association, Inc.

Notes on Use of Frenchay Activities Index

General

The aim is to record activities which require some initiative from the patient. It is important to concentrate upon the patient's actual frequency of activity over the recent past, not distant past performance nor potential performance. One activity can only score on one item.

Specific items

1. Needs to play a substantial part in the organization, preparation, and cooking of main meal. Not just making snacks.

continues

Exhibit A–21 continued

2. Must do it all or share equally; for example, washing or wiping and putting away. Not just rinsing an occasional item.
3. Organization of washing and drying of clothes, whether in washing machine, by hand wash, or at launderette.
4. Dusting; polishing; tidying small objects. Anything heavier is included in item 5.
5. All housework including making beds, cleaning floors and fires, moving chairs, etc.
6. Playing a substantial role in organizing and buying shopping, whether small or large amounts. Must go to shops and not just push a trolley.
7. Going out to clubs, church activities, cinema, theater, drinking, dinner with friends, etc. May be transported there, provided patient takes an active part once arrived. The common factor is activity, not travel.
8. Sustained walking for at least 15 min (allowed short stops for breath). About one mile. Can include walking to do shopping, provided walks far enough.
9. Must require some "active" participation and thought; for example, propagating plants in the house, knitting, painting, games, sports. Not just watching sport on television.
10. Must drive a car (not just be a passenger in a car) or get to a bus/coach and travel on it.
11. Coach or rail trips, or car rides, stop some place for pleasure. Not for a routine "social outing" (i.e. shopping, going to local friends). Must involve some organization and decision-making by the patient. Excludes trips organized passively by institution unless patient exercises choice on whether to go. The common factor is travel for pleasure.
12. Gardening outside:
    - Light: occasional weeding
    - Moderate: regular weeding, pruning, etc.
    - Heavy: all necessary work, including heavy digging
13. Household maintenance:
    - Light: repairing small items
    - Moderate: some painting/decorating, routine car maintenance
    - Heavy: most necessary household/car maintenance and repairs
14. Must be full length books; not magazines, periodicals, papers.
15. Work for which the patient is paid; not voluntary work.

Comment

This index was devised initially by a social worker (M. Holbrook) in order to help her in her clinical service. It has since been revised but its reliability needs further testing. However, it is clinically relevant and easy to perform and has been used in clinical research.

Source: Reproduced with permission from "Social activities after stroke: Measurement and natural history using the Frenchay Activities Index" by D.T. Wade, J. Legh-Smith, & R. L. Hewer, *International Rehabilitation Medicine, 7*, pp. 176–181, Copyright 1985, Eular Publishers.

Disability Rating Scale (Severe Head Trauma)

Another medical diagnosis–specific functional assessment instrument is the Disability Rating Scale (see Exhibit A–22), which was published by Rappaport, Hall, Hopkins, Belleza, and Cope in 1982. The authors' intent was to develop "a single instrument to provide quantitative information to chart the progress of severe head injury (HI) patients from coma to community, particularly through the midzone of the recovery spectrum, between early arousal from coma and early sentient functioning" (p. 118). It was designed to cover more variables than the Glasgow Coma Scale (Teasdale & Jennett, 1974) and Glasgow Outcome Scale (Jennett & Bond, 1975). In addition, several other extant instruments were reviewed, and none were found satisfactory for the particular purposes sought, which are described above.

The Disability Rating Scale was designed with eight items within the following four categories:

1. Arousability, awareness, and responsivity (Glasgow Coma Scale, modified from Teasdale & Jennett, 1974).
2. Cognitive ability for self-care activities (feeding, toileting, and grooming).
3. Dependence on others (adapted from Scranton, Fogel, & Erdman, 1970).
4. Psychosocial adaptability ("employability") for age-related work responsibilities (as employee, homemaker, or student).

Specific definitions are provided for terms used and ratings within each item. Initial standardization was performed by four trained professional raters directly observing 88 patients with head injury, as well as by interviews with nursing staff. Patients were evaluated at admission to a rehabilitation unit, approximately 12 months after injury, and at follow-up visits. Inter-rater correlations were high (.97–.98). Ratings also correlated significantly with brain-evoked potentials. Sensitivity to changes over time was demonstrated. The scale takes 5 to 15 minutes to complete if the rater is trained and can communicate with the nursing staff caring for the patient (Rappaport et al., 1982).

Since the development of the Disability Rating Scale, results from at least two major clinical studies—one with 162 and the other with 64 patients with closed head injury—have shown that the Disability Rating Scale is a useful measure for this population of patients (Fleming & Maas, 1994;

Thatcher, Cantor, McAlaster, Geisler, & Krause, 1991). Results of other studies have confirmed the scale's reliability, validity, and sensitivity (Eliason & Topp, 1984; Gouvier, Blanton, LaPorte, & Nepomuceno, 1987; Hall, Cope, & Rappaport, 1985). It also has been used successfully as an outcome measure in head injury research (Cope & Hall, 1982; Rappaport, Herrero-Backe, Rappaport, & Winterfield, 1989).

REFERENCES

Cope, D.N., & Hall, K. (1982). Head injury rehabilitation: Benefit of early intervention. *Archives of Physical Medicine and Rehabilitation, 63*(9), 433–437.

Eliason, M.R., & Topp, B.W. (1984). Predictive validity of Rappaport's Disability Rating Scale in subjects with acute brain dysfunction. *Physical Therapy, 64*(9), 1357–1360.

Fleming, J.M., & Maas, R. (1994). Prognosis of rehabilitation outcome in head injury using the Disability Rating Scale. *Archives of Physical Medicine and Rehabilitation, 75*(2), 156–163.

Gouvier, W.D., Blanton, P.D., LaPorte, K.K., & Nepomuceno, C. (1987). Reliability and validity of the Disability Rating Scale and Levels of Cognitive Functioning Scale in monitoring recovery from severe head injury. *Archives of Physical Medicine and Rehabilitation, 68*(2), 94–97.

Hall, K., Cope, D. N., & Rappaport, M. (1985). Glasgow Outcome Scale and Disability Rating Scale: Comparative usefulness in following recovery in traumatic head injury. *Archives of Physical Medicine and Rehabilitation, 66*(1), 35–37.

Jennett, B., & Bond, M. (1975). Assessment of outcome after severe brain damage: A practical scale. *Lancet, 1*(1905), 480–484.

Rappaport, M., Hall, K.M., Hopkins, K., Belleza, T., & Cope, D.N. (1982). Disability Rating Scale for severe head trauma patients: Coma to community. *Archives of Physical Medicine and Rehabilitation, 63*(3), 118–123.

Rappaport, M., Herrero-Backe, C., Rappaport, M.L., & Winterfield, K.M. (1989). Head injury outcome up to ten years later. *Archives of Physical Medicine and Rehabilitation, 70*(13), 885–892.

Scranton, J., Fogel, M.L., Erdman, W.J., II (1970). Evaluation of functional levels of patients during and following rehabilitation. *Archives of Physical Medicine and Rehabilitation, 51*(1), 1–21.

Teasdale, G., & Jennett, B. (1974). Assessment of coma and impaired consciousness: Practical scale. *Lancet, 2*(72), 81–84.

Thatcher, R.W., Cantor, D.S., McAlaster, R., Geisler, F., & Krause, P. (1991). Comprehensive predictions of outcome in closed head–injured patients. The development of prognostic equations. *Annals of the New York Academy of Sciences, 620*, 82–101.

Exhibit A–22 Disability Rating (DR) Scale for Severe Head Trauma Patients*

Name_____ Sex _____ Birthday_____ Brain Injury Date_____

Cause of Injury: _____ MVA/MCA**_____ Head Trauma*** _____ Infection _____ Stroke _____ Anoxia

_____ Developmental (Congenital) _____ Degenerative _____ Metabolic _____ Drowning

_____ Other (Specify) _____

**MVA = Motor Vehicle Accident; MCA = Motorcycle Accident. Circle one.

***Gun shot, blunt instrument, blow to head, fall, etc.

		DATE OF RATING							
CATEGORY	ITEM								
Arousability	Eye Opening[1]								
Awareness and	Communication Ability[2]†								
Responsivity••	Motor Response[3]								
Cognitive Ability for	Feeding[4]								
Self-Care	Toileting[4]								
Activities	Grooming[4]								
Dependence on Others•••	Level of Functioning[5]								
Psychosocial Adaptability	"Employable"[6]								

[2]*Communication Ability†*
Either Verbal; Writing or Letter Board; or Sign (viz. eye blink, head nod, etc.)

[1]*Eye Opening*

0 Spontaneous
1 To Speech
2 To Pain
3 None

0 Oriented
1 Confused
2 Inappropriate
3 Incomprehensible
4 None

[3]*Best Motor Resp.*

0 Obeying
1 Localizing
2 Withdrawing
3 Flexing
4 Extending
5 None

[4]*Cognitive Ability for Feeding, Toileting, Grooming (Does patient know how and when? Ignore motor disability.)*

0 Complete
1 Partial
2 Minimal
3 None

†In presence of tracheostomy (place T next to score); for voice or speech dysfunction (place D next to score if there is dysarthria, dysphonia, voice paralysis, aphasia, apraxia, etc.)

[5]*Level of Functioning*
(Consider both physical & cognitive disability)

0 Completely independent
1 Independent in special environment
2 Mildly dependent   - (a)
3 Moderately dependent   - (b)
4 Markedly dependent   - (c)
5 Totally dependent   - (d)

[6] *"Employability"* (As a full time worker, homemaker or student)

0 Not restricted
1 Selected jobs, competitive
2 Sheltered workshop, non-competitive
3 Not employable

Disability Categories

Total DR Score	Level of Disability
0	None
1	Mild
2–3	Partial
4–6	Moderate
7–11	Moderate severe
12–16	Severe
17–21	Extremely severe
22–24	Vegetative state
25–29	Extreme vegetative state
30	Death

a needs limited assistance (non-resident helper)
b needs moderate assistance (person in home)
c needs assistance with all major activities at all times
d 24-hour nursing care required

•Rappaport et al. Disability Rating Scale for Severe Head Trauma Patients: Coma To Community. *Arch Phys Med Rehab.* 63:118–123, 1982

••Modified from Teasdale, Jennett, *Lancet* 2:81-84, 1974

•••Modified from Scranton et al. *Arch Phys Med Rehab.* 51:1-21, 1970

continues

Exhibit A–22 continued

Item Definitions for Disability Rating Scale

Eye Opening

0—SPONTANEOUS: eyes open with sleep/wake rhythms indicating active arousal mechanisms; does not assume awareness.

1—TO SPEECH AND/OR SENSORY STIMULATION: a response to any verbal approach, whether spoken or shouted, not necessarily the command to open the eyes. Also, response to touch, mild pressure.

2—TO PAIN: tested by a painful stimulus.[1]

3—NONE: no eye opening even to painful stimulations.

Best communication ability (If patient cannot use voice because of tracheostomy or is aphasic or dysarthric or has vocal cord paralysis or voice dysfunction then estimate patient's best response and enter note under comments.)

0—ORIENTED: implies awareness of self and the environment. Patient able to tell you a) **who** he [sic] is; b) **where** he [sic] is; c) **why** he [sic] is there; d) year; e) season; f) month; g) day; h) time of day.

1—CONFUSED: attention can be held and patient responds to questions but responses are delayed and/or indicate varying degrees of disorientation and confusion.

2—INAPPROPRIATE: intelligible articulation but speech is used only in an exclamatory or random way (such as shouting and swearing); no sustained communication exchange is possible.

3—INCOMPREHENSIBLE: moaning, groaning or sounds without recognizable words; no consistent communication signs.

4—NONE: no sounds or communication signs from patient.

Best motor response

0—OBEYING: obeying command to move finger on best side. If no response or not suitable try another command such as "move lips," "blink eyes," etc. Do not include grasp or other reflex responses.

1—LOCALIZING: a painful stimulus[1] at more than one site causes a limb to move (even slightly) in an attempt to remove it. It is a deliberate motor act to move away from or remove the source of noxious stimulation. If there is doubt as to whether withdrawal or localization has occurred after 3 or 4 painful stimulations, rate as localization.

2—WITHDRAWING: any generalized movement away from a noxious stimulus that is more than a simple reflex response.

3—FLEXING: painful stimulation results in either flexion at the elbow, rapid withdrawal with abduction of the shoulder or a slow withdrawal with adduction of the shoulder. If there is confusion between flexing and withdrawing, then use pin prick on hands, then face.

4—EXTENDING: painful stimulation results in extension of the limb.

5—NONE: no response can be elicited. Usually associated with hypotonia. Exclude spinal transection as an explanation of lack of response; be satisfied that an adequate stimulus has been applied.

Cognitive ability for feeding, toileting and grooming. Rate each of the three functions separately. For each function answer the question, does the patient show *awareness of how* and *when* to perform each specified activity. *Ignore motor disabilities* that interfere with carrying out a function. (This is rated under Level of Functioning described below.) Rate best response for toileting based on bowel and bladder behavior. Grooming refers to bathing, washing, brushing of teeth, shaving, combing or brushing of hair and dressing.

0—COMPLETE: *continuously shows awareness that he* [sic] *knows how* to feed, toilet or groom self and can convey unambiguous information that he [sic] *knows when* this activity should occur.

1—PARTIAL: *intermittently shows awareness that he* [sic] *knows how* to feed, toilet or groom self and/or can intermittently convey reasonably clear information that he [sic] *knows when* the activity should occur.

2—MINIMAL: shows *questionable* or *infrequent awareness that he* [sic] *knows in a primitive way how* to feed, toilet or groom self and/or shows infrequently by certain signs, sound or activities that he [sic] is *vaguely aware when* the activity should occur.

3—NONE: shows *virtually no awareness at any time that he* [sic] *knows how* to feed, toilet or groom self and cannot *convey information by signs, sounds, or activity that he* [sic] *knows when* the activity should occur.

Level of functioning

0—COMPLETELY INDEPENDENT: able to live as he [sic] wishes, requiring no restriction due to physical, mental, emotional or social problems.

1—INDEPENDENT IN SPECIAL ENVIRONMENT: capable of functioning independently when needed requirements are met (mechanical aids).

2—MILDLY DEPENDENT: able to care for most of own needs but requires limited assistance due to physical, cognitive and/or emotional problems (e.g., needs nonresident helper).

3—MODERATELY DEPENDENT: able to care for self partially but needs another person at all times.

4—MARKEDLY DEPENDENT: needs help with all major activities and the assistance of another person at all times.

5—TOTALLY DEPENDENT: not able to assist in own care and requires 24-hour nursing care.

"Employability"

The psychosocial adaptability or "employability" item takes into account overall cognitive and physical ability to be an employee, homemaker, or student. This determination should take into account considerations such as the following:

continues

Exhibit A–22 continued

1. able to understand, remember and follow instructions; 2. can plan and carry out tasks at least at the level of an office clerk or in simple routine, repetitive industrial situations or can do school assignments; 3. ability to remain oriented, relevant and appropriate in work and other psychosocial situations; 4. ability to get to and from work or shopping centers using private or public transportation effectively; 5. ability to deal with number concepts; 6. ability to make purchases and handle simple money exchange problems; 7. ability to keep track of time schedules and appointments.

0—NOT RESTRICTED: can compete in the open market for a relatively wide range of jobs commensurate with existing skills; or can initiate, plan, execute and assume responsibilities associated with homemaking; or can understand and carry out most age relevant school assignments.

1—SELECTED JOBS, COMPETITIVE: can compete in a limited job market for a relatively narrow range of jobs because of limitations of the type described above and/or because of some physical limitations; or can initiate, plan, execute and assume many but not all responsibili-

ties associated with homemaking; or can understand and carry out many but not all school assignments.

2—SHELTERED WORKSHOP, NON-COMPETITIVE: cannot compete successfully in job market because of limitations described above and/or because of moderate or severe physical limitations; or cannot without major assistance initiate, plan, execute and assume responsibilities for homemaking; or cannot understand and carry out even relatively simple school assignments without assistance.

3—NOT EMPLOYABLE: completely unemployable because of extreme psychosocial limitations of the type described above; or completely unable to initiate, plan, execute and assume any responsibilities associated with homemaking; or cannot understand or carry out any school assignments.

Instructions: Place date of rating at top of column. Place appropriate rating next to each of the eight items listed. Add eight ratings to obtain total DR score.

[1]*Standard painful stimulus is the application of pressure across index fingernail of best side with wood of a pencil; for quadriplegics pinch nose tip and rate as 0, 1, 2, or 5.*

Source: Courtesy of Dr. Maurice Rappaport.

Quadriplegic Index of Function (QIF)

The Quadriplegic Index of Function (QIF) (Gresham et al., 1986) (see Exhibit A–23) was developed in 1980 for measurement of progress in patients with very high level spinal cord injury who were hospitalized at the Erie County Medical Center in Buffalo, New York. The interdisciplinary staff on the spinal cord unit recognized the limitations in measuring functional gains of persons with high quadriplegia with the available and widely used instruments for assessing activities of daily living. Although the Barthel Index has been used to examine outcomes in undifferentiated groups of persons with spinal cord injuries, this instrument was not sensitive nor comprehensive enough to measure small functional gains in quadriplegia (tetraplegia).

The 10 functional areas on the QIF are transfers, grooming, bathing, feeding, dressing, wheelchair mobility, bed activities, bladder program, bowel program, and understanding of personal care. Each category is divided into component parts and weighted. Total scores range from zero to 100. The categories and component parts were selected after review of other instruments used to measure activities of daily living and the literature related to these instruments, unstructured discussions with persons with spinal cord injury and their families, and group discussion and validation of individual professional team members' identification of categories and their component parts. The Barthel Index (Mahoney & Barthel, 1965) and Kenny Self-Care Evaluation (Schoening & Iversen, 1968) were used to illustrate percentage of differ-

ence in functional gain on admission and discharge as compared with findings on the QIF. The mean percentage of improvement in QIF scores between admission and discharge was 46, increasing from a mean of 3.9 on admission to a mean of 49.5 on discharge, whereas the mean percentages of improvement on the Kenny Self-Care Evaluation and Barthel Index were 30 and 20, respectively. Thus the QIF demonstrated greater sensitivity to positive change (Gresham et al., 1986).

Inter-rater reliability was established through the independent evaluation of 20 patients by three different raters with use of the QIF. Correlations for all ratings were statistically significant ($p < .001$) and ranged from .55 to .95 for 27 observations. Rehabilitation nurses used the instrument and found no problems in clarity of classification criteria or scoring instructions (Gresham et al., 1986).

The QIF has been compared with the Functional Independence Measure (FIM[SM] instrument) (Marino et al., 1993). When upper extremity motor scores (UEMS) on the Manual Muscle Test were used as a measure of neurological function to test the hypothesis that QIF scores were more closely related to motor power than FIM[SM] instrument scores, findings suggested that the QIF and FIM[SM] instrument showed significant and similar correlations to the UEMS on bathing and grooming. The QIF, however, had a significantly better correlation with the UEMS than the FIM[SM] instrument for the feeding category. Investigators concluded that the QIF detected changes in function that the FIM[SM] instrument may miss. Ditunno (1992) points out that "it may provide a more precise measure to link key muscles of the upper extremities to specific self-care tasks. . . . Its hypothetical advantage might be in linking key muscles of specific levels of quadriplegia such as C4, C5, or C6 complete lesions to self-care tasks such as drinking from a glass, feeding with a spoon, and other activities" (p. S303).

Strengths of the QIF are that it is sensitive to small changes in function, can be administered in 30 minutes, has inter-rater reliability, and includes the patient's understanding of his or her care. It is specific to persons with quadriplegia (tetraplegia).

REFERENCES

Ditunno, J.F. (1992). Functional assessment measures in CNS trauma. *Journal of Neurotrauma, 9*(Suppl. 1), S301–S305.

Gresham, G.E., Labi, M.L.C., Dittmar, S.S., Hicks, J.T., Joyce, S.Z., & Stehlik, M.A.P. (1986). The Quadriplegic Index of Function (QIF): Sensitivity and reliability demonstrated in a study of thirty quadriplegic patients. *Paraplegia, 24*(1), 38–44.

Mahoney, F.I., & Barthel, D.W. (1965). Functional evaluation: The Barthel Index. *Maryland State Medical Journal, 14*(2), 61–65.

Marino, R.J., Huang, M., Knight, P., Herbison, G.J., Ditunno, J.F., & Segal, M. (1993). Assessing self-care status in quadriplegia: Comparison of the Quadriplegic Index of Function (QIF) and the Functional Independence Measure (FIM^SM) instrument. *Paraplegia, 31*(4), 225–233.

Schoening, H.A., & Iversen, I.A. (1968). Numerical scoring of self-care status: A study of the Kenny Self-Care Evaluation. *Archives of Physical Medicine and Rehabilitation, 49*(4), 221–229.

Exhibit A–23 Quadriplegic Index of Function (QIF)

INTRODUCTION

The Quadriplegic Index of Function (QIF) was designed specifically for use in the functional assessment of persons with quadriplegia, as a means of monitoring their progress in rehabilitation and as an aid in determining specific problem areas as they develop during their program of rehabilitation.

Explanation of the FORMAT

The format was designed to be as objective as possible as well as convenient both for actual use and for subsequent data processing.

Record 1 contains baseline data on the patient. The codes for specific items are given on the same page as the items. Where the actual code used is less than the number of spaces provided, numbers must be written right-justified. For example, 9 spaces are provided for the ID #. If less than 9 numbers are used, the right hand–most columns are used first.

Records 2 and 3 contain the scores of the activities. Scores for TRANSFERS, GROOMING, BATHING, FEEDING, DRESSING, WHEELCHAIR MOBILITY, BED ACTIVITIES, BLADDER AND BOWEL PROGRAMS, are on Record 2. The scores for the UNDERSTANDING OF PERSONAL CARE are on Record 3.

- In the far left hand column are items or activities to be evaluated.
- The next column has printed the column numbers, and is primarily for key punching purposes.
- The next column to the right is blank. The appropriate score may be written in this column to facilitate key punching, or it may be circled if key punching is not a consideration.

COMPONENTS OF THE QIF

The QIF consists of 2 major parts. One is composed of specific activities which are grouped into 9 categories. Each activity under these categories is scored based on performance, from 0 to 4, in order of increasing independence. The criteria for these scores are:

4 = Patient completely independent, needs no assistive device.

3 = Patient independent with assistive device but requires no human supervision; patient must put assistive device on.

2 = Patient requires human supervision only; requires *no* lifting by another person.

1 = Patient requires physical contact which requires lifting of patient or part of patient's body by *one* other person.

0 = Patient completely dependent; does not do activity at all.

9 = Not applicable

It cannot be overemphasized that the QIF evaluates whether or not a patient *actually* does a specific maneuver, rather than whether or not the patient or evaluator feels the patient *can* do it. Thus, any maneuver which is not applicable (9) is usually not applicable because the activity is sex-related. Exceptions are to be noted in the space provided under Column 9. If a specific maneuver cannot be evaluated because the patient is in an artificially restricted environment, e.g. halo, then evaluation has to be postponed for that patient or the specific maneuver is considered as missing data.

The other part consists of a questionnaire aimed at assessing the quadriplegic's level of understanding of personal care variables. This understanding is considered an integral part of the person's program of rehabilitation. This questionnaire may have limited

continues

Exhibit A–23 continued

applicability to persons with head or cognitive injuries. The score for this part depends on the number of correct answers, according to the criteria.

The specific questionnaire included in the booklet contains questions deemed appropriate for patients in our particular center. If desired, these questions could be replaced by others that were believed to be more appropriate to a different setting. In this case, care would be required to ensure that final scoring for this section could be reduced to the 4, 3, 2, 1, 0, or 9 categories of each of the ten "Understanding of Personal Care" variables.

For questions, comments, inquiries, or requests for additional copies of this instrument, please address all correspondence to:

Sharon S. Dittmar, Ph.D., R.N.
School of Nursing
918 Kimball Tower
State University of New York at Buffalo
3435 Main St.
Buffalo, NY 14214

PATIENT'S DATA SHEET

	Identification No.									Evaluation		Record No.
Col. No.	1	2	3	4	5	6	7	8	9	10	11	1 12

	Sex	Marital Status	Education		Reporting Hospital	
Col. No.	13	14	15	16	17	18

	Date of Admission						Date of Birth						Date of Injury					
Col. No.	19	20	21	22	23	24	25	26	27	28	29	30	31	32	33	34	35	36

	Last Intact Motor Level			Degree	Last Intact Sensory Dermatome			Degree
Col. No.	37	38	39	40	41	42	43	44

CODING KEY

Column 13: *Sex*: Male = 1
                  Female = 2
Column 14: *Marital Status*: Single, never married = 0
                               Married = 1
                               Divorced = 2
                               Legally Separated = 3
                               Widowed = 4
                               Other = 8
                               Unknown = 9
Column 15–16: *Education*: Code number of completed years of schooling
Column 17–18: *Reporting Hospital*: Write name of participating hospital
Column 19–36: *Dates:* Code first 2 numbers of each *month, day, year* for each item. Code *month* first, *day* second and *year* last.
Column 37–39: *Motor Level*: Code letter and 2 digits of spinal segment, e.g. C01, C02, C03, etc.
Column 40: *Degree:* Complete = 0
                               Incomplete = 1
Column 41–44: Same Codes as Columns 37–39.

continues

Exhibit A–23 continued

COLUMN NUMBER	PATIENT IDENTIFICATION NUMBER	EVALUATION	RECORD NO.
	1 2 3 4 5 6 7 8 9	10 11	2 / 12

INSTRUCTIONS: Write in the appropriate number in the blank column or circle the number.
If *9* is circled, please specify reason why item is not applicable.

ACTIVITIES	Column Number	Completely independent; requires no assistive device	Independent with an assistive device, requires no human supervision; patient can put on assistive device	Requires human supervision only, with or without physical contact; requires *no* lifting by another person	Requires physical contact involving lifting of patient or part of patient's body by *one* person only	Completely dependent, patient cannot do activity at all	Not applicable (If checked, please specify reason)
I. *TRANSFERS* (16 points)		4	3	2	1	0	9
Bed—Chair	13	4	3	2	1	0	9
Chair—Bed	14	4	3	2	1	0	9
Chair—Toilet/Commode	15	4	3	2	1	0	9
Toilet/Commode—Chair	16	4	3	2	1	0	9
Chair—Vehicle	17	4	3	2	1	0	9
Vehicle—Chair	18	4	3	2	1	0	9
Chair—Shower/Tub	19	4	3	2	1	0	9
Tub/Shower—Chair	20	4	3	2	1	0	0
II. *GROOMING* (12 points)							
Brushing teeth/Managing Dentures	21	4	3	2	1	0	9
Brushing/Combing Hair	22	4	3	2	1	0	9
Shaving (for Men)	23	4	3	2	1	0	9
Managing tampon (for Women)	24	4	3	2	1	0	9

continues

Exhibit A–24 continued

ACTIVITIES	Column Number	Completely independent; requires no assistive device	Independent with an assistive device, requires no human supervision; patient can put on assistive device	Requires human supervision only, with or without physical contact; requires *no* lifting by another person	Requires physical contact involving lifting of patient or part of patient's body by *one* person only	Completely dependent, patient cannot do activity at all	Not applicable (If checked, please specify reason)
III. *BATHING* (8 points)							
Wash/Dry upper body	25	4	3	2	1	0	9
Wash/Dry lower body	26	4	3	2	1	0	9
Wash/Dry feet	27	4	3	2	1	0	9
Wash/Dry hair	28	4	3	2	1	0	9
(If patient takes bed bath, patient must obtain all needed materials)							
IV. *FEEDING* (24 points)							
Drink from cup/glass	29	4	3	2	1	0	9
Use spoon/fork	30	4	3	2	1	0	9
Cut food (meat)	31	4	3	2	1	0	9
Pour liquids out	32	4	3	2	1	0	9
Open carton/jar	33	4	3	2	1	0	9
Apply spreads to bread	34	4	3	2	1	0	9
Prepare simple meals	35	4	3	2	1	0	9
Apply adaptive equipment	36	4	3	2	1	0	9
V. *DRESSING* (20 points)							
Upper indoor clothes on	37	4	3	2	1	0	9
Upper indoor clothes off	38	4	3	2	1	0	9
Lower indoor clothes on	39	4	3	2	1	0	9
Lower indoor clothes off	40	4	3	2	1	0	9

continues

Exhibit A–23 continued

ACTIVITIES	Column Number	Completely independent; requires no assistive device	Independent with an assistive device, requires no human supervision; patient can put on assistive device	Requires human supervision only, with or without physical contact; requires *no* lifting by another person	Requires physical contact involving lifting of patient or part of patient's body by *one* person only	Completely dependent, patient cannot do activity at all	Not applicable (If checked, please specify reason)
Upper (heavy) outdoor clothes on	41	4	3	2	1	0	9
Upper (heavy) outdoor clothes off	42	4	3	2	1	0	9
Socks on/off	43	4	3	2	1	0	9
Shoes on/off	44	4	3	2	1	0	9
Fasteners	45	4	3	2	1	0	9
VI. *WHEELCHAIR MOBILITY* (28 points)							
Turn corners	46	4	3	2	1	0	9
Reverse direction	47	4	3	2	1	0	9
Lock WC brakes	48	4	3	2	1	0	9
Propel WC on rough/uneven surface	49	4	3	2	1	0	9
Propel WC on an incline	50	4	3	2	1	0	9
Move and position in chair	51	4	3	2	1	0	9
Maintain sitting balance	52	4	3	2	1	0	9
VII. *BED ACTIVITIES* (20 points)							
Supine—Prone	53	4	3	2	1	0	9
Lying to long sitting	54	4	3	2	1	0	9
Supine—side	55	4	3	2	1	0	9
Side—side	56	4	3	2	1	0	9
Maintain long sitting balance	57	4	3	2	1	0	9

continues

Exhibit A–23 continued

VIII. *BLADDER PROGRAM* (28 points)

Please use the scoring criteria for each routine on pages x–x. Score inapplicable routine as *9*.

				4	3	2	1	0	9
A.	1.	Voluntary Voiding:	Toilet	58	4	3	2	1	0	9
	2.	Voluntary Voiding:	Commode	59	4	3	2	1	0	9
B.		Intermittent Catheterization Program (ICP)		60		3	2	1	0	9
C.		Automatic Bladder Program		61		3	2	1	0	9
D.		Indwelling Catheter		62		3	2	1	0	9
E.		Ileal Diversion		63		3	2	1	0	9
F.		Credé		64		3	2	1	0	9

IX. *BOWEL PROGRAM* (24 points)

Please use the scoring criteria for each routine on pages x–xx. Score inapplicable routines as *9*.

			4	3	2	1	0	9
A.	1. Complete Control: Toilet	65	4	3	2	1	0	9
	2. Complete Control: Commode	66		3	2	1	0	9
B.	1. Suppository: Toilet	67	4	3	2	1	0	9
	2. Suppository: Commode/Bed/Chux Pad	68		3	2	1	0	9
C.	1. Digital Disimpaction: Toilet	69	4	3	2	1	0	9
	2. Commode/Bed Disimpaction	70		3	2	1	0	9
D.	1. Digital or Mechanical Stimulation: Toilet	71	4	3	2	1	0	9
	2. Digital or Mechanical Stimulation: Commode/Bed	72		3	2	1	0	9

VIII. *BLADDER PROGRAM*: SCORING CRITERIA

A. Voluntary Voiding
   1. Toilet
      4 = Patient is completely independent i.e. needs no help in transfer, managing clothes and in cleaning self afterwards.
      3 = Patient is independent in transfers but may require assistance in *only* one of the following: managing clothes or cleaning self afterwards.
      2 = Patient is independent in transfers but requires assistance in managing clothes and in cleaning self afterwards.
      1 = Patient needs help in transfers *and* in *one* of the following: managing clothes or cleaning self afterwards.
      0 = Patient cannot do *any* of the above. Completely dependent.

   2. Commode
      3 = Patient is independent, i.e. can get commode, requires no assistance in managing clothes or cleaning self afterwards.
      2 = Patient can prepare commode but requires assistance in either managing clothes or cleaning afterwards but not both.
      1 = Patient can prepare commode but requires assistance in managing clothes *and* in cleaning afterwards.
      0 = Patient cannot do any of the above.
B. ICP
   3 = Patient needs *no* assistance in preparing, positioning and disposing of equipment, manages clothes and cleans self afterwards.
   2 = Patient can manage clothes but needs assistance in *only* one of the following: preparing, positioning and disposing of equipment, and in cleaning self afterwards.

continues

Exhibit A–23 continued

1 = Patient needs help in all of the above but is able to instruct others in the necessary procedure.

0 = No bladder program at all or patient does not possess sufficient knowledge to instruct others in the necessary procedure.

C. Automatic Bladder Program

3 = Patient is completely independent, i.e. he [sic] manages clothes, prepares, applies and removes external device *and* cleans self afterwards without help.

2 = Patient manages clothes but needs help in one of the following: preparing, applying and removing external device and cleaning self afterwards.

1 = Patient cannot do any of the above but can instruct someone in the necessary procedure.

0 = Patient cannot do any of the above.

D. Indwelling Catheter

3 = Patient needs no help in managing clothes, changing bags, catheters, positioning and in cleaning self afterwards.

2 = Patient needs help in no more than two of the following: managing clothes, preparing catheters, changing bags, positioning, and cleaning self.

1 = Patient needs help in three or more of the above areas *but* can instruct someone in the necessary procedure.

0 = Completely dependent and cannot instruct someone in the necessary procedure.

E. Ileal Diversion

3 = Patient needs no help in managing clothes, changing bags and cleaning self afterwards.

2 = Patient needs help in one of the above.

1 = Patient needs help in two or more of the above *but* can also instruct someone in the necessary procedure.

0 = Patient cannot instruct someone in the necessary procedure.

F. Credé

3 = Patient needs no help in managing clothes, preparing supplies, credéing and cleaning afterwards.

2 = Patient needs help in (only) *one* of the above.

1 = Patient needs help in two or more of the above but can also instruct someone in necessary procedure.

0 = Patient cannot instruct someone in the necessary procedure.

IX. *BOWEL PROGRAM*: SCORING CRITERIA

A. 1. Complete Control: *Toilet*

4 = Patient is completely independent, i.e. needs no help in transfer, managing clothes and cleaning self afterwards.

3 = Patient is independent in transfers but requires assistance either in managing clothes *or* in cleaning self afterwards, but not both.

2 = Patient is independent in transfers but requires assistance in managing clothes, and cleaning self afterwards.

1 = Patient needs help in transfers and in *one* of the following: managing clothes, and cleaning self afterwards.

0 = Patient needs help in all of the above.

2. Complete Control: *Commode*

3 = Patient is independent, i.e. requires no assistance in managing clothes, getting commode and cleaning self afterwards.

2 = Patient can prepare commode but requires assistance either in managing clothes or cleaning self afterwards, but not both.

1 = Patient can prepare commode but requires assistance in both managing clothes *and* in cleaning self afterwards.

0 = Patient cannot do any of the above. Total dependence.

B. Suppository

1. Toilet

4 = Patient is completely independent, i.e. needs no help in transfers, managing clothes, inserting suppository and cleaning afterwards.

3 = Patient is independent in transfers, but needs assistance in *one* of the following: inserting suppository, managing clothes or cleaning afterwards.

2 = Patient is independent in transfers but needs assistance in two of the following: inserting suppository, managing clothes or cleaning afterwards.

1 = Patient needs help in all of the above but can instruct others in necessary procedure

or

1 = Patient can transfer but needs help in all the others.

0 = Patient cannot do any of the above, i.e. patient is incontinent.

2. Commode/Bed/Chux Pad

3 = Patient is independent in preparing materials, inserting suppository and in cleaning self.

2 = Patient needs help either in obtaining and inserting suppository but not both.

1 = Patient needs help in both areas but can instruct others in the necessary procedure.

0 = Patient cannot do any of the above.

C. Digital Disimpaction

1. Toilet Disimpaction

4 = Patient is independent in transfers, managing clothes; performs disimpaction by himself [sic] and cleans self afterwards.

3 = Patient is independent in transfers, but requires assistance with *one* (only) of the following: managing clothes, disimpacting or cleaning self afterwards.

2 = Patient is independent in transfers but requires assistance in *two* of the following: managing clothes, disimpacting or cleaning self afterwards.

1 = Patient needs help in all of the above but can instruct someone in necessary procedure

or

1 = Patient is independent in transfer but needs assistance in all the other procedures.

continues

Exhibit A–23 continued

0 = Patient does not do anything. Total dependence.
2. Commode/Bed Disimpaction
3 = Patient can get needed materials for disimpaction, performs disimpaction, manages clothes and cleans self afterwards.
2 = Patient needs help in *one* of the following: getting materials for disimpaction, managing clothes, disimpacting and cleaning.
1 = Patient needs help in *two* of the following: getting materials, managing clothes, disimpacting or cleaning.
0 = Patient needs help in everything.

D. Digital or Mechanical Stimulation
1. Toilet
4 = Patient is completely independent, i.e. needs no help in transfers, managing clothes, performing digital stimulation and cleaning afterwards.
3 = Patient is independent in transfers, but needs assistance in *one* of the following: performing digital stimulation, managing clothes or cleaning afterwards.
2 = Patient is independent in transfers but needs assistance in *two* of the following: performing digital stimulation, managing clothes or cleaning afterwards.
1 = Patient needs help in all of the above but can instruct others in necessary procedure.
or
1 = Patient can transfer but needs help in all other areas.
0 = Patient cannot do any of the above.
2. Commode/Bed
3 = Patient is independent, i.e. performs digital stimulation, manages clothes and cleans afterwards.
2= Patient performs digital stimulation but needs assistance in one of the following: managing clothes or cleaning afterwards.
1 = Patient needs assistance in stimulation, managing clothes *and* in cleaning afterwards but can instruct others in the necessary procedure.
0 = Patient cannot do any of the above.

X. UNDERSTANDING OF PERSONAL CARE: QUESTIONNAIRE
(The following multiple-choice questions are currently being used at Erie County Medical Center to "test" understanding of personal care variables by persons with quadriplegia. They may have limited applicability to persons with head or cognitive injuries.)

A. *SKIN CARE*
1. Skin pressure should be relieved:
a) every 15 minutes in wheelchair, every 2 hours when in bed
b) every 2 hours both when in bed and in wheelchair
c) every 2 hours in wheelchair, every 4 hours in bed
d) 3 times a day

2. Which of the following equipment should you *not* use to relieve skin pressure?
a) alternating pressure mattresses (air mattresses)
b) wheelchair cushions
c) doughnuts (rubber rings)
d) sheepskin

3. What should you *avoid* in order to prevent skin pressure sores?
a) relieving pressure at frequent intervals
b) checking skin frequently for reddened areas
c) sitting for long periods
d) keeping skin dry and clean

4. Checking your skin, relieving pressure at regular intervals and making decisions regarding your skin care are the responsibilities of your
a) attendant
b) family member
c) friend
d) self

B. *DIET/NUTRITION*
1. An appropriate diet/nutrition program is important to someone with spinal cord injury as a means of:
a) maintaining an adequate bowel program
b) preventing deep vein thrombosis (blood clots in the veins of the legs)
c) preventing upper respiratory infections
d) relieving skin pressure

2. Which of the following *don't you need* in your daily diet:
a) cereals, bread, pasta
b) doughnuts, pastry, ice cream
c) fruits and green vegetables
d) meat, fish or poultry

C. *MEDICATION*
1. Please list one medication you are taking, indicating the purpose, the specific time and dosage you are to take.
Name   Purpose   Dosage   Frequency

2. What should you do if you run out of your medication, because your prescription has expired?
a) stop taking medication
b) obtain more medication as soon as it is convenient
c) call your doctor for additional prescription
d) substitute any handy medication which is similar to your own until you can get more of the original medication

D. *EQUIPMENT*
1. Resting splints are used to:
a) protect hands from injury
b) prevent muscle contracture
c) maintain joints, muscles and ligaments in a

continues

Exhibit A–23 continued

functional position
   d) b & c
   e) a & b
2. Reddened areas on the skin after removal of splints indicate a pressure area. You should contact your O.T. for splint adjustment if the redness does not disappear in:
   a) one hour
   b) one day
   c) twenty minutes
   d) immediately
3. Your plastic splints may be cleaned with
   a) mild soap and cool/lukewarm water
   b) hot water and strong detergent
   c) hot water and mild soap
   d) they will not hold up if immersed in water
4. If your splints break or are lost, what should you do?
   a) buy a similar one from your drug store
   b) contact the O.T. Department
   c) have a handy person make a similar one for you
   d) call the County's Social Services Department
5. Your wheelchair can be serviced by:
   a) yourself or under your supervision
   b) a family member or friend
   c) the vendor from whom the chair was purchased
   d) all of the above
6. Adaptive equipment should be obtained through
   a) recommendations by O.T. with prescription from the physician for commercially-made equipment
   b) direct purchase from the vendor
   c) custom design by O.T. with prescription from the physician
   d) a & c
7. Splints, if left in the car on a hot day may:
   a) crack
   b) melt
   c) be stolen
   d) none of the above

E. *RANGE OF MOTION*
1. What do range of motion (ROM) exercises do for your body?
   a) increase muscle strength
   b) assist circulation
   c) prevent infection
   d) maintain length of soft tissue and muscles surrounding joints
   e) both b & d
2. What is most important to remember about ROM exercises?
   a) that they're done on a regular basis
   b) that the entire body from fingers to toes is exercised
   c) that professional help is obtained when problems arise
   d) that force should be applied gently but firmly at

end of motion
   e) all of the above
3. What will cause limitation in normal range of motion?
   a) hypertension
   b) bladder infections
   c) swelling of arms or legs
   d) spinal shock
4. How should someone exercise very spastic legs?
   a) quickly with fast jerky movements
   b) slowly with slow but deliberately long movements
   c) only when spasticity stops
   d) don't bother exercising them at all

F. *AUTONOMIC DYSREFLEXIA* (AUTONOMIC HYPER-REFLEXIA)
1. Autonomic Dysreflexia:
   a) is overactive reflex activity which is uncontrollable
   b) is underactive reflex activity which is uncontrollable
   c) usually occurs anytime after the stage of spinal shock in persons with lesions *below* T-6
   d) all of the above
2. Dysreflexia can be caused by:
   a) bladder distention, urologic procedures
   b) bowel distention
   c) spasms, infection, bladder stones
   d) all of the above
3. Signs and symptoms of dysreflexia are:
   a) pounding headache
   b) slow pulse
   c) increase in blood pressure
   d) all of the above
4. If you think you might be having dysreflexia, which of the following should be done?
   a) sit up and check blood pressure
   b) make sure bladder is emptying properly
   c) check for fecal impaction
   d) all of the above
   e) none of the above

G. *UPPER RESPIRATORY INFECTION*
1. What are the symptoms of a respiratory infection?
   a) general ill feeling
   b) slight fever
   c) possible muscle pain
   d) rattling sound in chest
   e) all of the above
2. How can deep breathing and assisted coughing aid in prevention of upper respiratory infection (URI)?
   a) by increasing size of chest muscles
   b) by strengthening stomach (abdominal) muscles
   c) by increasing the blood supply to the heart
   d) by keeping airway passages open
3. Why does the resultant paralysis in quadriplegia increase the possibility of developing an upper respiratory infection?
   a) decreased activity and pooling of secretions in

continues

Exhibit A–23 continued

areas of lungs
b) increased bladder tone
c) lungs become paralyzed
d) decreased force in coughing
e) both a & d

4. When should you seek medical assistance with a suspected URI?
   a) symptoms are serious and/or prolonged
   b) chest is painful
   c) cough blood or rusty colored sputum
   d) inability to bring up secretions
   e) rapidly rising temperature
   f) all of the above.

H. *URINARY TRACT INFECTION*

1. Which of the following are symptoms of urinary tract infection?
   a) Fever
   b) Chills
   c) Cloudy, foul smelling urine
   d) Increased spasticity
   e) All of the above

2. What would you do if you suspect that you have a urinary tract problem?
   a) obtain a urine specimen and take it to your doctor
   b) increase your level of activity
   c) stop taking all medications
   d) increase your intake of dairy products

3. To help prevent urinary tract problems, which of these should you *not* do:
   a) do your caths at different times each day in order to train the bladder to retain more fluid
   b) regulate your intake of body fluids
   c) comply with your regimen of medication
   d) none of these

I. *DEEP VEIN THROMBOSIS* (Blood clots in veins of legs)

1. The most important thing to do if your leg(s) become swollen is:
   a) stay in bed
   b) call the doctor
   c) cross your legs
   d) all of the above

2. Deep vein thrombosis is a complication of
   a) immobility
   b) overeating
   c) poor fluid intake
   d) exercise

3. Which of the following are helpful in preventing deep vein thrombosis?
   a) elastic stockings, properly fitted and applied
   b) regular range of motion exercises to legs

c) proper body positioning
d) all of the above
e) none of the above

J. *OBTAINING HUMAN SERVICES*

1. For which of the following problems can you get help from your nearest spinal cord injury rehabilitation center?
   a) questions about payment for different types of equipment or services
   b) feelings of depression that persist and do not get better
   c) problems with your bladder or bowel program
   d) all of the above
   e) none of the above

2. Which of the following is *not* a "third party" program that pays for health care?
   a) Medicaid
   b) Blue Cross/Blue Shield (or other insurance company)
   c) Med. Tech.
   d) Medicare

3. Which of the following would *not* be a wise procedure if you became acutely ill and could not reach your own physician?
   a) go to the nearest hospital emergency room
   b) call an ambulance or your local police/fireman to take you to a hospital
   c) go to the emergency room at the hospital where you were originally rehabilitated (provided it is nearby)
   d) just "tough it out" until you can reach your own physician, no matter how long it takes

4. Which of the following agencies might be helpful to a quadriplegic living in the community?
   a) Visiting Nurse Service
   b) Office of Vocational Rehabilitation
   c) County Health Department
   d) all of the above
   e) none of the above

5. "Prior approval" to ensure payment for equipment or supplies is required to prevent:
   a) somebody getting cheated
   b) the doctor for losing money
   c) your getting something inappropriate
   d) your managing your own affairs

6. If you have a problem you haven't been able to solve, you should:
   a) keep calling appropriate people and agencies
   b) quit talking to every one and give up
   c) find a way to punish people for their indifference
   d) put it out of your mind and hope it will resolve itself

continues

Exhibit A–23 continued

UNDERSTANDING OF PERSONAL CARE: SCORING INSTRUCTIONS

A. Scoring Criteria: Check the answers to the questionnaire against the key provided on page xx.

1. For *Skin Care, ROM, Autonomic Dysreflexia, Upper Respiratory Infection,* and *Obtaining Needed Human Services,* final score corresponds to the number of correct answers on the diagnostic test. Thus, if a patient gets all 4 questions right, his [sic] score for the item is 4. If he [sic] gets 3 right, his [sic] score is 3, etc.

2. For *Urinary Tract Infection* and *Deep Vein Thrombosis,* final score is as follows:

3 correct answers	= 4 points
2 correct answers	= 3 points
1 correct answer	= 2 points
no correct answers	= 0

3. For *Equipment,* final score is determined as follows:

7 correct answers	= 4
5–6 correct answers	= 3
3–4 correct answers	= 2
1–2 correct answers	= 1
no correct answers	= 0

4. For *Diet*: If patient gets both answers correct, score equals 4. One correct answer equals a score of 2.

5. *Medication*: Score for this variable is determined as follows:

4 = Patient answers all the questions correctly and accurately, i.e. name, dosage and frequency of medication must be answered correctly.
3 = Patient answers question 2 correctly, but question 1 is only partly correct.
2 = Patient answers question 1 correctly and accurately, but not question 2.
1 = Patient answers *only* question 2 correctly.
0 = Patient cannot answer either question correctly.

B. To compute the overall score for the *Understanding of Personal Care* variables, add the scores for each category, e.g. Skin Care, Urinary Tract Infection, etc. and note on the tally sheet on page xx.

PATIENT IDENTIFICATION NUMBER	EVALUATION	RECORD NO.
__ __ __ __ __ __ __ __ __	__ __	3
1 2 3 4 5 6 7 8 9	10 11	12

X. *UNDERSTANDING OF PERSONAL CARE*

Please use scoring criteria above.

		`	4	3	2	1	0	9
A.	SKIN CARE	13	4	3	2	1	0	9
B.	DIET/NUTRITION	14	4	3	2	1	0	9
C.	MEDICATION	15	4	3	2	1	0	9
D.	EQUIPMENT	16	4	3	2	1	0	9
E.	RANGE OF MOTION	17	4	3	2	1	0	9
F.	AUTONOMIC DYSREFLEXIA (HYPERREFLEXIA)	18	4	3	2	1	0	9

continues

Exhibit A–23 continued

G.	UPPER RESPIRATORY TRACT INFECTION	19	4	3	2	1	0	9
H.	URINARY TRACT INFECTION	20	4	3	2	1	0	9
I.	DEEP VEIN THROMBOSIS	21	4	3	2	1	0	9
J.	OBTAINING NEEDED HUMAN SERVICES	22	4	3	2	1	0	9

TOTAL RAW SCORE: _____

Q I F: SCORING GUIDE

Determine the score for each of the QIF component variables (e.g. transfers, dressing, etc.) using the following guide:

ACTIVITIES	SCORE
A. *Transfers*: Add the scores for each of the items under this category and then divide the sum by 2. There should be 8 individual items, each item being scored from 0–4. Therefore, the final *transfer* score will range from 0–16.	_____
B. *Grooming*: The score is equal to the sum of the scores for the three activities. Final *grooming* score will range from 0–12.	_____
C. *Bathing*: The final score is the sum of the scores for the four items divided by 2. Final *bathing* score will range from 0–8.	_____
D. *Dressing*: There are 9 items under this category. Add items 5 and 6 and multiply the sum by 1.5. Compute the sum of items 1 through 4, 7 through 9, plus the subscore computed for items 5 and 6. Divide the total by 2 for the final *dressing* score which will range from 0–20.	_____
E. *Feeding*: Multiply the sum of the 8 items under this category by .75. Final *feeding* score will range from 0–24.	_____
F. *Wheelchair Mobility*: Add the scores for the 7 items under *Wheelchair Mobility*. Final *wheelchair mobility* score will range from 0–28.	_____
G. *Bed Activities*: Add the scores for the 5 items. Final *bed activities* score will range from 0–20.	_____
H. *Bladder Program*: Multiply the score for the appropriate applicable routine by 7. Final *bladder program* score will range from 0–28.	_____
I. *Bowel Program*: Multiply the score for the appropriate applicable routine by 6. Final *bowel program* score will range from 0–24.	_____
J. *Understanding of Personal Care*: Divide overall raw score by 2. Final score will range from 0–20.	_____
TOTAL POINTS:	_____
QIF SCORE: $\dfrac{TOTAL\ SCORE \times 100}{200}$	_____

continues

Exhibit A–23 continued

Functional Assessment Instruments Used with Specific Age Groups

WeeFIM® Functional Independence Measure For Children

The Functional Independence Measure for Children (WeeFIM® instrument) (Braun, Msall, & Granger, 1991) (see Exhibit A–24), a pediatric functional assessment instrument, was developed by researchers at the Uniform Data System for Medical Rehabilitation, State University of New York at Buffalo in 1987. This instrument is an adaptation of the Functional Independence Measure (FIM℠ instrument), the adult version that was developed previously for the Uniform Data System. The WeeFIM® instrument was designed to assess and track functional independence in children ages six months to seven years and is used across health, developmental, educational, and community settings (Msall, DiGaudio, Duffy, et al., 1994). Key characteristics of the FIM℠ instrument (discussed earlier in this Appendix) and WeeFIM® instrument are the minimal data set, emphasis on consistent actual performance, and discipline-free (can be done by any reliable rehabilitation clinical professional) pa-

tient observation and collection of data in a variety of settings (Msall, DiGaudio, & Duffy, 1993).

The WeeFIM® instrument contains 18 items in the content domains of self-care, sphincter control, mobility, locomotion, communication, and social cognition. A seven-level ordinal scoring system ranging from one for total assistance to seven for complete independence is used. A score between one and five indicates need for some amount of assistance from another person to complete an activity. A score of six indicates that the individual can complete an activity independently but may require an assistive device, need more than the normal amount of time, or require monitoring for safety.

To ensure appropriate administration, use, and scoring, training in administration of the WeeFIM® instrument is required. Those familiar with the adult FIM℠ instrument will find the WeeFIM® easy to learn. A guide is available in English for all users (Braun et al., 1991). Other training can be accomplished by either watching an introductory video (Msall, Braun, & Granger, 1990) or attending workshops on the WeeFIM® instrument.

The WeeFIM® instrument is based on two conceptual models (Braun & Granger, 1991): the World Health Organization (1980) model of disablement and the concept of "burden of care." The WeeFIM® instrument is an indicator of severity of disability. It is presumed that a better quality of life is achieved when attention is focused on gains in function, rather than on impairment, in a child's environment. Burden of care refers to the amount of assistance required to perform a given activity. It is a reflection of social and economic resources. Braun and Granger (1991) state that "the ultimate goal of the WeeFIM® is to measure changes in function over time and to weigh the burden of care in terms of physical, technologic, and financial resources" (p. 47).

Validity and reliability for the WeeFIM® instrument have been determined. Content validity was established by a panel of eight interdisciplinary experts (nurses, occupational and physical therapists, a physician, and a psychologist) with an average of 13 years of work experience (McCabe & Granger, 1990).

Results of a pilot study conducted with a sample of 111 children with no known disability demonstrated a strong correlation between WeeFIM® scores and age (Braun & Granger, 1991; McCabe, 1991). Test items seemed to demonstrate a developmental sequence. The WeeFIM® instrument was administered to the children before and after returning from camp and by the counselors while at camp. Test–retest reliability and inter-rater agreement were satisfactory. Criterion-related validity (extra time/help) demonstrated that scores were more representative of amount of helper effort required than amount of time required, suggesting that the WeeFIM® instrument identifies the burden of care of a disability. Test–retest and inter-rater reliability were also demonstrated (Heinemann, Hamilton, Granger, Linacre, & Wright, 1992; McCabe, 1991).

Forty-two premature infants with a mean gestational age of 25.9 weeks and mean birth weight of 870 g were monitored at age four to five years (Msall, Mallen, Rogers, Catanzaro, & Duffy, 1991). Blinded neurodevelopmental, psychometric, and functional assessments were performed. Cerebral palsy was diagnosed in 9.5% of the children; mental retardation, in 9.5%; multiple handicaps, in 4.8%; and freedom from major impairments, in 76.2%. Children with a major impairment had significantly lower WeeFIM® instrument scores than children with no impairment. Children whose parents perceived their health status as poor had significantly lower WeeFIM® instrument scores than children whose parents perceived their children were healthy. The family's socioeconomic status and neonatal complications were not correlated with the WeeFIM® instrument scores. Normative sampling and use with children of various disabilities have also been done (Msall, DiGaudio, Duffy, et al., 1994; Msall, DiGaudio, Rogers, et al., 1994).

REFERENCES

Braun, S., Msall, M.E., & Granger, C.V. (1991). *Manual for the Functional Independence Measure for Children (WeeFIM®)* (version 1.4). Buffalo, NY: Center for Functional Assessment Research, Uniform Data System for Medical Rehabilitation, State University of New York.

Braun, S.L., & Granger, C.V. (1991). A practical approach to functional assessment in pediatrics. *Occupational Therapy Practice, 2*(2), 46–51.

Heinemann, A.W., Hamilton, B.B., Granger, C.V., Linacre, M.J., & Wright, B.D. (1992). *Rehabilitation efficacy for brain and spinal injury* (Final Report). Chicago: Rehabilitation Institute of Chicago. (Grant No. R49/CCR503609)

McCabe, M.A. (1991). *Evaluating the validity and reliability of the pediatric functional independence measure.* Unpublished doctoral dissertation, Rush University, Chicago.

McCabe, M.A., & Granger, C.V. (1990). Content validity of a pediatric functional independence measure. *Applied Nursing Research, 3*(3), 120–121.

Msall, M.E., Braun, S., & Granger, C.V. (1990). Use of the Functional Independence Measure for Children (WeeFIM®): An interdisciplinary training tape [Abstract]. *Developmental Medicine and Child Neurology, 32*(Suppl. 62), 46.

Msall, M.E., DiGaudio, K.M., & Duffy, L.C. (1993). Use of functional assessment in children with disabilities. *Physical Medicine and Rehabilitation Clinics of North America, 4*(3), 517–527

Msall, M.E., DiGaudio, K., Duffy, L.C., LaForest, S., Braun, S., & Granger, C.V. (1994). WeeFIM® normative sample of an instrument for tracking functional independence in children. *Clinical Pediatrics, 33*(7), 431–438.

Msall, M.E., DiGaudio, K., Rogers, B.T., LaForest, S., Catanzaro, N.L., Campbell, J., Wilcenski, F., & Duffy, L.C. (1994). The Functional Independence Measure for Children (WeeFIM®): Conceptual basis and pilot use in children with developmental disabilities. *Clinical Pediatrics, 33*(7), 421–430.

Msall, M.E., Mallen, S., Rogers, B.T., Catanzaro, N., & Duffy, L.C. (1991). Pilot use of a functional status measure at age 4–5 years in extremely premature infants after surfactant [Abstract]. *Developmental Medicine and Child Neurology, 33*(Suppl. 64), 15–16.

World Health Organization. (1980). *International classification of impairments, disabilities, and handicaps: A manual of classification relating to the consequences of disease.* Geneva: Author.

Exhibit A–24   Guide for the Uniform Data Set for Medical Rehabilitation (WeeFIM® Instrument) Inpatient—Case Coding Sheets

WeeFIM® INSTRUMENT CASE CODING SHEET

Rehabilitation Patient

1a. Facility Code

1b. Facility Care Class   (Pediatric Care Only)
       2-Inpatient   6-Clinic   7-Home   8-School

2. Patient Code

3. Birth Date
    MONTH   DAY   YEAR

4. ZIP/Postal Code   (home)

5. Gender
    1-Male   2-Female

6. Ethnicity
    1-White   2-Black   3-Asian
    4-Native American   5-Other   6-Hispanic

7. English Language
    1-Yes   2-No   3-Partial

8. Marital Status (Not Applicable)

Dates

9. Admission Date
    MONTH   DAY   YEAR

10. Admission Class   1-Initial Rehabilitation
    2-Short Stay   3-Readmission   4-Outpatient

11. Discharge Date
    MONTH   DAY   YEAR

12. Program Interrupted?   Check if program is interrupted. and enter Transfer and Return Dates.

13. Program Interruption Dates

1st Interruption
a. Transfer Date   **b. Return Date**
MONTH DAY YEAR   MONTH DAY YEAR

2nd Interruption
c. Transfer Date   **d. Return Date**
MONTH DAY YEAR   MONTH DAY YEAR

3rd Interruption
e. Transfer Date   **f. Return Date**
MONTH DAY YEAR   MONTH DAY YEAR

Payment Source and Rehabilitation Charges

14. Payment Source
    1-Blue Cross   2-Medicare
    3-Medicaid/Welfare
    4-Commercial Insurance
    5-HMO   6-Workers' Compensation
    7-Crippled Children's Service
    8-Developmental Disabilities Service.
    9-State Vocational Rehabilitation   10-Private Pay
    11-Employee Courtesy   12-Unreimbursed   13-CHAMPUS
    14-Other   15-None (only for Secondary)
    16-State Education Department (only for Outpatient)

Primary

Secondary

15. Gross Rehabilitation Charges

a. Total   (Dollars only) $

b. Physician Fee   1-Included   2-Not Included

16. Net Rehabilitation Charges

a. Total   (Dollars only) $

b. Physician Fee   1-Included   2-Not Included

Diagnosis

17. Impairment Group
(Condition requiring admission to rehabilitation)

18. Date of Onset
    MONTH   DAY   YEAR

19. Etiologic Diagnosis   (ICD-9 Code)

20. ASIA Impairment Scale   (Traumatic SCI only)
    A-Complete   B-Sensory Preserved
    C-Motor Nonfunctional   D-Motor Functional   E-Normal

continues

Exhibit A–24 continued

WeeFIM® ASSESSMENT CODING SHEET

Rehabilitation Patient

1a. Facility Code ☐☐☐☐☐

1b. Facility Care Class (Pediatric Care Only)
2-Inpatient 6-Clinic 7-Home 8-School ☐

2. Patient Code ☐☐☐☐☐☐☐☐

9. Admission Date ☐☐ ☐☐ ☐☐
MONTH   DAY   YEAR

Assessment

21. Assessment Type 1-Admit 2-Interim 3-Discharge 4-Followup ☐

22. Assessment Date ☐☐ ☐☐ ☐☐
MONTH   DAY   YEAR

23. Admit From Setting (Same as item 24) ☐☐

24. Living Setting ☐☐
1-Home 2-Acute Unit of own facility 3-Acute Unit of other facility
4-Chronic Hospital 5-Rehabilitation Facility 6-School Based Program
7-Home Care 8-Alternate Level of Care 9-Board and Care
10-Transitional Living 11-Intermediate Care 12-Skilled Nursing 13-Other 14-Died

25. Living With (Only if item 24 is coded 1-Home) ☐
1-Two Parents 2-One Parent 3-Relatives
4-Foster Care 5-Shelter 6-Other

26. Educational Category ☐
1-Not a student 2-Early Intervention Program
3-Pre-School 4-Regular School 5-Other

27. Educational Setting (Only if item 26 is coded 2,3 or 4) ☐
1-Regular Class 2-Special Class 3-Home Based
4-Day Care/Nursery School (Only if item 26 is 2 or 3)

28. Information Source (Only for followup or outpatient) ☐
1-Patient 2-Family 3-Other 4-Clinician

29. Assessment Method (Only for followup or outpatient) ☐
1-In person 2-Telephone 3-Mailed questionnaire

30. Health Maintenance (Only for followup or outpatient)
1-Own care
2-Unpaid person or family   Primary ☐
3-Paid attendant or aide
4-Paid, skilled professional   Secondary ☐

31. Therapy (Only for discharge, followup or outpatient) ☐
1-None 2-Outpatient therapy 3-Home based paid professional therapy
4-Both 2 &3 5-Inpatient Hospital 6-Long-term care facility
7-Other Combinations 8-School based

32. Therapy Services (Only for discharge, followup or outpatient) ☐
1-None 2-Physical Therapy 3-Occupational Therapy
4-Speech Therapy 5-Physical & Occupational
6-Physical, Occupational & Speech 7-Other Combinations of 2, 3 or 4

33. Other Diagnoses (ICD-9 codes)
a. ☐☐☐.☐☐   d. ☐☐☐.☐☐
b. ☐☐☐.☐☐   e. ☐☐☐.☐☐
c. ☐☐☐.☐☐   f. ☐☐☐.☐☐
g. ☐☐☐.☐☐

34. Functional Independence Measure (FIM)

MOTOR

Self-Care
A. Eating ☐
B. Grooming ☐
C. Bathing ☐
D. Dressing-Upper Body ☐
E. Dressing-Lower Body ☐
F. Toileting ☐

Sphincter Control
G. Bladder Management ☐
H. Bowel Management ☐

Transfers
I. Chair, Wheelchair ☐
J. Toilet ☐
K. Tub, Shower ☐

Locomotion
L. Walk/Wheelchair/Crawl ☐   { ◯ Walk ◯ Wheelchair ◯ Crawl ◯ Combination }
M. Stairs ☐

COGNITIVE

Communication
N. Comprehension ☐   { ◯ Auditory ◯ Visual ◯ Both }
O. Expression ☐   { ◯ Vocal ◯ Nonvocal ◯ Both }

Social Cognition
P. Social Interaction ☐
Q. Problem Solving ☐
R. Memory ☐

(NOTE: Leave no blanks; enter 1 if not testable due to risk)

FIM LEVELS

NO HELPER

7 Complete Independence (Timely, Safely)
6 Modified Independence (Device)

HELPER

Modified Dependence
5 Supervision
4 Minimal Assistance (Subject = 75 % +)
3 Moderate Assistance (Subject = 50 % +)

Complete Dependence
2 Maximal Assistance (Subject = 25 % +)
1 Total Assistance (Subject = 0 % +)

Source: Reprinted with permission of Dr. Carl V. Granger, Copyright 1993, Uniform Data System for Medical Rehabilitation, UB Foundation Activities, Inc.

Exhibit A–24 continued

Guide for the Uniform Data Set for Medical Rehabilitation (WeeFIM® Instrument) Inpatient—Norm Tables

Tables which appear on the following pages present norms for the WeeFIM® instrument for the Motor, the Cognitive Subscale and the Total WeeFim® instrument. These norms reflect the results of extensive research efforts on our norming sample, including examination of item, subscale and total scores across age groups.

Our research has shown that WeeFIM® instrument normative scores are well-predicted by a child's chronological age, and are even better predicted by using the logarithm of a child's age. Since the relationship between normal children's chronological age and WeeFIM® instrument scores is curvilinear, using the log of a child's age allows for a stronger linear prediction of WeeFIM® instrument norm scores. The norm tables on the following pages thus are based upon a simple prediction equation using the log age of each child in the norm study to determine the WeeFIM® instrument Motor, Cognitive and Total Norms. This unique approach to the norms yields individual predicted norms of each child in the norming study by using his or her exact chronological age in the prediction formula. These predicted norms were then averaged across children in the age groupings presented in the tables to form norms, with standard deviations and confidence intervals to form ranges of normal for each age interval.

The norm tables are presented in four-month age intervals for normal children and reflect the close correspondence between chronological age and WeeFIM® instrument scores in normal

children. The norms begin at the chronological age of 6-7 months, where normal children are expected to be quite dependent in function (scores of 1 in all WeeFIM® Instrument items), and progress in age and WeeFIM® Instrument scores to the age of 92-95 months, where normal children are expected to be functionally independent (all 7's).

Rasch analyses on the WeeFIM® instrument (Heinemann, 1992; McCabe, 1991) have identified two individual dimensions upon which the individual items of the WeeFIM® instrument fall. These two dimensions, Motor and Cognitive, comprise the first 13 and the last 5 items of the WeeFIM® instrument, respectively. The tables which follow thus include separate Motor and Cognitive norms. However, individual item norms are also possible resulting from the Rasch analyses.

Rasch analyses of the norming sample determined the order of item difficulty of each of the 18 items on the WeeFIM® instrument. An important advantage of this approach was the ability to define a hierarchy of item difficulties from low to high, and to use this hierarchy to calculate individual item norms in addition to the Motor, Cognitive and Total norms presented on the following pages. Individual item norms vary according to the formula for age and predicted WeeFIM® instrument scores. Thus, these are individually calculated and are too numerous to present here. However, by computerized formulae, they are automatically calculated for the user in FIM ware, and appear as the Norm Column in the WeeFIM® instrument Profile Screen. They also form the basis for comparisons with the most recent WeeFIM® instrument assessment in each individual Patient Tracking Report.

WeeFIM® Motor Subscale Norms

Age Groups in Months	WeeFIM® Mean Ratings	Standard Deviation	95% Confidence Interval		
6–7	13.00	.00	13.00	to	13.00
8–11	17.84	3.67	16.52	to	19.17
12–15	29.96	3.35	28.61	to	31.32
16–19	39.26	2.23	38.19	to	40.34
20–23	46.07	2.34	44.77	to	47.36
24–27	50.63	1.56	49.94	to	51.33
28–31	56.23	1.48	55.34	to	57.13
32–35	60.41	1.14	59.90	to	60.91
36–39	64.39	1.12	63.91	to	64.87
40–43	67.24	1.03	66.70	to	67.77
44–47	70.71	.77	70.31	to	71.10
48–51	73.06	.81	72.77	to	73.36
52–55	76.04	.73	75.74	to	76.34
56–59	78.64	.50	78.36	to	78.93
60–63	80.33	.48	80.11	to	80.55
64–67	83.25	.46	82.86	to	83.64
68–71	84.88	.33	84.71	to	85.05
72–75	86.27	.47	85.96	to	86.59
76–79	88.14	.36	87.93	to	88.35
80–83	89.93	.83	89.45	to	90.41
84–87	91.00	.00	91.00	to	91.00
88–91	91.00	.00	91.00	to	91.00
92–95	91.00	.00	91.00	to	91.00
Total	61.90	23.38	59.59	to	64.21

continues

Exhibit A–25 continued

WeeFIM® Cognitive Subscale Norms

Age Groups in Months	WeeFIM® Mean Ratings	Standard Deviation	95% Confidence Interval		
6–7	5.00	.00	5.00	to	5.00
8–11	6.13	1.26	5.67	to	6.58
12–15	10.50	1.27	9.99	to	11.01
16–19	13.95	.71	13.61	to	14.29
20–23	17.20	.94	16.88	to	17.72
24–27	18.77	.75	18.44	to	19.11
28–31	21.00	.71	20.57	to	21.43
32–35	22.36	.49	22.15	to	22.58
36–39	24.22	.42	24.04	to	24.40
40–43	25.41	.51	25.15	to	25.67
44–47	26.53	.51	26.26	to	26.79
48–51	27.71	.46	27.54	to	27.88
52–55	28.76	.44	28.58	to	28.94
56–59	29.79	.43	29.54	to	30.03
60–63	30.71	.46	30.50	to	30.93
64–67	31.63	.52	31.19	to	32.06
68–71	32.18	.39	31.97	to	32.38
72–75	33.00	.00	33.00	to	33.00
76–79	33.64	.50	33.36	to	33.93
80–83	34.29	.47	34.02	to	34.56
84–87	35.00	.00	35.00	to	35.00
88–91	35.00	.00	35.00	to	35.00
92–95	35.00	.00	35.00	to	35.00
Total	23.28	9.17	22.37	to	24.18

WeeFIM® Total Scale Norms

Age Groups in Months	WeeFIM® Mean Ratings	Standard Deviation	95% Confidence Interval		
6–7	18.00	.00	18.00	to	18.00
8–11	23.97	4.86	22.22	to	25.72
12–15	40.46	4.62	38.59	to	42.33
16–19	53.21	2.92	51.80	to	54.62
20–23	63.27	3.28	61.45	to	65.09
24–27	69.41	2.30	68.39	to	70.43
28–31	77.23	2.17	75.92	to	78.54
32–35	82.77	1.60	82.06	to	83.48
36–39	88.61	1.47	87.97	to	89.24
40–43	92.65	1.50	91.88	to	93.42
44–47	97.23	1.25	96.59	to	97.88
48–51	100.77	1.23	100.32	to	101.23
52–55	104.80	1.12	104.34	to	105.26
56–59	108.43	.85	107.94	to	108.92
60–63	111.05	.80	110.68	to	111.41
64–67	114.87	.83	114.18	to	115.57
68–71	117.06	.56	116.77	to	117.34
72–75	119.27	.47	118.96	to	119.59
76–79	121.79	.70	121.38	to	122.19
80–83	124.21	1.25	123.49	to	124.94
84–87	126.00	.00	126.00	to	126.00
88–91	126.00	.00	126.00	to	126.00
92–95	126.00	.00	126.00	to	126.00
Total	85.17	32.55	81.95	to	88.39

Source: Copyright © 1993, Dr. Carl V. Granger, Uniform Data System for Medical Rehabilitation, UB Foundation Activities.

Pediatric Evaluation of Disability Inventory (PEDI)

The *Pediatric Evaluation of Disability Inventory (PEDI)* (Haley, Coster, Ludlow, Haltwanger, & Andrellos, 1992) (see Exhibit A–25) began as the Tufts Assessment of Motor Performance (TAMP) (Haley, Hallenborg, & Gans, 1989). The *PEDI* was developed to provide a clear description of functional status and evaluate change as a result of rehabilitation intervention in infants and young children. The World Health Organization's (1980) model of impairment, disability, and handicap was used as a conceptual basis. Reid, Boschen, and Wright (1993) believe that the authors of this instrument try to provide "an approach for a functional assessment that is more objective and comprehensive than in previously developed measures" (p. 57).

The *PEDI* is a comprehensive clinical tool for use with children six months to 7.5 years of age and children older than 7.5 whose functional abilities are below what is expected of children this age without disabilities (Haley, Coster, Ludlow, et al., 1992). The Rasch model organizes items into hierarchical ability scales that provide congruence between a child's clinical score and expected level of performance represented by the summary score (Haley, Ludlow, & Coster, 1993). The child's capabilities and performance of functional activities are measured in three content domains: self-care (15 items), mobility (13 items), and social function (13 items). These 41 items are scored on a six-point scale with zero for total assistance and five for independent (Basmajian, 1994). Measurement dimensions include the child's performance, amount of caregiver assistance needed, and modifications or equipment required (Reid et al., 1993).

Cronbach's alphas were calculated for the three domains and three dimensions to yield coefficients ranging from .95 to .99, indicating high internal consistency for each of the scales. Inter-rater reliability in the normative sample was very high, as indicated by intraclass correlation coefficients for the Caregiver Assistance scales. Agreement on the Modifications scales was also high, although the intraclass correlation coefficient dropped to .79 (Reid et al., 1993). Inter-rater reliability in a clinical sample was high (.84–1.00) for the Caregiver Assistance and Modifications dimensions. No information was reported for the Functional Skills items (Haley et al., 1992; Reid et al., 1993).

Content validity was also satisfactory as a result of Rasch technology used to eliminate or adjust items when their content or scoring led to scaling difficulties. Construct validity of the *PEDI* pilot version discriminated effectively between disabled and nondisabled children (Feldman, Haley, & Coryell, 1990). Feldman and others (1990) supported concurrent validity by finding a moderate correlation (.70–.80) between the BATTELLE Development Inventory Screening Test (BDIST) and the *PEDI* pilot version. Reid and others (1993) report correlations ranging from .62–.97 among the *PEDI*, BDIST, and Wee-FIM®. Finally, the *PEDI*'s discriminative validity results showed that summary scores "could be used to accurately predict a child's correct group status between the normative and clinical samples" (Reid et al., 1993, p. 75).

The *PEDI* is designed for use by special educators, nurses, occupational and physical therapists, and other professionals. Professionals can complete the *PEDI* by using direct observation, professional judgments, parent report, or structured interview. The amount of time required to administer the *PEDI* depends on the method of administration and the child's age and level of disability. Reported administration times vary from 20 minutes to one hour (Reid et al., 1993). Results can be reported as normative standard scores, scaled scores, and frequency counts. A software program is also available for scoring purposes.

A manual that provides basic administrative and scoring information, along with the conceptual framework, applications, administrative guidelines, scoring instructions, and technical support, accompanies the instrument. Currently, the *PEDI* is published only in English (Haley & Coster, 1993).

The *PEDI* can be used to help identify goals for Individual Family Service Plans and Individual Educational Plans; identify functional deficits or delays in self-care, mobility, and social skills; monitor progress; and measure outcomes for program evaluation. Refinement of the instrument is ongoing (Haley & Coster, 1993).

REFERENCES

Basmajian, J. (Ed.) (1994). *Physical rehabilitation outcome measures.* Toronto, Ontario, Canada: Canadian Physiotherapy Association in co-operation with Health and Welfare Canada Communications Group.

Feldman, A.B., Haley, S.M., & Coryell, J. (1990). Concurrent and construct validity of the Pediatric Evaluation of Disability Inventory. *Physical Therapy, 70*(10), 602–610.

Haley, S.M., & Coster, W.J. (1993). Response to Reid DT et al.'s critique of the Pediatric Evaluation of Disability Inventory. *Pediatric and Occupational Therapy in Pediatrics, 13*(4), 89–93.

Haley, S.M., Coster, W.J., Ludlow, L.H., Haltiwanger, J.T., & Andrellos, P.J. (1992). *Pediatric Evaluation of Disability Inventory (PEDI).* Boston: New England Medical Center.

Haley, S.M., Hallenborg, S.C., & Gans, B.M. (1989). Functional assessment in young children with neurological impairments. *Topics in Early Childhood Special Education, 9*(1), 106–126.

Haley, S.M., Ludlow, L.H., & Coster, W.J. (1993). Pediatric Evaluation of Disability Inventory: Clinical interpretation of summary scores using Rasch rating scale methodology. *Physical Medicine and Rehabilitation Clinics of North America, 4*(3), 529–540.

Reid, D.T., Boschen, K., & Wright, V. (1993). Critique of the Pediatric Evaluation of Disability Inventory (PEDI). *Physical and Occupational Therapy in Pediatrics, 13*(4), 57–87.

World Health Organization. (1980). *International classification of impairments, disabilities, and handicaps.* Geneva: Author.

Exhibit A–25 *Pediatric Evaluation of Disability Inventory (PEDI) Score Form*

SCORE FORM

ABOUT THE CHILD   ID# _____

Name _____

Sex M ☐ F ☐ Ethnic group or race _____

Age   Year   Month   Day

  Interview Date   _____   _____   _____

  Birth Date   _____   _____   _____

  Chronological age _____   _____   _____

Diagnosis (if any) _____

ICD-9 code(s)   _____ _____ _____
                  primary   additional

CURRENT STATUS OF CHILD

  ☐ hospital inpatient   ☐ lives at home

    ☐ acute care   ☐ lives in residential facility

    ☐ rehabilitation

other (specify) _____

School or other facility _____

Grade placement _____

ABOUT THE RESPONDENT (Parent or Guardian)

Name _____

Sex M ☐ F ☐

Relationship to child _____

Type of work (be specific) _____

Years of education _____

ABOUT THE INTERVIEWER

Name _____

Position _____

Facility _____

ABOUT THE ASSESSMENT

Referred by _____

Reason for the assessment

_____

_____

_____

Notes _____

_____

GENERAL DIRECTIONS

Below are the general guidelines for scoring. All the items have specific descriptions. Consult the Manual for individual item scoring criteria.

PART I Functional Skills: 197 discrete items of functional skills

Self-care, Mobility, Social Function

0 = unable, or limited in capability, to perform item in most situations

1 = capable of performing item in most situations, or item has been previously mastered and functional skills have progressed beyond this level

PART II Caregiver Assistance: 20 complex functional activities

Self-care, Mobility, Social Function

5 = Independent

4 = Supervise/Prompt/Monitor

3 = Minimal Assistance

2 = Moderate Assistance

1 = Maximal Assistance

0 = Total Assistance

PART III Modifications: 20 complex functional activities.

Self-care, Mobility, Social Function

N = No Modifications

C = Child-oriented (non-specialized) Modifications

R = Rehabilitation Equipment

E = Extensive Modifications

PLEASE BE SURE YOU HAVE ANSWERED ALL ITEMS.

PEDI **PEDI Research Group**, c/o Stephen M. Haley, Department of Rehabilitation Medicine, New England Medical Center Hospital, # 75K/R, 750 Washington St, Boston MA 02111-1901 • Phone (617) 956-5031, Fax (617) 956-5353

Source: Reprinted with permission from S.M. Haley, W.J. Coster, L.H. Ludlow, et al., *Pediatric Evaluation of Disability Inventory (PEDI)*, © 1992, New England Medical Center.

Older Adults Resources and Services (OARS)

The Older Adults Resources and Services (OARS) Social Resources Scale (see Exhibit A–26) was developed at Duke University Center for the Study of Aging and Human Development (1978) as a multidimensional instrument designed to obtain information about the functional status of the community-dwelling older person. The OARS was constructed to elicit information about basic activities of daily living and instrumental activities of daily living in combination, rather than separately.

Five domains are scored in the OARS: social resources, economic resources, mental health, physical health, and activities of daily living. A trained rater makes a subjective assessment about level of function in each of the domains by using a structured interview (Robinson, Lund, Keller, & Cuervo, 1986). The Social Resource scale contains items related to family structure (marital status, living companions, frequency of family visits), contact with friends, availability of a confidant, satisfaction with the social interaction pattern, and availability of someone to help when a person is sick or disabled (Matteson & McConnell, 1988).

Items within the five domains are scored on a six-point scale, with one being excellent function and six being totally impaired. The ratings for each domain can be combined in a variety of ways. The six-point scale can be collapsed into a dichotomous scale in which individuals judged one to three are considered to function adequately and individuals judged four to six are considered impaired for that dimension. When dichotomous scales are used, scores range from five (no impairment in any domain) to 30 (all domains totally impaired) (Kane & Kane, 1981).

Test–retest reliability was established by using the larger parent instrument, which was administered to 30 community residents representative of those older than 65 years in the Durham, North Carolina, area. They were retested over a three- to six-week interval. Correlation coefficients for each domain ranged from 0.32 for mental health to 0.82 for physical health and activities of daily living. Inter-rater reliability was established by using data from 17 community surveys. Eight questionnaires were rated by 10 different raters and nine questionnaires by eight raters. Coefficients of concordance ranged from .38 for economic resources to .88 for physical health. All other correlations were .65 or greater. Intra-rater reliability was established by using eight community survey questionnaires rated again 12 to 18 months later by seven of the original 10 testers.

The OARS can also discriminate among different populations, and the authors claim discriminant validity by comparing means for community, clinic, and institutional populations. Means demonstrate progressive direction as expected whereby community residents would be the most functional and institutional residents the least functional. No problems have been found in applying the five categories, although no reliability or validity studies have been done on the categories (Kane & Kane, 1981).

The Social Resource scale has been used to predict mortality in an older population 30 months after initial assessment (Blazer, 1982). The complete OARS instrument has been used in large community surveys to identify the need for supportive services and to assess communities.

A shorter streamlined form of the OARS exists as the Functional Assessment Inventory.* This version takes only 30 minutes to complete and provides a numerical score in each of the five domains described above. The Functional Assessment Inventory has been used in a variety of service settings, including adult congregate living facilities, nursing homes, adult day care centers, and senior centers. It is used to describe differences in service need and population characteristics (Pfeiffer, Johnson, & Chiofolo, 1981).

---

*Not to be confused with the Functional Assessment Inventory of Crewe and Athelstan (1978). (See description of their Functional Assessment Inventory later in this Appendix.)

REFERENCES

Blazer, D.G. (1982). Social support and mortality in an elderly community population. *American Journal of Epidemiology, 115*(5), 684–693.

Duke University Center for the Study of Aging and Human Development. (1978). *Functional assessment: The OARS methodology.* Durham, NC: Duke University.

Kane, R.A., & Kane, R.L. (1981). *Assessing the elderly: A practical guide to measurement.* Lexington, MA: Lexington Books.

Matteson, M.A., & McConnell, E.S. (1988). *Gerontological nursing: Concepts and practice.* Philadelphia: Saunders.

Pfeiffer, E., Johnson, T., & Chiofolo, F. (1981). Functional assessment of elderly subjects in four service settings. *Journal of the American Geriatric Society, 29*(10), 433–436.

Robinson, B.E., Lund, C.A., Keller, D., & Cuervo, C.A. (1986). Validation of the Functional Assessment Inventory against a multidisciplinary home care team. *Journal of the American Geriatric Society, 34*(12), 851–854.

Exhibit A–26 Older Adults Resources and Services (OARS) Social Resource Scale

Now, I'd like to ask you some questions about your family and friends.

Are you single, married, widowed, divorced, or separated?

1 Single   3 Widowed   5 Separated

2 Married   4 Divorced   — Not answered

If "2" ask following

Does your spouse live here also?

1 Yes

2 No

—Not answered

Who lives with you

(Check "yes" or "no" for each of the following.)

Yes	No	
_____	_____	No one
_____	_____	Husband or wife
_____	_____	Children
_____	_____	Grandchildren
_____	_____	Parents
_____	_____	Grandparents
_____	_____	Brothers and sisters
_____	_____	Other relatives (does not include in-laws covered in the above categories)
_____	_____	Friends
_____	_____	Nonrelated paid help (includes free room)
_____	_____	Others (specify) _____
		_____

In the past year how often did you leave here to visit your family and/or friends for weekends or holidays or to go on shopping trips or outings?

1 Once a week or more

2 1-3 times a month

3 Less than once a month or only on holidays

4 Never

— Not answered

How many people do you know well enough to visit with in their homes?

3 Five or more

2 Three to four

1 One to two

0 None

— Not answered

About how many times did you talk to someone—friends, relatives or others—on the telephone in the past week (either you called them or they called you)? (If subject has no phone, question still applies).

3 Once a day or more

2 Twice

1 Once

0 Not at all

— Not answered

How many times during the past week did you spend some time with someone who does not live with you, that is, you went to see them, or they came to visit you or you went out to do things together?

How many times in the past week did you visit with someone, either with people who live here or people who visited you here?

3 Once a day or more

2 Two to six

1 Once

0 Not at all

— Not answered

Do you have someone you can trust and confide in?

2 Yes

0 No

— Not answered

Do you find yourself feeling lonely quite often, sometimes, or almost never?

0 Quite often

1 Sometimes

2 Almost never

— Not answered

Do you see your relatives and friends as often as you want to, or are you somewhat unhappy about how little you see them?

1. As often as wants to

2. Somewhat unhappy about how little

— Not answered

Is there someone (*outside this place*) who would give you any help at all if you were sick or disabled, for example, your husband/wife, a member of your family, or a friend?

1 Yes

0 No one willing and able to help

— Not answered

If "yes" ask a and b.

a. Is there someone (outside this place) who would take care of you as long as needed, or only for a short time, or only someone who would help you now and then (for example, taking you to the doctor, or fixing lunch occasionally, etc.)?

1 Someone who would take care of subject indefinitely (as long as needed)

2 Someone who would take care of subject for a short time (a few weeks to 6 months)

3 Someone who would help subject now and then (taking to the doctor or fixing lunch, etc.)

— Not answered

b. Who is this person?

Name_____

Relationship_____

continues

Exhibit A–26 continued

RATING SCALE
Rate the current social resources of the person being evaluated along the 6-point scale presented below. Circle the one number that best describes the person's present circumstances.

1. **Excellent Social Resources:** Social relationships are very satisfying and extensive; at least one person would take care of him (her) indefinitely.

2. **Good Social Resources:** Social relationships are fairly satisfying and adequate and at least one person would take care of him (her) indefinitely, or
Social relationships are very satisfying and extensive, and only short-term help is available.

3. **Mildly Socially Impaired:** Social relationships are unsatisfactory, of poor quality, few; but at least one person would take care of him (her) indefinitely, or

Social relationships are fairly satisfactory and adequate, and only short-term help is available.

4. **Moderately Socially Impaired:** Social relationships are unsatisfactory, of poor quality, few; and only short-term care is available, or
Social relationships are at least adequate or satisfactory, but help would only be available now and then.

5. **Severely Socially Impaired:** Social relationships are unsatisfactory, of poor quality, few; and help would be available only now and then, or
Social relationships are at least satisfactory or adequate, but help is not available even now and then.

6. **Totally Socially Impaired:** Social relationships are unsatisfactory, of poor quality, few; and help is not available even now and then.

Note: Italicized questions apply to those living in institutions.

Source: Copyright © 1978 Dr. Harvey Jay Cohen, Duke University Center for the Study of Aging and Human Development.

Rapid Disability Rating Scale

The Rapid Disability Rating Scale (Linn, 1967) was developed in the context of geriatrics/gerontology and "especially for research purposes" (p. 211). Although initially designed for use by nursing personnel, it can be administered by any clinician or trained lay person familiar with the patient.

The Rapid Disability Rating Scale contains 16 items:

1. Eating
2. Diet
3. Medication
4. Speech
5. Hearing
6. Sight
7. Walking
8. Bathing
9. Dressing
10. Incontinence
11. Shaving
12. Safety supervision
13. Confined to bed
14. Mentally confused
15. Uncooperative
16. Depression

Each item is rated on a three-level ordinal scale. Total scores can range from 16 to 48. It provides, as its title implies, a quick overview of relevant functional disabilities in the older patient.

Initial standardization was done on 100 cases. Ratings should be performed by a clinician familiar with the overall condition of the patient being assessed. Time required is "about two minutes" (Linn, 1967, p. 213). Reliability and concurrent validity were documented (Linn, 1967).

The Rapid Disability Rating Scale was used by Homma and colleagues in a study comparing various ways of evaluating dementia in 246 patients (Homma, Niina, Ishii, & Hasegawa, 1991; Homma, Niina, Ishii, Hirata, & Hasegawa, 1989). Vida, Gauthier, & Gauthier (1989) used the scale in a study of two pharmacologic agents in the treatment of Alzheimer's disease.

Linn and Linn (1982) published a revised version of the scale, the Rapid Disability Rating Scale-2 (see Exhibit A–27). They described the revisions as follows:

> Item definitions were sharpened and directions expanded to indicate that ratings are based upon the patient's performance in regard to behavior and that prostheses normally used by the patient should be included in the assessment. Three items have been added to increase the breadth of the scale [*mobility*, *adaptive tasks*, and *toileting*]. Response items have been changed from three-point to four-point ratings in order to increase group discrimination and make the scale more sensitive to changes in treatment. The new appraisals of reliability, factor structure and validity were reported, along with the potential uses of the scale. (Linn & Linn, 1982, p. 378)

The following information is from a form letter sent out to explain the scale further:

> Item ratings require some subjectivity. This is intentional, based on the fact that clinicians make

such judgments with a certain degree of face validity. If categories are rigidly defined, new circumstances will inevitably arise that were not defined. The question is whether good overall reliability can be achieved with some subjectivity.

A. *Mobility*: Refers to movement inside or outside of a building. A *bed*bound patient would receive a 4. The idea is ability to "get around" regardless of physical handicaps.

B. *Bathing*: If a patient requires some degree of personal or mechanical assistance in order to bathe (whether tub, shower, bed baths), he [sic] receives a 2 or 3, depending on the *amount* of assistance required.

C. *Adaptive Tasks*: The bottom line is "ability" whether from physical *or* mental capacity.

D. *Medication*: Refers to "amount" required (not ability to self-administer). It represents a measure of severity of condition.

E. *Mental Confusion*: Again, it is the "degree" of confusion that is rated whether it is from lack of orientation and/or short-term memory loss.

F. *Scale Points*: Ideally, one would hope to have an equal interval scale that rated no disability to complete disability; therefore, "a little" would describe the individual who needed some personal or mechanical help; had some noticeable (but minimal) problems with communication, hearing, etc.; or some *minimal* confusion, etc. In other words, one would not be able to say "none" for the item, but neither would it be classified as "a lot" (considerable). "A lot" should be thought of as requiring more than minimal assistance but less than total assistance for the first eight items and moderately incapacitating in regard to the other items. Perhaps it would help to think of the categories as reflecting "none, minimal, moderate, or severe" as scale points. You might have different interviewers rate a few of the same individuals and see how closely they agree on their ratings. Most clinicians agree on the distinctions between a little and a lot based on intensity of need for assistance. One other suggestion (if you have enough lead time) is to establish more specific definitions for the scales based on your own population. This could be very useful if you are trying to identify subtle changes in function. (P.A. Mugar, former secretary to Dr. M.W. Linn, personal communication, June 4, 1996)

REFERENCES

Homma, A., Niina, R., Ishii, T., & Hasegawa, K. (1991). Behavioral evaluation of Alzheimer disease in clinical trials: Development of the Japanese version of the GBS Scale. *Alzheimer Disease and Associated Disorders, 5*(Suppl. 1), 40–48.

Homma, A., Niina, R., Ishii, T., Hirata, N., & Hasegawa, K. (1989). Reliability and validity of the Japanese version of the GBS Scale (Japanese). *Nippon Ronen Igakkai Zasshi—Japanese Journal of Geriatrics, 26*(6), 617-623.

Linn, M.W. (1967). A rapid disability rating scale. *Journal of the American Geriatrics Society, 15*(2), 211–214.

Linn, M.W., & Linn, B.S. (1982). The Rapid Disability Rating Scale-2. *Journal of the American Geriatrics Society, 30*(6), 378–382.

Vida, S., Gauthier, L., & Gauthier, S. (1989). Canadian collaborative study of tetrahydroaminoacridine (THA) and lecithin treatment of Alzheimer's disease: Effect on mood. *Canadian Journal of Psychiatry—Revue Canadieene de Psychiatrie, 34* (3), 165–170.

Exhibit A–27 Rapid Disability Rating Scale-2 (RDRS-2)

Directions: Rate what the person does to reflect current behavior. Circle one of the four choices for each item. Consider rating with any aids or prostheses normally used. None = completely independent or normal behavior. Total = that person cannot, will not, or may not (because of medical restriction) perform a behavior or has the most severe form of disability or problem.

Assistance with activities of daily living

Eating	None	A little	A lot	Spoon-feed; intravenous tube
Walking (with cane or walker if used)	None	A little	A lot	Does not walk
Mobility (going outside and getting about with wheelchair, etc., if used)	None	A little	A lot	Is housebound
Bathing (include getting supplies, supervising)	None	A little	A lot	Must be bathed
Dressing (include help in selecting clothes)	None	A little	A lot	Must be dressed
Toileting (include help with clothes, cleaning, or help with ostomy, catheter)	None	A little	A lot	Uses bedpan or unable to care for ostomy/catheter
Grooming (shaving for men, hairdressing for women, nails, teeth)	None	A little	A lot	Must be groomed
Adaptive tasks (managing money/possessions; telephoning; buying newspaper, toilet articles, snacks)	None	A little	A lot	Cannot manage

Degree of disability

Communication (expressing self)	None	A little	A lot	Does not communicate
Hearing (with aid if used)	None	A little	A lot	Does not seem to hear
Sight (with glasses, if used)	None	A little	A lot	Does not see
Diet (deviation from normal)	None	A little	A lot	Fed by intravenous tube
In bed during day (ordered or self-initiated)	None	A little (<3 hrs)	A lot	Most/all of time
Incontinence (urine/feces, with catheter or prosthesis, if used)	None	Sometimes	Frequently (weekly +)	Does not control
Medication	None	Sometimes	Daily, taken orally	Daily; injection; (+ oral if used)

Degree of special problems

Mental confusion	None	A little	A lot	Extreme
Uncooperativeness (combats efforts to help with care)	None	A little	A lot	Extreme
Depression	None	A little	A lot	Extreme

Source: Department of Veterans Affairs, Medical Center, Miami, Florida.

CATEGORIES OF FUNCTIONAL ASSESSMENT INSTRUMENTS TO MEASURE SOCIETAL LIMITATION

Family Functioning

McMaster Family Assessment Device

The McMaster Family Assessment Device (see Exhibit A–28) was developed to function as a screening instrument for identifying problem areas in family function. It is designed to collect information on various dimensions of the family system directly from family members (Epstein, Baldwin, & Bishop, 1983). It is based on the McMaster Model of Family Functioning (MMFF), which is a clinical conceptualization of families designed to measure structure, function, and transactions of family groups and distinguish between healthy and unhealthy families (Epstein, Sigal, & Rakoff, 1962; Westley & Epstein, 1969).

There are seven scales within the McMaster Family Assessment Device: problem solving, communication, roles, affective responsiveness, affective involvement, behavior control, and general functioning. The device consists of 53 items within these seven scales. Each item has four alternative responses: strongly agree, agree, disagree, and strongly disagree. Family members rate their agreement or disagreement with how well an item describes their family. The questionnaire takes approximately 15 to 20 minutes to complete and can be filled out by all family members older than age 12 years.

Five-hundred and three individuals participated in the development of the McMaster Family Assessment Device. In this group, 294 individuals came from a group of 112 families. The group included four families of children in a psychiatric day hospital, six families of patients in a stroke rehabilitation unit, and nine families of students in an advanced psychology course. The other ninety-three families in this group each had one member who was an inpatient in an adult psychiatric hospital. The inpatients had many different diagnoses.

In developing the McMaster Family Assessment Device, the MMFF was used to define the domains the instrument was to assess and cover the areas of family functioning previously found to be important. To develop the item pool covering the six dimensions of the MMFF, goal attainment scale point descriptions from a previous outcome study were used (Woodward, Santa Barbara, Levin, Epstein, & Streiner, 1977; Woodward et al., 1975). Additional items were added to cover all areas of each dimension. Furthermore, all items were revised so that (1) each applied to a single dimension of the MMFF and (2) an equal number of items existed to describe healthy and unhealthy families. The dimension of General Functioning was added to assess overall health/pathology of the family. Reliability of the seven scales ranged from .72 to .92. Correlations between the seven dimensions ranged from .4 to .7. When General Functioning was excluded, correlations ranged from .4 to .6 among the remaining six dimensions.

The McMaster Family Assessment Device includes a Family Information Form to elicit information about the background of each family member. Included are family role, first name, religion, age, sex, education, and medical/psychiatric problems for those living, and not living, in the home. Also elicited is information about the marital status of heads of household, family income, ethnic group, race, and type of work and kind of organizations in which the respondent is engaged, as well as his or her most important or major activities/duties at work.

The General Functioning subscale has been used alone for survey research in which a global assessment of family functioning is required. Validity has been assessed by hypothesizing relationships expected between scores on this subscale and those on other family variables included in the Ontario Child Health Study. Reliability was measured by Cronbach's alpha and split-half correlation. Results indicated good reliability, and all hypotheses of validity were supported (Byles, Byrne, Boyle, & Offord, 1988).

The McMaster Family Assessment Device has been used in studies of prevalence of poor adjustment and family dysfunction among chronically ill clinic patient populations (Arpin, Fitch, Browne, & Corey, 1990), of family functioning of male alcoholics and their female partners (Liepman et al., 1989), of impact of a child's liver transplant on the family (LoBiondo-Wood, Bernier-Henn, & Williams, 1992), and to evaluate the sensitivity of this instrument with Hawaiian-American and Japanese-American families (Morris, 1990).

REFERENCES

Arpin, K., Fitch, M., Browne, G.B., & Corey, P. (1990). Prevalence and correlates of family dysfunction and poor adjustment of chronic illness in specialty clinics. *Journal of Clinical Epidemiology, 43*(4), 373–383.

Byles, J., Byrne, C., Boyle, M.H., & Offord, D.R. (1988). Ontario Child Health Study: Reliability and validity of the general functioning subscale of the McMaster Family Assessment Device. *Family Process, 27*(1), 97–104.

Epstein, N.B., Baldwin, L.M., & Bishop, D.S. (1983). The McMaster Family Assessment Device. *Journal of Marital and Family Therapy, 9*(2), 171–180.

Epstein, N.B., Sigal, J., & Rakoff, V. (1962). Family categories schema. Unpublished manuscript, Jewish General Hospital, Montreal, Canada.

Liepman, M.R., Nirenberg, T.D., Doolittle, R.H., Begin, A.M., Broffman, T.E., & Babich, M.E. (1989). Family functioning of male alcoholics and their female partners during periods of drinking and abstinence [Review]. *Family Process, 28*(2), 239–249.

LoBiondo-Wood, G., Bernier-Henn, M., & Williams, L. (1992). Impact of the child's liver transplant on the family: Maternal perspective [journal, CEU, exam questions, research, tables/charts]. *Pediatric Nursing, 18*(5), 461–471.

Morris, T.M. (1990). Culturally sensitive family assessment: An evaluation of the Family Assessment Device used with Hawaiian-American and Japanese-American families. *Family Process, 29*(1), 105–116.

Westley, W.A., & Epstein, N.B. (1969). *The silent majority.* San Francisco: Jossey-Bass.

Woodward, C.A., Santa Barbara J., Levin, S., Epstein, N.B., & Streiner, D. (1977). *The McMaster family therapy outcome study. 3: Client and treatment characteristics significantly contributing to clinical outcomes.* Paper presented at the 54th annual meeting of the American Orthopsychiatric Association, New York City, NY.

Woodward, C.A., Santa Barbara, J., Levin, S., Goodman, J., Streiner, D., & Epstein, N.B. (1975). *Client and therapist characteristics related to family therapy outcome, closure, and follow-up evaluation.* Paper presented at the meeting of the Society for Psychotherapy Research, Boston, MA.

Exhibit A–28 Items and Subscales of the McMaster Family Assessment Device

PROBLEM SOLVING

We usually act on our decisions regarding problems.
After our family tries to solve a problem, we usually discuss whether it worked or not.
We resolve most emotional upsets that come up.
We confront problems involving feelings.
We try to think of different ways to solve problems.

COMMUNICATION

When someone is upset the others know why.
You can't tell how a person is feeling from what they are saying.
People come right out and say things instead of hinting at them.
We are frank with each other.
We don't talk to each other when we are angry.
When we don't like what someone has done, we tell them (sic).

ROLES

When you ask someone to do something, you have to check that they (sic) did it.
We make sure members meet their family responsibilities.
Family tasks don't get spread around enough.
We have trouble meeting our bills.
There's little time to explore personal interests.
We discuss who is to do household jobs.
If people are asked to do something, they need reminding.
We are generally dissatisfied with the family duties assigned to us.

AFFECTIVE RESPONSIVENESS

We are reluctant to show our affection for each other.
Some of us just don't respond emotionally.
We do not show our love for each other.
Tenderness takes second place to other things in our family.
We express tenderness.
We cry openly.

AFFECTIVE INVOLVEMENT

If someone is in trouble, the others become too involved.
You only get the interest of others when something is important to them.

We are too self-centered.
We get involved with each other only when something interests us.
We show interest in each other when we can get something out of it personally.
Our family shows interest in each other only when they can get something out of it.
Even though we mean well, we intrude too much into each other's lives.

BEHAVIOR CONTROL

We don't know what to do when an emergency comes up.
You can easily get away with breaking the rules.
We know what to do in an emergency.
We have no clear expectations about toilet habits.
We have rules about hitting people.
We don't hold to any rules or standards.
If the rules are broken, we don't know what to expect.
Anything goes in our family.
There are rules about dangerous situations.

GENERAL FUNCTIONING

Planning family activities is difficult because we misunderstand each other.
In times of crisis we can turn to each other for support.
We cannot talk to each other about the sadness we feel.
Individuals are accepted for what they are.
We avoid discussing our fears and concerns.
We can express feelings to each other.
There are lots of bad feelings in the family.
We feel accepted for what we are.
Making decisions is a problem for our family.
We are able to make decisions about how to solve problems.
We don't get along well together.
We confide in each other.

Each family member rates his or her agreement or disagreement with how well an item describes their (sic) families by selecting among four alternative responses: strongly agree, agree, disagree, and strongly disagree. The questionnaire takes approximately fifteen to twenty minutes to complete.

Source: Reprinted from Volume (9), Number (2), of the *Journal of Marital and Family Therapy*, Copyright © 1983, The American Association for Marriage and Family Therapy. Reprinted with permission.

Vocational Function

Functional Assessment Inventory

The Functional Assessment Inventory was developed for "diagnostic use in vocational rehabilitation" (Crewe & Athelstan, 1981, p. 299). In preliminary form (designed for research only), the Functional Assessment Inventory contained 31 items, each scored from zero to three, with zero being no significant impairment and three being item-specific major impairment. Ratings were to be made on known function or actual performance (Crewe & Athelstan, 1978). The instrument was the result of careful effort to build from a comprehensive and practical theoretical base but to have the resulting instrument be useful for vocational rehabilitation

(Crewe, Athelstan, & Meadows, 1975). The number of items was subsequently reduced to 25, and a pilot study of 18 former medical rehabilitation patients was carried out with an average inter-rater reliability of 69%.

Crewe and Athelstan next used the instrument—then increased to 30 items with groupings of motor, social and biographical, psychological and intellectual, and sensory and environmental (Crewe & Athelstan, 1981)—to study 351 vocational rehabilitation clients. Extensive data analysis showed concurrent validity with the clinical judgment of vocational counselors. Mysiw, Corrigan, Hunt, Cavin, and Fish (1989) used the instrument, along with the Rancho Los Amigos Levels of Cognitive Functioning, Mini-Mental Status Examination, and Glasgow Outcome Scale, to study 76 survivors of traumatic brain injury. They concluded that "the FAI composite score has the greatest discriminating power in screening the vocational readiness of this population" (Mysiw et al., 1989, p. 27). The vocationally oriented Functional Assessment Inventory is not to be confused with an instrument by the same name devised by Cairl and colleagues for use in evaluating geriatric inpatient groups (Cairl, Pfeiffer, Keller, Burke, & Samis, 1983).

REFERENCES

Cairl, R.E., Pfeiffer, E., Keller, D.M., Burke, H., & Samis, H.V. (1983). An evaluation of the reliability and validity of the Functional Assessment Inventory. *Journal of the American Geriatrics Society, 31*(10), 607–612.

Crewe, N.M., & Athelstan, G.T. (1978). Appendix II. Functional Assessment Inventory. In B. Bolton & D.W. Cook (Eds.), *Rehabilitation client assessment* (pp. 289–296). Minneapolis: University of Minnesota.

Crewe, N.M., & Athelstan, G.T. (1981). Functional assessment in vocational rehabilitation: A systematic approach to diagnosis and goal setting. *Archives of Physical Medicine and Rehabilitation, 62*(7), 299–305.

Crewe, N.M., Athelstan, G.T., & Meadows, M.A. (1975). Vocational diagnosis through assessment of functional limitations. *Archives of Physical Medicine and Rehabilitation, 56*(12), 513–516.

Mysiw, W.J., Corrigan, J.D., Hunt, M., Cavin, D., & Fish, T. (1989). Vocational evaluation of traumatic brain injury patients using the functional assessment inventory. *Brain Injury, 3*(1), 27–34.

Community Integration

CHART: Craig Handicap Assessment and Reporting Technique

The CHART: Craig Handicap Assessment and Reporting Technique (Whiteneck, Charlifue, Gerhart, Overholser, & Richardson, 1992b) (see Exhibit A–29) is a weighted measure based on the World Health Organization's (1980) conceptualization of impairment, disability, and handicap. This instrument is designed to measure handicap (societal limitation) including five of six dimensions identified by the World Health Organization as components of handicap (societal limitation). Both individual characteristics and social limitation were viewed as aspects of handicap (societal limitation).

The CHART is designed as an interview tool and uses measurable behavioral terms to compare persons with spinal cord injuries with able-bodied members of society in terms of functional norms for society (Whiteneck, Charlifue, Gerhart, Overholser, & Richardson, 1992a). Psychometric properties have been established with persons who have spinal cord injuries. Norms were set with able-bodied friends (proxies) identified by persons with spinal cord injuries. After testing psychometric properties, item weights and six alternative weights were examined for correlation and found to be highly intercorrelated.

The six dimensions in the description of the CHART—identified by the World Health Organization (1980) as components of what is currently referred to as societal limitation—are orientation, physical independence, mobility, occupation, social integration, and economic self-sufficiency. The CHART measures all dimensions except orientation, which is still being developed. Each dimension is weighted in accordance with how the general population views specific social roles. Only productive roles are given weights. Weights are assigned this way because nonproductive roles, such as sleeping and watching TV (if scored), would be scored as zero and would not affect the total score except for time taken away from productive activities. For example, the dimension of occupation contains seven items, but the first four items were given twice the weight of the last three because of the lesser value placed on volunteer work, recreational activities, and other self-improvement activities by the general population.

The CHART is composed of 27 items, including three for the physical independence dimension, nine for the mobility dimension including transportation, seven for the occupation dimension, six for social integration, and two for economic self-sufficiency. Maximum attainable scores for each of the dimensions is 100, with a maximum score for all dimensions of 500. Scores less than 100 on any dimension indicated that time was not spent in ways generally expected of able-bodied members of society. Scoring directions are given for calculating scores on each dimension (Whiteneck, Charlifue, Gerhart, et al., 1992a).

Test-retest reliability coefficients with a one-week interval were as follows: total CHART score, .93; physical independence, .92; mobility, .95; occupation, .89; economic self-sufficiency, .80; and social integration, .81. Proxies were asked to respond to the same items on the CHART, and resulting subject–proxy correlations were as follows: total CHART scores, .83; physical independence, .80; mobility, .84; occupation, .81; economic self-sufficiency, .69; and social integration, .28. The low correlation for social integration increased to .58 when only spouses were queried. This increase was attributed to better agreement when proxy and subject were more closely related.

Validity was established by a panel of rehabilitation professionals asked to judge level of social role limitation. Significant differences between subjects with high and low scores on total and subscale CHART scores supported validity. The instrument was subjected to Rasch analyses for further evaluation of measurement characteristics. Results indicated the scale was well calibrated, had a relatively good fit of data to the mathematical model, and demonstrated a good fit within subscale clusters (Whiteneck, Charlifue, Gerhart, et al., 1992b).

The weighting scheme was then tested with 243 persons, including rehabilitation professionals, persons with spinal cord injury, and lay persons. They were asked to compare and rate the relative importance of the CHART's items in determining the extent of social role limitation. Original item weights and six alternative weights were highly intercorrelated and yielded similar scores regardless of which set of value orientations and items was used. Therefore the initial weighting technique was retained (Whiteneck, Charlifue, Gerhart, et al., 1992b).

The CHART was initially used with 342 former patients of a regional spinal cord injury system. Findings were as follows:

1) the 90th percentile score in the groups with paraplegia and incomplete quadriplegia (American Spinal Cord Injury Association motor index score [1992] >49) was 500. It could be concluded that at least 10% of this group had no social role limitation.

2) median scores of groups with paraplegia and incomplete quadriplegia were 100 on the dimensions of physical independence, mobility, social integration, and economic self-sufficiency.

3) the more severe the impairment, the more significant the social role limitation in all 5 dimensions of the CHART.

4) there was great variability in social role limitation among individuals with similar impairments.

5) scores among various spinal cord injured groups were lowest on the dimension of occupational role limitation.

6) the median total chart score for all able-bodied subjects was 500. (Whiteneck et al., 1992b)

Fuhrer, Rintala, Hart, Clearman, and Young (1993) used the CHART to study depressive symptoms in a community-based sample of 100 men and 40 women with spinal cord injury. The reported test–retest reliability for the CHART's mobility, social integration, and occupation dimensions was supported with coefficients of .95, .81, and .89, respectively. Women reported being less mobile than men, but mobility was inversely related to depression scores. That is, decreased mobility was associated with endorsing more items indicative of a depressive symptom. Direction of causation was by no means clear. That is, restricted mobility may contribute to depressive symptoms or be a reflection of them. The same situation was reported for the dimensions of social integration and occupation, although these variables did not differentiate between men and women.

In another report of this study done by Fuhrer, Garber, Rintala, Clearman, & Hart (1993), findings showed that persons with more severe pressure ulcers incurred their injury later in life and had significantly lower scores in occupation and mobility dimensions of the CHART. In this same cohort, the Life Satisfaction Index—A associated positively with the social integration, occupation, and mobility dimensions of the CHART. Findings suggested that life satisfaction of persons with spinal cord injury seems to be influenced, albeit indirectly, by selective aspects of their social role performance (handicap), but not their degree of impairment or disability (Fuhrer, Rintala, Hart, Clearman, & Young, 1992).

Results of a study by Menter et al. (1991) of 205 patients with spinal cord injury at Craig Hospital, with use of the Functional Independence Measure (FIM^SM) as a measure of disability and the CHART as a measure of handicap (societal limitation) showed there were significant increases in disability and societal limitation in older individuals. When chronological age was added to the number of years after injuries, significant increases in disability, handicap (societal limitation), and costs of care were noted at all levels.

The CHART does measure handicap (societal limitation) and thus contributes significantly to the rehabilitation field because few instruments exist to measure this classification.

There are five strengths of the CHART:

1. It has high test–retest reliability.

2. There is good agreement between ratings of subjects and their proxies except on the dimension of social integration, for which degree of agreement was related to how closely the proxy knew the subject.
3. Evidence of validity is demonstrated by success in differentiating groups of subjects globally evaluated by rehabilitation professionals as having high or low handicap (societal limitation).
4. There is good fit of items and persons to the CHART's data, as demonstrated by Rasch analysis.
5. Scoring is robust and relatively insensitive to variations in item weights that reflect the range of values commonly held in the population.

Thus, all these findings "support the psychometric soundness of the instrument" (Whiteneck, Charlifue, Gerhart, et al., 1992b, p. 523).

Other advantages of the CHART include that it

- is a simple objective index to measure dimensions of social role outlined by the World Health Organization (1980)
- measures the outcome of limitations in social role without any attempt to measure the causes
- does not attempt to measure disability along with social role limitations and
- is useful for rehabilitation program evaluation because it documents rehabilitation outcomes.

REFERENCES

American Spinal Cord Injury Association, International Medical Society of Paraplegia. (1992). *International standards for neurological and functional classification of spinal cord injury.* Chicago: American Spinal Cord Injury Association.

Fuhrer, M.J., Garber, S.L., Rintala, D.H., Clearman, R., & Hart, K.A. (1993). Pressure ulcers in community resident persons with spinal cord injury: Prevalence and risk factors. *Archives of Physical Medicine and Rehabilitation, 74*(11), 1172–1177.

Fuhrer, M.J., Rintala, D.H., Hart, K.A., Clearman, R., & Young, M.E. (1992). Relationship of life satisfaction to impairment, disability, and handicap among persons with spinal cord injury living in the community. *Archives of Physical Medicine and Rehabilitation, 63*(6), 552–557.

Fuhrer, M.J., Rintala, D.H., Hart, K.A., Clearman, R., & Young, M.E. (1993). Depressive symptomatology in persons with spinal cord injury who reside in the community. *Archives of Physical Medicine and Rehabilitation, 74*(3), 255–260.

Menter, R.R., Whiteneck, G.G., Charlifue, S.W., Gerhart, K., Solnick, S.J., Brooks, C.A., & Hughes, L. (1991). Impairment, disability, and handicap and medical expenses of persons aging with spinal cord injury. *Paraplegia, 29*(9), 613–619.

Whiteneck, G.G., Charlifue, S.W., Gerhart, K.A., Overholser, J.D., & Richardson, G.N. (1992a). *Guide for use of the CHART: Craig Handicap Assessment and Reporting Technique.* Englewood, CO: Craig Hospital.

Whiteneck, G.G., Charlifue, S.W., Gerhart, K.A., Overholser, J.D., & Richardson, G.N. (1992b). Quantifying handicap: A new measure of long-term rehabilitation outcomes. *Archives of Physical Medicine and Rehabilitation, 73*(6), 519–526.

World Health Organization. (1980). *International classification of impairments, disabilities, and handicaps.* Geneva: Author.

Exhibit A–29 CHART Questions

What Assistance Do You Need?

1. How many hours in a typical 24-hour day do you have someone with you to provide assistance? (hours paid/hours unpaid)
2. Not including any regular care as reported above, how many hours in a *typical month* do you occasionally have assistance with such things as grocery shopping, laundry, housekeeping, or infrequent medical needs like catheter changes?
3. Who takes responsibility for instructing and directing your attendants and/or caregivers?

Are You Up and About Regularly?

4. On a *typical day*, how many hours are you out of bed?
5. In a typical *week*, how many days do you get out of your house and go somewhere?
6. In the last *year*, how many nights have you spent away from your home (excluding hospitalization)? (none); (1–2); (3–4); (5 or more)
7. Can you enter and exit your home without any assistance from someone? (yes) (no)
8. In your home, do you have independent access to your sleeping area, kitchen, bathroom, telephone, and TV (or radio)? (yes) (no)

Is Your Transportation Adequate?

9. Can you use your transportation independently? (yes) (no)
10. Does your transportation allow you to get to all the places you would like to go? (yes) (no)
11. Does your transportation let you get out whenever you want? (yes) (no)
12. Can you use your transportation with little or no advance notice? (yes) (no)

How Do You Spend Your Time?

13. How many hours per week do you spend working in a job for which you get paid?
14. How many hours per week do you spend in school working toward a degree or in an accredited technical training program? (Hours in class or studying)

15. How many hours per week do you spend in active home-making including parenting, housekeeping, and food preparation?
16. How many hours per week do you spend in home maintenance activities such as yard work, house repairs, or home improvement?
17. How many hours per week do you spend in ongoing volunteer work for an organization?
18. How many hours per week do you spend in recreational activities such as sports, exercise, playing cards, or going to movies? Please do not include time spent watching TV or listening to the radio.
19. How many hours per week do you spend in other self-improvement activities such as hobbies or leisure reading? Please do not include time spent watching TV or listening to the radio.

With Whom Do You Spend Time?

20. Do you live alone, or with, a spouse or significant other; children (how many); other relatives (how many); roommate (how many); attendant (how many)?
21. If you don't live with a spouse or significant other are you involved in a romantic relationship? (Yes) (No)
22. How many relatives (not in your household) do you visit, phone, or write to at least once a month?
23. How many business or organizational associates do you visit, phone, or write to at least once a month?
24. How many friends (nonrelatives contacted outside business or organizational settings) do you visit, phone, or write to at least once a month?
25. With how many strangers have you initiated a conversation in the last month (for example, to ask information or place an order)? (none); (1–2); (3–5); (6 or more)

What Financial Resources Do You Have?

26. Approximately what was the combined annual income of **all family members in your household?** (consider all sources including wages and earnings, disability benefits, pensions and retirement income, income from court settlements, investments and trust funds, child support and alimony, contributions from relatives, and any other source.)
27. Approximately how much did you pay last year for medical care expenses? (Consider any amounts paid by yourself or the family members in your household and not reimbursed by insurance or benefits.)

Source: Reprinted with permission from G.G. Whiteneck et al., Quantifying Handicap: A New Measure of Long-Term Rehabilitation Outcomes, *Archives of Physical Medicine and Rehabilitation,* Vol. 73, pp. 519–526, © 1992, W.B. Saunders.

Activity Pattern Indicators

The Activity Pattern Indicators (APIs) are the third set of Rehabilitation Indicators and were developed to measure behavioral output. The Rehabilitation Indicators are a package of four constituent instruments:

1. Skill Indicators, which indicate behavioral strengths and weaknesses in diverse areas of functioning
2. Status Indicators, which measure behavioral output at varying levels of detail
3. Activity Pattern Indicators, which document the person's functioning according to typical patterns and temporal characteristics of participation in activities
4. Environmental Indicators, which were never completely developed but were to be designed to measure factors outside the client that are relevant to the person's ability to function optimally

Only the APIs are discussed here because they are a measure of community integration (Brown, Gordon, & Diller, 1984). All these instruments were developed at New York University Medical Center with support from the National Institute of Handicapped Research (now the National Institute on Disability and Rehabilitation Research) to define what a person can do in reality and document what a person does within the client's actual environment.

Activity Pattern Indicators (Brown et al., 1984) are analyzed according to activity clusters and document dimensions of a client's daily activities such as the following:

• Mobility, as measured for example by percentage of time spent out of residence, diversity of away-from residence activities, and percentage of time spent in travel.
• Activity Level, as measured for example by diversity of activities, tempo of activities (e.g., occurrences each day), and percentage of time spent in inactivity as well as passive recreation.
• Independence and community involvement, as measured for example by amount of time spent in activities in which assistance was received, amount of time spent working or in school, and diversity of activities occurring away from residence.
• Social/recreational involvement, as measured for example by frequency of engaging in active recreation, and percentage of time spent with people.

Many approaches are used in gathering data to determine activity patterns. The individual who is studied may keep a diary or the investigator may administer an interview or a questionnaire. Activity Pattern Indicators data can also be obtained through observation. Consequently, many different formats exist, and time for administration also varies from 10 to 20 minutes (shortest range) to 40 to 60 minutes (longest range) of a client's time. Because of these variations, it is difficult to obtain validity and reliability data (Brown et al., 1984).

There are many reasons that collection of reliable and valid data at the individual level is difficult. "Test–retest measures for reliability are of questionable use" (Brown et al., 1984, p. 196) because this form of reliability assumes whatever is measured is relatively stable, and test–retest variation is a function of measurement error, rather than of any real behavior change. However, activities of daily living may vary on a weekly basis concurrent with variation in the accuracy of the rater. Obtaining across-recorder measures is also difficult because most people do not like to have one or two observers in the home to determine reliability of self-report or reliability of observers. Thus there have been two ways to determine reliability and validity of APIs.

The first method is to examine other studies in which activity data were obtained with similar approaches to assessment to those of APIs, and results of which have indicated reliability of activity data can be quite high (Bishop, Jeanrenaud, & Lawson, 1975; Bratfisch, 1972; Converse, 1972; Dougherty, 1977; Robinson, 1977; Stephens, Norris-Baker, & Willems, 1983; Widmer, 1978). The second method is to seek construct validity in groups of clients. Expected differences were compared to actual differences in functioning for two or more groups or one group at two or more times. These studies have been repeated with consistent corroboration of predicted differences, so that researchers concluded that APIs were a valid tool for group interpretation. The validity, however, of individual client functioning varies largely as a function of factors that contribute to reliability. Therefore "some of the API approaches, such as those requiring a shorter period of recall, are better choices whenever a user needs client-specific information" (Brown et al., 1984, p. 197).

The Rehabilitation Indicators have been used to study many disabilities and limitations in social role. The Activity Indicators tool for the Rehabilitation Indicators has been used to study time allocation in activities, such as socializing, household tasks, personal care, TV, quiet recreation, active recreation, vocational activities, inactivity, and travel in groups with spinal cord injury vs. groups classified as able-bodied (Brown, Gordon, & Ragnarsson, 1985). They have also been used to study adults with mental retardation in institutions and communities (O'Neill, Brown, Gordon, Schonhorn, & Greer, 1981) and impact of electronic assistive devices on quality of life for persons with high level quadriplegia (Efthimiou, Gordon, Sell, & Stratford, 1981).

REFERENCES

Bishop, D., Jeanrenaud, C., & Lawson, K. (1975). Comparison of time diary and recall questionnaire for surveying leisure activities. *Journal of Leisure Research, 7*, 73–80.

Bratfisch, O. (1972). Time estimations of the main activities of university students. *Catalog of Selected Documents in Psychology, 2*, 29–30.

Brown, M., Gordon, W.A., & Diller, L. (1984). Rehabilitation indicators. In A.S. Halpern & M.S. Fuhrer (Eds.), *Functional assessment in rehabilitation* (pp. 187–203). Baltimore: Paul H. Brookes.

Brown, M., Gordon, W.A., & Ragnarsson, K. (1985, September). *Unhandicapping the disabled: What is possible?* Paper presented at the annual meeting of the American Congress of Rehabilitation Medicine, Kansas City, MO.

Converse, P.E. (1972). Country differences in time use. In A. Szalai (Ed.), *The use of time.* The Hauge, Mouton.

Dougherty, T.W. (1977). *Development and evaluation of a self-recorded diary for measuring job behavior.* Unpublished master's thesis, University of Houston, TX.

Efthimiou, M.S.J., Gordon, W.A., Sell, G.H., & Stratford, C. (1981). Electronic assistive devices: Their impact on the quality of life of high level quadriplegic persons. *Archives of Physical Medicine and Rehabilitation, 62*(3), 131–134.

O'Neill, J., Brown, M., Gordon, W., Schonhorn, R., & Greer, E. (1981). Activity patterns of mentally retarded adults in institutions and communities: A longitudinal study. *Applied Research in Mental Retardation, 2*(4), 367–379.

Robinson J.P. (1977). *How Americans use time.* New York: Praeger.

Stephens, M.A., Norris-Baker, C., & Willems, E.P. (1983). Patient behavior monitoring through self-reports. *Archives of Physical Medicine and Rehabilitation, 64*(4), 167–171.

Widmer, M.L. (1978). *Telephone contact as a method of gathering data on everyday behavior of noninstitutionalized adults.* Unpublished master's thesis, University of Houston, TX.

Community Integration Questionnaire (CIQ)

The Community Integration Questionnaire (see Exhibit A–30) was developed at the State University of New York, University at Buffalo by a research team within the Rehabilitation Research and Training Center for Community Integration of Persons with Traumatic Brain Injury. This 15-item instrument was designed to assess home integration, social integration, and productive activity in persons with acquired brain injury (Corrigan & Deming, 1995; Willer, Ottenbacher, & Coad, 1994).

To develop the questionnaire, a two-day conference was convened in 1990. Fourteen experts with experience in various aspects of rehabilitation and research related to traumatic brain injury and consumers of rehabilitation, namely persons challenged by traumatic brain injury, were asked to identify items for inclusion. Experts were divided into three groups. Each group was asked to focus on home integration, social roles, or productive activity, respectively. The version of the Community Integration Questionnaire developed as a result of this consensus conference contained 47 items. Thus the instrument has a high likelihood of content validity (Willer et al., 1994).

A pilot test with administration of the instrument to 35 men and 14 women (age range, 16 to 79 years; mean, 36.40; *SD*, 13.86) resulted in reduction of items to 15. Redundant items and items that did not reach a threshold correlation coefficient with the subscale total score were eliminated. Principal components analysis with use of varimax rotation was applied to reassign or drop items that did not factor consistent with the original expert assignment. Final factors remained consistent with the three identified domains of community integration. The final form contains five items associated with home integration, six items related to social integration, and four items dealing with productive activities.

Test–retest reliability was established by administering the instrument to 16 individuals with acquired brain injury and the family members identified as most knowledgeable about the individual's health and social situation (Willer, Rosenthal, Kreutzer, Gordon, & Rempel, 1993). Reliability coefficients were high for individuals with traumatic brain injury ($r = .91$) and family members or caregivers ($r = .97$). Reliability coefficients on subscales ranged from a low of .83 (individual's rating of productive activities) to .97 (family member's assessment of productive activities). Inter-rater reliability has not been established for this instrument. Comparisons of a separate sample of 59 patients and their family members, however, resulted in correlation coefficients of .81 for home integration, .74 for social integration, and .96 for productive activity (Willer et al., 1994). Scoring guidelines are shown in Exhibit A–30.

The instrument is usually completed by the person being assessed. However, an interviewer may be present and assist with interpretation of specific items. At times, because of physical, cognitive, or behavioral problems, the person with the head injury may not be able to complete the questionnaire. In these instances, a person familiar with the individual with traumatic brain injury may complete the instrument. Computerized as well as paper-and-pencil versions of the Community Integration Questionnaire are available from Dr. B. Willer, Departments of Psychiatry and Rehabilitation Medicine, State University of New York, University at Buffalo, 3435 Main St., Buffalo, NY 14214, or from the Ontario Brain Injury Association.

The Community Integration Questionnaire is a relatively new instrument and warrants further tests of reliability as well as the further determination of inter-rater reliability. It is one of the few instruments that measures outcomes in terms of societal limitations.

REFERENCES

Corrigan, J.D., & Deming, R. (1995). Psychometric characteristics of the community integration questionnaire: Replication and extension. *Journal of Head Trauma Rehabilitation, 10*(4), 41–53.

Willer, B., Ottenbacher, K.J., & Coad, M.L. (1994). The Community Integration Questionnaire. *American Journal of Physical Medicine and Rehabilitation, 73*(2), 103–111.

Willer, B., Rosenthal, M., Kreutzer, J., Gordon, W., & Rempel, R. (1993). Assessment of community integration following rehabilitation for traumatic brain injury. *Journal of Head Trauma Rehabilitation, 8*(2), 75–87.

Exhibit A–30 Community Integration Questionnaire

Name: _____ ID Number: _____

Education: _____ Sex: _____ Marital Status: _____

Occupation: _____

Address: _____

_____

Date of Birth: _____/_____/_____

Date of Test: _____/_____/_____

Age: _____

Did a proxy complete the questionnaire? Yes: _____ No: _____

CIQ Score:

Home Integration Scale: _____

Social Integration Scale: _____

Productivity Scale: _____

CIQ Total Score: _____

Direct Correspondence to:

Ontario Brain Injury Association
Centre for Training and Education
P.O. Box 2338
St. Catharines, ON
L2M 7M7
Ph: (905) 641–8877 FAX: (905) 641–0323

continues

Exhibit A–30 continued

1. Who usually does shopping for groceries or other necessities in your household?
   - ❏ yourself alone
   - ❏ yourself and someone else
   - ❏ someone else

2. Who usually prepares meals in your household?
   - ❏ yourself alone
   - ❏ yourself and someone else
   - ❏ someone else

3. In your home, who usually does normal everyday housework?
   - ❏ yourself alone
   - ❏ yourself and someone else
   - ❏ someone else

4. Who usually cares for the children in your home?
   - ❏ yourself alone
   - ❏ yourself and someone else
   - ❏ someone else
   - ❏ not applicable/no children under 17 in the home

5. Who usually plans social arrangements such as get-togethers with family and friends?
   - ❏ yourself alone
   - ❏ yourself and someone else
   - ❏ someone else

6. Who usually looks after your personal finances, such as banking or paying bills?
   - ❏ yourself alone
   - ❏ yourself and someone else
   - ❏ someone else

Can you tell me approximately how many times a month you now usually participate in the following activities outside your home:

7. Shopping
   - ❏ Never   ❏ 1–4 times   ❏ 5 or more

8. Leisure activities such as movies, sports, restaurants, etc.
   - ❏ Never   ❏ 1–4 times   ❏ 5 or more

9. Visiting friends or relatives
   - ❏ Never   ❏ 1–4 times   ❏ 5 or more

10. When you participate in leisure activities, do you usually do this alone or with others?
    - ❏ mostly alone
    - ❏ mostly with friends who have head injuries
    - ❏ mostly with family members
    - ❏ mostly with friends who do not have head injuries
    - ❏ with a combination of family and friends

11. Do you have a best friend with whom you confide?
    - ❏ yes
    - ❏ no

12. How often do you travel outside the home?
    - ❏ almost every day
    - ❏ almost every week
    - ❏ seldom/never (less than once per week)

13. Please choose the answer below that best corresponds to your current (during the past month) work situation:
    - ❏ full-time (more than 20 hours per week)
    - ❏ part-time (less than or equal to 20 hours per week)
    - ❏ not working, but actively looking for work
    - ❏ not working, not looking for work
    - ❏ not applicable, retired due to age

14. Please choose the answer below that best corresponds to your current (during the past month) school or training program situation:
    - ❏ full-time
    - ❏ part-time
    - ❏ not attending school or training program

15. In the past month, how often did you engage in volunteer activities?
    - ❏ never
    - ❏ 1–4 times
    - ❏ 5 or more

Source: Copyright © Barney S. Willer, PhD.

Community Integration Questionnaire Administration and Scoring Guidelines Background and Rationale

The Community Integration Questionnaire (CIQ) is intended as a brief, reliable measure of an individual's level of integration into the home and community. The CIQ was developed by a small group of experts interested in assessing community integration for persons who have experienced traumatic brain injury. These experts met together to establish a consensus on what characterizes an individual's experience in the community, especially after the acute rehabilitation phase.

It is important to note that this questionnaire represents a finite set of indicators of community integration, and as such does not encompass all possible indicators of integration. Therefore, it is recommended that the CIQ be used in concert with similar assessments of impairment, disability, environmental barriers, and demographic descriptors.

Although the CIQ was designed specifically for individuals with traumatic brain injury, it is applicable to all individuals, disabled or not, living outside institutions.

Administration

The CIQ is normally completed by the individual being assessed. In most cases an interviewer should be present to assist with interpretation of specific items. In certain instances, the individual being assessed may not be able to complete the questionnaire (e.g., due to expressive or receptive language deficits, memory impairment, physical disabilities, etc.). In these instances, a person who is familiar with the individual being assessed may complete the form, provided that the individual being assessed is present when the form is completed.

continues

Exhibit A–30 continued

Most of the questions are directed to how the individual performs a specific activity within the household or the community. Responses usually indicate that the individual performs the activity alone, with another person, or that the activity is typically performed by someone else. For some responses, the individual being assessed may find it difficult to decide which response fits best with how a particular activity is performed. In these instances, the individual should be encouraged by the examiner to choose the response reflecting the usual or typical performance of that activity.

Scoring Guidelines

The CIQ consists of a total of 15 questions. The overall score, which represents a summation of the scores from individual questions, can range from 0 to 29. A higher score indicates greater integration, and lower score reflects less integration. The CIQ can be further divided into three subscores, corresponding to integration in the home, social integration, and productivity. Procedures for deriving the subscores are outlined on the scoring sheet.

The following guidelines provide scoring information for specific items or groups of items.

Items 1 to 6
Score:
2 = The activity is performed alone
1 = The activity is performed with someone else
0 = The activity is performed by someone else
  Note: For item 4, if there are no children under 17 in the home, the average (mean) score for items 1 through 3 and item 5 should be substituted.

Items 7 to 9
Score:
2 = The activity was performed 5 or more times in the past month
1 = The activity was performed 1–4 times in the past month
0 = The activity was not performed in the past month

Item 10
Score:
2 = Mostly with friends without head injury or combination of family and friends
1 = Mostly with friends who have head injuries or with family
0 = Mostly alone

Item 11
Score:
2 = Yes response
0 = No response

Item 12
Score:
2 = Almost every day
1 = Almost every week
0 = Seldom/never (less than once per week)

Items 13 to 15
Although these items are collected individually, they will be combined to form one variable, Productivity. The scoring of this variable is dependent on the combination of answers to questions 13, 14 and 15. Following is a listing of answer sets to these questions and their associated score.

Scoring of the Productivity variable

Question #13 Work		Question #14 School		Question #15 Volunteer Work	Score
Not working/not looking	+	No school	+	No Volunteering	= 0
Not working/not looking	+	No school	+	1–4 times/month	= 1
Not working/not looking	+	No school	+	5 or more times/month	= 1
Not working/looking	+	No school	+	No Volunteering	= 0
Not working/looking	+	No school	+	1–4 times/month	= 2
Not working/looking	+	No school	+	5 or more times/month	= 2
Retired due to age	+	No school	+	No Volunteering	= 0
Retired due to age	+	No school	+	1–4 times/month	= 2
Retired due to age	+	No school	+	5 or more times/month	= 3
Retired due to age	+	Part-time	+	No Volunteering	= 4
Retired due to age	+	Part-time	+	1–4 times/month	= 5
Retired due to age	+	Part-time	+	5 or more times/month	= 5
Retired due to age	+	Full-time	+	Any answer	= 5
Not working	+	Part-time	+	Any answer	= 3
Not working	+	Full-time	+	Any answer	= 4
Part-time	+	No school	+	Any answer	= 3
Part-time	+	Part-time	+	Any answer	= 4
Part-time	+	Full-time	+	Any answer	= 5
Full-time	+	No school	+	Any answer	= 4
Full-time	+	Part-time	+	Any answer	= 5

continues

Exhibit A–30 continued

Subscales

Subscales have been developed to allow an analysis of integration within specific domains of everyday life. Items have been grouped with respect to their association with: 1) activities primarily related to the home; 2) activities associated with socialization; and 3) educational or vocational activities. These groupings have been made both logically and on the basis of principal components analysis of items which cluster together. Separate home integration, social integration, and productivity subscale scores are derived as following:

Home Integration: Summation of items 1 through 5
Social Integration: Summation of items 6 through 11
Productivity: Summation of item 12 and the Productivity variable

The overall CIQ score is the additive sum of items 1 through 12 and the Productivity variable.

Community Integration Questionnaire Scoring Sheet

Item Number	Description	Score	
1	Shopping	_____	
2	Prepare meals	_____	
3	Housework	_____	
4	Caring for Children	_____	
5	Social Arrangement	_____	
	HOME INTEGRATION SUBSCALE		_____
6	Personal Finances	_____	
7	Shopping (times/month)	_____	
8	Leisure activities (times/month)	_____	
9	Visiting friends or relatives	_____	
10	Leisure activities (with whom)	_____	
11	Having a best friend	_____	
	SOCIAL INTEGRATION SUBSCALE		_____
12	Travel outside of home	_____	
13,14,15	Productivity	_____	
	PRODUCTIVITY SUBSCALE		_____
	CIQ TOTAL SCORE		_____

Direct Correspondence to:
Ontario Brain Injury Association
Centre for Training and Education
P.O. Box 2338
St. Catharines, ON
L2M 7M7
Ph: (905) 641–8877 Fax: (905) 641–0323

Quality of Life

Sickness Impact Profile (SIP)™

The Sickness Impact Profile (SIP)™ (see Exhibit A–31) is a behaviorally based instrument (Bergner, Bobbitt, Carter, & Gilson, 1981) that is broadly applicable across types and severity of illness, as well as across demographically and cul-turally diverse groups. It was developed to provide an appropriate and sensitive measure of health status to assess the outcome of health care services. Measurement does not depend on diagnostic criteria. Modifications were made and described by Deyo (1976, 1986, 1988), Deyo and Diehl (1983), and Roland and Morris (1983). No considerations related to prognosis have been incorporated in this instrument (Gilson et al., 1975).

The SIP™ contains 136 items scored according to 12 categories: sleep and rest, eating, work, home management, recreation and pastime, ambulation, mobility, body care and movement, social interaction, alertness/intellectual functioning, emotional behavior, and communication. Of the 12 categories, five are independent, three represent physical, and four represent psychosocial dimensions (Hulsebos, Beltman, dos Reis Miranda, & Spangenberg, 1991). Scores fall within two domains: physical health and psychological health. The SIP™ scores range from zero to 100 (Weinberger, Samsa, Tierney, Belyea, & Hiner, 1992).

In developing the instrument, more than 1,000 professional and lay persons were asked to describe sickness-related changes in behavior specifically. In addition, functional assessment instruments designed to evaluate specific patient groups were reviewed for descriptions of behavior. This procedure yielded 1,250 specific statements of behavioral change that, after standard grouping techniques according to defined criteria, yielded 312 unique statements, each "describing a behavior or activity and specifying a dysfunction" (Gilson et al., 1975, p. 1307). Fourteen categories were identified. Later revisions for the population with low back pain resulted in 136 items divided into 12 categories (Deyo, 1986).

Before the SIP™ was field tested, a standardized and structured interview was developed. This interview included "the 312 items, several questions about the personal characteristics of the subject and a request that the subject list any additional changes in his [or her] behavior that were related to his [or her] health and were not covered by the items" (Gilson et al., 1975, p. 1307). As a result of positive responses to items that described these subjects (they were asked to respond positively only to those items that described them related to their health), a detailed profile or protocol was developed.

To provide a basis for scoring, SIP™ items were rated by 25 judges, including graduate nursing students, medical students, health services administrators, and physicians. Judges were asked to rate each item on an 11-point scale, ranging from minimally dysfunctional to severely dysfunctional and then to place items judged most and least dysfunctional within each category on a single 15-point scale. There was a high level of agreement between judges in both steps of this process (Gilson et al., 1975). Four groups of 25 judges each were then used to validate the construct of dysfunction and to determine the relationship of SIP™ scores to a more global assessment of dysfunction. Again, there was a high level of

agreement among judges who rated 50 protocols of subjects obtained in a field trial of the SIP™. Both the profile method of scoring and the permanent scoring method were retained (Gilson et al., 1975). Items checked by respondents or interviewers are counted, and the weighted total of each category is calculated. According to Basmajian (1994), "the sum is divided by the maximum possible score of the SIP™ and multiplied by 100 to give a total SIP™ score. Physical and psychosocial dimensions are calculated from the appropriate categories" (p. 86).

Test–retest reliability was established for total scores (Bergner, Bobbitt, Pollard, Martin, & Gilson, 1976; Deyo, 1976, 1988; Follick, Smith, & Ahern, 1985; Gilson et al., 1975) and values ranged from .73 to .88. Reliability of actual items was established (Bergner et al., 1976; Follick et al., 1985) and ranged from .45 to .89. Bergner, Bobbitt, Kressel, and colleagues (1976) report high inter-rater reliability.

The SIP™ has been used with several populations. Weinberger and colleagues (1992) found the SIP™ and Arthritis Impact Measurement Scales to be significantly correlated (physical domain, .75 to .76; psychological health, .37 to .40; total health, .70 to .73) when used in a longitudinal study of patients with knee or hip arthritis. Longstreth, Nelson, Linde, and Munoz (1992) found Parkinson's disease–specific scales correlated well with the physical domain but less well with the psychosocial domain when these instruments were administered to 44 clinic patients with Parkinson's disease and 44 age- and sex-matched control subjects. The SIP™ has also been used to measure quality of life in women with urinary incontinence (Hunskaar & Vinsnes, 1991), as well as health status in noncognitively impaired nursing home residents (Rothman, Hedrick, & Inui, 1989) and elderly veterans (Weinberger et al., 1991). The instrument has also been modified for use with persons who are head injured without "increased ability to classify subjects correctly into head injury or TC [*trauma control*] groups." (Temkin, Dikmen, Machamer, & McLean, 1989, p. 549).

The SIP™ is available in English and Spanish versions. It can be self-administered or administered by interview. Administration takes 20 to 30 minutes, and scoring takes 5 to 10 minutes with a calculator. An interviewer's manual and the instrument may be obtained from M. Bergner or B. Gilson, Department of Health Services, School of Public Health and Community Medicine, SC-37, University of Washington, Seattle, Washington 98195.

REFERENCES

Basmajian, J. (Ed.). (1994). *Physical rehabilitation outcome measures.* Toronto, Ontario, Canada: Canadian Physiotherapy Association.

Bergner, M., Bobbitt, R.A., Carter, W.B., & Gilson, B.S. (1981). The Sickness Impact Profile: Development and final revision of a health status measure. *Medical Care, 19*(8), 787–805.

Bergner, M., Bobbitt, R.A., Kressel, S., Pollard, W.E., Gilson, B.S., & Morris, J.R. (1976). The Sickness Impact Profile: Conceptual formulation and methodology for the development of a health status measure. *International Journal of Health Services, 6*(3), 393–415.

Bergner, M., Bobbitt, R.A., Pollard, W.E., Martin, D.P., & Gilson, B.S. (1976). The Sickness Impact Profile: Validation of a health measure. *Medical Care, 14*(1), 57–67.

Deyo, R.A. (1976). Pitfalls in measuring the health status of Mexican Americans: Comparative validity of the English and Spanish Sickness Impact Profile. *Health Services Research, 11*(4), 516–528.

Deyo, R.A. (1986). Comparative validity of the Sickness Impact Profile and shorter scales for functional assessment on low-back pain. *Spine, 11*(9), 951–954.

Deyo, R.A. (1988). Measuring the functional status of patients with low back pain. *Archives of Physical Medicine and Rehabilitation, 69*(12), 1044–1053.

Deyo, R.A., & Diehl, A.K. (1983). Measuring physical and psychosocial function in patients with low back pain. *Spine, 18*(6), 635–642.

Follick, M.J., Smith, T.W., & Ahern, D.K. (1985). The Sickness Impact Profile: A global measure of disability in chronic low back pain. *Pain, 21*(1), 67–76.

Gilson, B.S., Gilson, J.S., Bergner, M., Bobbitt, R.A., Kressel, S., Pollard, W.E., & Vesselago, M. (1975). The Sickness Impact Profile. *American Journal of Public Health, 65*(12), 1304–1310.

Hulsebos, R.G., Beltman, F.W., dos Reis Miranda, D., & Spangenberg, J.F.A. (1991). Measuring quality of life with the Sickness Impact Profile. *Intensive Care Medicine, 17*(5), 285–288.

Hunskaar, S., & Vinsnes, A. (1991). The quality of life in women with urinary incontinence as measured by the Sickness Impact Profile. *Journal of the American Geriatrics Society, 39*, 378–382.

Longstreth, W.T., Nelson, L., Linde, M., & Munoz, D. (1992). Utility of the Sickness Impact Profile in Parkinson's disease. *Journal of Geriatric Psychiatry and Neurology, 5*(3), 142–148.

Roland, M., & Morris, R. (1983). A study of the natural history of back pain. Part 2: Development of guidelines for trials of treatment in primary care. *Spine, 8*(2), 145–150.

Rothman, M.L., Hedrick, S., & Inui, T. (1989, March). The Sickness Impact Profile as a measure of the health status of noncognitively impaired nursing home residents. *Medical Care, 27*(Suppl. 3), S157–S167.

Temkin, N.R., Dikmen, S., Machamer, J., & McLean, A. (1989). General versus disease-specific measures. Further work on the Sickness Impact Profile for head injury. *Medical Care, 27*(Suppl. 3), S44–S53.

Weinberger, M., Samsa, G.P., Hanlon, J.T., Schmader, K., Doyle, M.E., Cowper, P.A., Uttech, K.M., Cohen, H.J., & Feussner, J.R. (1991). Evaluation of a brief health status measure of elderly veterans. *Journal of the American Geriatrics Society, 39*(7), 691–694.

Weinberger, M., Samsa, G.P., Tierney, W.M., Belyea, M.J., & Hiner, S.L. (1992). Generic versus disease specific health status measures: Comparing the Sickness Impact Profile and the Arthritis Impact Measurement Scales. *The Journal of Rheumatology, 19*(4), 543–546.

Exhibit A–31 Sickness Impact Profile (SIP™)

Please respond to (check) *only* those statements that you are sure describe you today and are related to your state of health.

1. I spend much of the day lying down in order to rest _____
2. I sit during much of the day _____
3. I am sleeping or dozing most of the time—day and night _____
4. I lie down more often during the day in order to rest _____
5. I sit around half-asleep _____
6. I sleep less at night, for example, wake up too early, don't fall asleep for a long time, awaken frequently _____
7. I sleep or nap more during the day _____

1. I say how bad or useless I am, for example, that I am a burden to others _____
2. I laugh or cry suddenly _____
3. I often moan and groan in pain or discomfort _____
4. I have attempted suicide _____
5. I act nervous or restless _____
6. I keep rubbing or holding areas of my body that hurt or are uncomfortable _____
7. I act irritable and impatient with myself, for example, talk badly about myself, swear at myself, blame myself for things that happen _____
8. I talk about the future in a hopeless way _____
9. I get sudden frights _____

1. I make difficult moves with help, for example, getting into or out of cars, bathtubs _____
2. I do not move into or out of bed or chair by myself but am moved by a person or mechanical aid _____
3. I stand only for short periods of time _____
4. I do not maintain balance _____
5. I move my hands or fingers with some limitation or difficulty _____
6. I stand up only with someone's help _____
7. I kneel, stoop, or bend down only by holding on to something _____
8. I am in a restricted position all the time _____
9. I am very clumsy in body movements _____

continues

Exhibit A–31 continued

10. I get in and out of bed or chairs by grasping something for support or using a cane or walker   _____
11. I stay lying down most of the time   _____
12. I change position frequently   _____
13. I hold on to something to move myself around in bed   _____
14. I do not bathe myself completely, for example, require assistance with bathing   _____
15. I do not bathe myself at all, but am bathed by someone else   _____
16. I use bedpan with assistance   _____
17. I have trouble getting shoes, socks, or stockings on   _____
18. I do not have control of my bladder   _____
19. I do not fasten my clothing, for example, require assistance with buttons, zippers, shoelaces   _____
20. I spend most of the time partly undressed or in pajamas   _____
21. I do not have control of my bowels   _____
22. I dress myself, but do so very slowly   _____
23. I get dressed only with someone's help   _____

This group of statements has to do with any work you usually do in caring for your home or yard. Considering just those things that you do, please respond to (check) only those statements that you are *sure* describe you today and are related to your state of health.   _____

1. I do work around the house only for short periods of time or rest often   _____
2. I am doing **less** of the regular daily work around the house than I would usually do   _____
3. I am not doing **any** of the regular daily work around the house that I would usually do   _____
4. I am not doing **any** of the maintenance or repair work that I would usually do in my home or yard   _____
5. I am not doing **any** of the shopping that I would usually do   _____
6. I am not doing **any** of the house cleaning that I would usually do   _____
7. I have difficulty doing handwork, for example, turning faucets, using kitchen gadgets, sewing, carpentry   _____
8. I am not doing **any** of the clothes washing that I would usually do   _____
9. I am not doing heavy work around the house   _____
10. I have given up taking care of personal or household business affairs, for example, paying bills, banking, working on budget   _____

Please respond to (check) *only* those statements that you are *sure* describe you today and are related to your state of health.

1. I am getting around only within one building   _____
2. I stay within one room   _____
3. I am staying in bed more   _____
4. I am staying in bed most of the time   _____
5. I am not now using public transportation   _____
6. I stay home most of the time   _____
7. I am only going to places with restrooms nearby   _____
8. I am not going into town   _____
9. I stay away from home only for brief periods of time   _____
10. I do not get around in the dark or in unlit places without someone's help   _____

1. I am going out less to visit people   _____
2. I am not going out to visit people at all   _____
3. I show less interest in other people's problems, for example, don't listen when they tell me about their problems, don't offer to help   _____
4. I often act irritable toward those around me, for example, snap at people, give sharp answers, criticize easily   _____
5. I show less affection   _____
6. I am doing fewer social activities with groups of people   _____
7. I am cutting down the length of visits with friends   _____
8. I am avoiding social visits from others   _____
9. My sexual activity is decreased   _____

continues

Exhibit A–31 continued

10. I often express concern over what might be happening to my health   _____
11. I talk less with those around me   _____
12. I make many demands, for example, insist that people do things for me, tell them how to do things   _____
13. I stay alone much of the time   _____
14. I act disagreeable to family members, for example, I act spiteful, I am stubborn.   _____
15. I have frequent outbursts of anger at family members, for example, strike at them, scream, throw things at them   _____
16. I isolate myself as much as I can from the rest of the family   _____
17. I am paying less attention to the children   _____
18. I refuse contact with family members, for example, turn away from them   _____
19. I am not doing the things I usually do to take care of my children or family   _____
20. I am not joking with family members as I usually do   _____

1. I walk shorter distances or stop to rest often   _____
2. I do not walk up or down hills   _____
3. I use stairs only with mechanical support, for example, handrail, cane, crutches   _____
4. I walk up or down stairs only with assistance from someone else   _____
5. I get around in a wheelchair   _____
6. I do not walk at all   _____
7. I walk by myself but with some difficulty, for example, limp, wobble, stumble, have stiff leg   _____
8. I walk only with help from someone   _____
9. I go up and down stairs more slowly, for example, one step at a time, stop often   _____
10. I do not use stairs at all   _____
11. I get around only by using a walker, crutches, cane, walls, or furniture   _____
12. I walk more slowly   _____

1. I am confused and start several actions at a time   _____
2. I have more minor accidents, for example, drop things, trip and fall, bump into things   _____
3. I react slowly to things that are said or done   _____
4. I do not finish things I start   _____
5. I have difficulty reasoning and solving problems, for example, making plans, making decisions, learning new things   _____
6. I sometimes behave as if I were confused or disoriented in place or time, for example, where I am, who is around, directions, what day it is   _____
7. I forget a lot, for example, things that happened recently, where I put things, appointments   _____
8. I do not keep my attention on any activity for long   _____
9. I make more mistakes than usual   _____
10. I have difficulty doing activities involving concentration and thinking   _____

1. I am having trouble writing or typing   _____
2. I communicate mostly by gestures, for example, moving head, pointing, sign language   _____
3. My speech is understood only by a few people who know me well   _____
4. I often lose control of my voice when I talk, for example, my voice gets louder or softer, trembles, changes unexpectedly   _____
5. I don't write except to sign my name   _____
6. I carry on a conversation only when very close to the other person or looking at him   _____
7. I have difficulty speaking, for example, get stuck, stutter, stammer, slur my words   _____
8. I am understood with difficulty   _____
9. I do not speak clearly when I am under stress   _____

The next group of statements has to do with any work you usually do other than managing your home. By this we mean anything you regard as work that you do on a regular basis.

Do you usually work other than managing your home   YES_____   NO_____
If YES skip to next section; if NO then:
    Are you retired: YES_____   NO_____
    If you are retired, was your retirement related to your health?   YES_____   NO_____
    If you are not retired, but are not working, is this related to your health?   YES_____   NO_____

continues

Exhibit A–31 continued

If you are not working and it is not because of your health, please skip this section.

Now consider the work you do and respond to (check) only those statements that you are sure describe you today and are related to your state of health. (If today is a Saturday or Sunday or some other day that you would usually have off, please respond as if today were a working day.)

1. I am not working at all   _____

If you checked this statement, skip to the next section

2. I am doing part of my job at home   _____
3. I am not accomplishing as much as usual at work   _____
4. I often act irritable toward my work associates, for example, snap at them, give sharp answers, criticize easily   _____
5. I am working shorter hours   _____
6. I am doing only light work   _____
7. I work only for short periods of time or take frequent rests   _____
8. I am working at my usual job but with some changes, for example, using different tools or special aids, trading some tasks with other workers   _____
9. I do not do my job as carefully and as accurately as usual   _____

This group of statements has to do with activities you usually do in your free time. These activities are things that you might do for relaxation, to pass the time, or for entertainment. Please respond to (check) *only* those statements that you are *sure* describe you today and are related to your state of health.

1. I do my hobbies and recreation for shorter periods of time   _____
2. I am going out for entertainment less often   _____
3. I am cutting down on **some** of my usual inactive recreation and pastimes, for example, watching TV, playing cards, reading   _____
4. I am not doing **any** of my usual inactive recreation and pastimes, for example, watching TV, playing cards, reading   _____
5. I am doing more inactive pastimes in place of my other usual activities   _____
6. I am doing fewer community activities   _____
7. I am cutting down on **some** of my usual physical recreation or activities   _____
8. I am not doing **any** of my usual physical recreation or activities   _____

Please respond to (check) *only* those statements that you are sure describe you today and are related to your state of health.

1. I am eating much less than usual   _____
2. I feed myself but only by using specially prepared food or utensils   _____
3. I am eating special or different food, for example, soft food, bland diet, low-salt, low-fat, low-sugar   _____
4. I eat no food at all but am taking fluids   _____
5. I just pick or nibble at my food   _____
6. I am drinking less fluids   _____
7. I feed myself with help from someone else   _____
8. I do not feed myself at all, but must be fed   _____
9. I am eating no food at all, nutrition is taken through tubes or intravenous tubes   _____

Functional Assessment Resources

BOOKS

Asher, I.E. (1989). *An annotated index of occupational therapy evaluation tools.* Bethesda, MD: American Occupational Therapy Association.

Basmajian, J. (Ed.)., Cole, B., Finch, E., Gowland, C., Mayo, N. (Working Group). (1994). *Physical rehabilitation outcome measures.* Toronto, Ontario, Canada: Canadian Physiotherapy Association in cooperation with Health and Welfare Canada and the Canada Communications Group.

Cushman, L.A., & Scherer, M.J. (Eds.). (1995). *Psychological assessment in medical rehabilitation.* Washington, DC: American Psychological Association.

Granger, C.V., & Gresham, G.E. (Eds.). (1984). *Functional assessment in rehabilitation medicine.* Baltimore: Williams & Wilkins.

Halpern, A.S., & Fuhrer, M.J. (Eds.). (1984). *Functional assessment in rehabilitation.* Baltimore: Paul H. Brookes.

Harrison, D.K., Garnett, J.M., & Watson, A.L. (1981). *Client assessment measures in rehabilitation.* Ann Arbor, MI: University of Michigan Rehabilitation Research Institute.

Kane, R.A., & Kane, R.L. (1981). *Assessing the elderly: A practical guide to measurement.* Lexington, MA: Lexington Books.

Lubinski, R., & Frattali, C. (1995). *Professional issues in speech-language pathology and audiology.* San Diego, CA: Singular Publishing Group.

Sawin, K.J., & Harrigan, M.P. (Authors), Woog, P. (Ed.). (1995). *Measures of family functioning for research and practice.* New York: Springer.

Streiner, D.L., & Norman, G.R. (1995). *Health measurement scales: A practical guide to their development and use* (2nd ed.). New York: Oxford University Press.

Wade, D.T. (1992). *Measurement in neurological rehabilitation.* New York: Oxford University Press.

GOVERNMENT PUBLICATION

U.S. Department of Health and Human Services. (1993). *Research plan for the National Center for Medical Rehabilitation Research* (NIH Publication No. 93-3509). Rockville, MD: National Institutes of Health, National Institute of Child Health and Human Development.

JOURNALS

Granger, C.V., & Gresham, G.E. (Guest Eds.). (1993). New developments in functional assessment. *Physical Medicine and Rehabilitation Clinics of North America, 4*(3), 417–611. Published four times per year. Available from:
Accounting and Circulation Offices
6277 Sea Harbor Drive
Orlando, FL 32887–4800

American Journal of Physical Medicine and Rehabilitation. Published bimonthly. Available from:
Williams & Wilkins
351 West Camden St.
Baltimore, MD 21201–2436

American Rehabilitation. Published quarterly. Available from:
Superintendent of Documents
U.S. Government Printing Office
Washington, DC 20402

Archives of Physical Medicine and Rehabilitation. Published monthly. Available from:
Accounting and Circulation Offices
6277 Sea Harbor Drive
Orlando, FL 32887–4800

International Journal of Rehabilitation Research. Published quarterly. Available from:

> USA/Canada
> Journals Promotion Department
> Chapman & Hall, Inc.
> 115 Fifth Ave.
> New York, NY 10003
> Tel: 1–212/564–1060
> FAX: 1–212/564–1505

Journal of Head Trauma Rehabilitation. Published six times per year. Available from:

> Fulfillment
> Aspen Publishers, Inc.
> 7201 McKinney Circle
> Frederick, MD 21704
> 1–800–638–8437

Journal of Occupational Therapy. 10 issues per year. Available from:

> The American Occupational Therapy Association, Inc.
> 4720 Montgomery Lane
> Bethesda, MD 20814–3425

Journal of Rehabilitation Outcomes Measurement. Published six times per year. Available from:

> Fulfillment
> Aspen Publishers, Inc.
> 7201 McKinney Circle
> Frederick, MD 21704
> 1–800–638–8437

Journal of Rehabilitation Research and Development. Published quarterly. Available from:

> Superintendent of Documents Depositories
> U.S. Government Printing Office
> Washington, DC 20402
>
> Single articles available on request from:
> Congressional Information Services
> Bethesda, MD 20814

Journal of Speech and Hearing Research. Published six times per year. Available from:

> Subscription Sales Coordinator
> ASHA
> 10801 Rockville Pike
> Rockville, MD 20852–3279
> Tel: 301–897–5700, Ext 218

NeuroRehabilitation. Available from:

> Elsevier Science Ireland Ltd.
> Customer Relations Manager
> Bay 15K
> Shannon Industrial Estate
> Shannon, Co.
> Clare, Ireland
> Tel: (+353–61) 471844
> FAX: (+353–61) 472144

Rehabilitation Counseling Bulletin. Published quarterly. Available from:

> PP&F
> ACA Subscriptions
> P.O. Box 2513
> Birmingham, AL 35201-2513
> 1–800–633–4931

Rehabilitation Nursing. Published six times a year. Available from:

> Association of Rehabilitation Nurses
> 4700 W. Lake Avenue
> Glenview, IL 60025–1485
> Tel: 1–800–229–7530
> E-mail arn@amctec.com

Rehabilitation Psychology. Published quarterly. Available from:

> Springer Publishing Company
> 536 Broadway
> New York, NY 10012
> Tel: 1–212–431–4370
> FAX: 1–212–941–7842

The Journal of Rehabilitation. Published quarterly. Available from:

> *Journal of Rehabilitation*
> 633 South Washington St.
> Alexandria, VA 22314
> Tel: 703–836–0850
> FAX: 703–836–0848

Topics in Geriatric Rehabilitation. Published quarterly. Available from:

> Fulfillment
> Aspen Publishers, Inc.
> 7201 McKinney Circle
> Frederick, MD 21704
> 1–800–638–8437

Topics in Language Disorders. Published quarterly. Available from:

> Fulfillment
> Aspen Publishers, Inc.
> 7201 McKinney Circle
> Frederick, MD 21704
> 1–800–638–8437

Topics in Spinal Cord Injury Rehabilitation

> Specifically:

Ditunno, J.F. (Issue Editor). (1996, Spring). Functional assessment. *Topics in Spinal Cord Injury Rehabilitation, 1*(4), Total issue. Available from:

> Fulfillment
> Aspen Publishers, Inc.
> 7201 McKinney Circle
> Frederick, MD 21704
> 1–800–638–8437

Topics in Stroke Rehabilitation. Published quarterly. Available from:

> Fulfillment
> Aspen Publishers, Inc.
> 7201 McKinney Circle
> Frederick, MD 21704
> 1–800–638–8437

PROFESSIONAL ORGANIZATIONS

American Academy of Physical Medicine and Rehabilitation (AAPM&R)
122 South Michigan Ave.
Suite 1300
Chicago, IL 60603–6107

American Congress of Rehabilitation Medicine (ACRM)
4700 W. Lake Ave.
Glenview, IL 60025–1485

American Geriatrics Society (AGS)
770 Lexington Ave.
Suite 300
New York, NY 10021

American Occupational Therapy Association (AOTA)
P. O. Box 31220
4720 Montgomery Lane
Bethesda, MD 20824–1220
Tel: 1–301–652–2682

American Physical Therapy Association (APTA)
1111 North Fairfax St.
Alexandria, VA 22314

American Psychological Association
750 First St., NE
Washington, DC 20002

American Rehabilitation Counseling Association (ARCA)
5999 Stevenson Ave.
Alexandria, VA 22304

American Speech-Language-Hearing Association (ASHA)
10801 Rockville Pike
Rockville, MD 20852
Voice or TDD: 301–897–5700
FAX: 301–571–1457

Association of Rehabilitation Nurses (ARN)
4700 W. Lake Ave.
Glenview, IL 60025–1485
Tel: 708–375–4710
1–800–229–7530

Association of Academic Physiatrists
5987 E. 71st St.
Suite 112
Indianapolis, IN 46220
Tel: 317–845–4200
FAX: 317–845–4299

International Federation of Physical Medicine and Rehabilitation (IFPMR)
600 University Ave.
Suite 1160
Toronto, Ontario M5G 1X5
Canada

International Rehabilitation Medicine Association (IRMA)
1333 Moursund Ave.
Suite A–221
Houston, TX 77030

ONLINE SOURCES OF INFORMATION AND INSTRUMENTS (SOURCE—THE INTERNET)

ABLEDATA Database Program—**BRS/ABLE
Macro International
8455 Colesville Rd.
Suite 935
Silver Spring, MD 10910–3319
Database of commercially available rehabilitation products from more than 1,900 companies. Includes personal care, therapeutic sensory, educational, vocational, and transportation aids. Produced by Adaptive Equipment Center, Newington Children's Hospital, 181 East Cedar St., Newington, CT 06111; 203–667–5437.

AgeLine—**BRS/AARP
Produced by:
American Association of Retired Persons
National Gerontology Resource Center
1919 K St., NW
Washington, DC 20049
Provides access to citations and abstracts for materials concerning the sociopsychological, economic, health-related, and political aspects of aging. Types of documents covered include journal articles, books, reports, government documents, and book chapters.

AGRICOLA BRS/CAIN
DIALOL/10,110
Produced by:
National Agricultural Library
U.S. Department of Agriculture
10301 Baltimore Blvd.
Beltsville, MD 20705
301–344–3813
Includes worldwide coverage of journals and monographs on agriculture and related topics. Focuses on rural training. Rehabilitation topics include disabled homemaking and farming.

COMPENDEX **BRS/COMP
>Produced by:
>Engineering Information, Inc.
>345 East 47th St.
>New York, NY 10067
>212–705–7615
>800–221–1044

Online counterpart to Engineering Index, contains bibliographic information on journal articles, books, conference papers, and reports in the areas of engineering technology. Includes materials dealing with the environment, geology, petroleum, computers, etc., including rehabilitation engineering.

ERIC Clearinghouse on Disabilities and Gifted Education (ERIC/EC)
>Council for Exceptional Children (CEC)
>1920 Association Dr.
>Reston, VA 22091

Handicapped Users' Database-HUD **COMPUSERVE
>Produced by:
>Georgia Griffith
>Rear 4
>Furry Court
>Lancaster, OH 43130

Contains articles for and about people with disabilities, lists of organizations servicing people with disabilities, educational materials, current news stories, and a reference library.

Health and Psychosocial Instruments **BRS/HAPI
>Produced by:
>Behavioral Measurement Data Base Services (BMDS)

Contains information on national and international instruments, published in the English language, for researchers, practitioners, educators, administrators, and evaluators in the health fields, the psychosocial sciences and organizational behavior/human resources. Includes questionnaires, interview schedules, observation checklists/manuals, etc.

ISMEC—Information Services in Mechanical Engineering **DIALOG/14
>Produced by:
>Cambridge Scientific Abstracts
>5161 River Rd.
>Bethesda, MD 20816
>301–951–1400
>800–368–8076

Indexes articles from international mechanical engineering journals, books, reports, and conferences. Contains citations in the area of assistive devices, biomedical engineering, and training for disabled persons.

REHABDATA **BRS/NRIC
>Produced by:
>NARIC
>8455 Colesville Rd.
>Silver Spring, MD 20910
>800–346–2742
>301–588–9284

Database of rehabilitation literature reflecting the collection of the National Rehabilitation Information Clearinghouse (NARIC). Includes research reports from projects funded by National Institute of Disability and Rehabilitation Research (NIDRR) and Rehabilitation Services Administration (RSA). Also includes commercial publications, journal articles, and other government documents. A sampling of subject areas includes disability management, functional evaluation, independent living, placement, and transportation.

Resources in Vocational Education **BRS/RIVE
>Produced by:
>National Center for Research/Vocational Education
>University of California at Berkeley

Includes information on state and federally administered research, curriculum development, and professional development projects in vocational education.

SPORT Database **BRS/SFDB
>Produced by:
>Sport Information Resource Center
>1600 James Naismith Dr.
>Gloucester, Ontario KIB5N4
>Canada
>613–748–5658

Standards and Specifications **DIALOG/113
>Produced by:
>National Standards Association

Cites government and industry standards, specifications, testing safety, terminology, performance, and materials. Includes standards for buildings and equipment for the disabled.

OTHER SOURCES OF INFORMATION AND INSTRUMENTS

Agency for Health Care Policy and Research
Public Health Service
U.S. Department of Health and Human Services
Executive Office Center
Suite 501
2101 East Jefferson St.
Rockville, MD 20852

Commission on Accreditation of Rehabilitation Facilities (CARF)
101 North Wilmot Rd.
Suite 500
Tucson, AZ 85711

Department of Veterans Affairs
810 Vermont Ave. NW
Washington, DC 20410

Disability Statistics Rehabilitation Research and Training Center Institute for Health and Aging, UCSF
Box 0646, Laurel Heights
San Francisco, CA 94143–0646

Joint Commission on Accreditation of Healthcare Organizations
1 Renaissance Plaza
Oakbrook, IL 60181
1–630–792–5000

Medical Outcomes Trust
20 Park Plaza
Suite 1014
Boston, MA 02116–4313

Model Spinal Cord Injury System
Thomas Jefferson University
Jefferson Medical College
11th and Walnut Sts.
Philadelphia, PA 19107

Model System of Comprehensive Rehabilitation for Persons with TBI
Virginia Commonwealth University
Medical College of Virginia
Department of Physical Medicine and Rehabilitation
MCV Station, Box 542
Richmond, VA 23298–0542

National Center for Medical Rehabilitation Research (NCMRR)
6100 Executive Blvd.
Room 2A03
Rockville, MD 20852

National Council on Aging (NCOA)
409 3rd St. SW
Washington, DC 20024

National Council on Disability
1331 F St. NW
Suite 1040
Washington, DC 20004–1107

National Council on Independent Living (NCIL)
2111 Wilson Blvd.
Suite 405
Arlington, VA 22201

National Head Injury Foundation, Inc. (NHIF)
1776 Massachusetts Ave. NW
Suite 100
Washington, DC 20036

National Institute of Neurological and Communicative Disorders and Stroke (NINCDS)
National Institutes of Health
U.S. Department of Health and Human Services
Building 31, Room 8A 06
9000 Rockville Pike
Bethesda, MD 20892

National Rehabilitation Association (NRA)
633 South Washington St.
Alexandria, VA 22314–4193

National Rehabilitation Information Clearinghouse (NARIC)
8455 Colesville Rd.
Suite 935
Silver Spring, MD 20910–3319

National Technical Information Service (NTIS)
U.S. Department of Commerce
5285 Port Royal Rd.
Springfield, VA 22161

Rehabilitation Research and Training Center on Aging with Spinal Cord Injury
Craig Hospital
University of Colorado Health Science Center
Research Department
3425 South Clarkson
Englewood, CO 80110

Rehabilitation Research and Training Center on Functional Assessment and Rehabilitation Outcomes
State University of New York at Buffalo
School of Medicine and Biomedical Sciences
232 Parker Hall, SUNY South Campus
Buffalo, New York 14214–3007
Tel: 716–829–2076
FAX: 716–829–2080

Resource Unit for Information and Education (RU-Northwestern University REC)
345 East Superior St.
Room 1441
Chicago, IL 60611

RESNA Technical Assistance Project
1700 N. Moore St.
Suite 1540
Arlington, VA 22209–1903

The Rehabilitation Engineering Research Center on Aging
UB Center for Assistive Technology
515 Kimball Tower
State University of New York at Buffalo
Buffalo, NY 14214
Tel: 1–716–829–3141
FAX: 1–716–829–3217

Trace Research & Development Center
S-151 Waisman Center
1500 Highland Ave.
Madison, WI 53705–2280

Index

Page numbers in *italics* denote exhibits and figures; those followed by "t" denote tables.